Understanding Balance

The mechanics of posture and locomotion

Tristan D.M. Roberts

Formerly Reader in Physiology
University of Glasgow
UK

CHAPMAN & HALL
London · Glasgow · Weinheim · New York · Tokyo · Melbourne · Madras

Published by Chapman & Hall, 2–6 Boundary Row, London SE1 8HN, UK

Chapman & Hall, 2–6 Boundary Row, London SE1 8HN, UK

Blackie Academic & Professional, Wester Cleddens Road, Bishopbriggs, Glasgow G64 2NZ, UK

Chapman & Hall GmbH, Pappelallee 3, 69469 Weinheim, Germany

Chapman & Hall USA, 115 Fifth Avenue, New York, NY 10003, USA

Chapman & Hall Japan, ITP-Japan, Kyowa Building, 3F, 2-2-1 Hirakawacho, Chiyoda-ku, Tokyo 102, Japan

Chapman & Hall Australia, 102 Dodds Street, South Melbourne, Victoria 3205, Australia

Chapman & Hall India, R. Seshadri, 32 Second Main Road, CIT East, Madras 600 035, India

Distributed in the USA and Canada by Singular Publishing Group Inc., 4284 41st Street, San Diego, California 92105

First edition 1995

© 1995 Tristan D.M. Roberts

Dr T.D.M. Roberts has asserted his right to be identified as the author of this book.

Typeset in 10/12 Palatino by Best-set Typesetter Ltd., Hong Kong
Printed in Great Britain by TJ Press (Padstow) Ltd, Cornwall

ISBN 0 412 60160 5   1 56593 416 4 (USA)

A catalogue record for this book is available from the British Library

Library of Congress Catalog Card Number: 94-74684

∞ Printed on permanent acid-free text paper, manufactured in accordance with ANSI/NISO Z39.48-1992 and ANSI/NISO Z39.48-1984 (Permanence of Paper).

Contents

Preface

This book is the outcome of a lifetime's research. Since balance, in man as well as in animals, clearly depends on muscular activity, and since the muscles are controlled by the nervous system, I set out originally with the idea that a detailed understanding would depend on knowing something about the neurophysiology of the subject. Indeed, I wrote a book about this, called *The Neurophysiology of Postural Mechanisms*, the second edition of which appeared in 1978 (London: Butterworths). It is long since out of print.

At the time of writing that book I had come to the conclusion that everything to do with balance came down to a problem in recognition. For example, if one is to make corrective movements to avoid over-balancing, one must be able, on some level, to recognize that the moment has arrived at which such corrective movements are called for. Orthodox neurophysiological teaching could, at that time, offer no clue as to how the brain could carry out acts of recognition of any sort, in spite of the fact that recognition processes clearly form an important feature of everyday experience. I felt I had arrived at an impasse.

The activities of balance and locomotion are not the only features of common experience that we take for granted but which are hard to explain in terms of the behaviour of individual neurons. Two other important examples are the notions of spatial contiguity and of temporal succession. Both of these are involved in detecting trends of change in the environment such as form the basis for formulating patterns of motor activity. In discussing these processes we find ourselves embroiled in philosophical questions of consciousness and 'voluntary' behaviour. It may be that all these difficulties will be soluble in terms of a mechanism for gestalt perception.

A fundamental difficulty is that each single neuron, out of all the thousands of millions of neurons in the nervous system, behaves as an independent individual. We urgently require some scheme to account for the way these individual cell activities are linked together in co-operation. Edelman's recent Theory of Neuronal Group Selection provides one such scheme, now backed up by effective computer simulations. I present an account of a modification of his scheme in my concluding chapter.

The earlier chapters prepare the ground by dealing with various aspects of balancing behaviour from the point of view of what can be directly observed. In treating the actions of the forces involved I have preferred to speak in terms of classical Newtonian mechanics, and to avoid the treacherous oversimplifications of conventional schoolroom physics. This has involved a restatement of certain basic principles that are often overlooked or misunderstood.

Some readers, such as professional academic physiologists and the like, may find certain elementary passages rather laboured. Others, with a different background of expertise but perhaps more directly concerned with the practical problems of individual patients and athletes, may, on the other hand, find some sections heavy going. In each case, patience is appropriate since a full understanding requires at least a nodding acquaintance with each of the various topics treated. The concepts involved form an interlacing network. In the linear pro-gress of a continuous narrative it is necessary to visit certain nodes in the network more than once, some of the relevant features being restated each time as a reminder to the reader who can then better appreciate their interactions.

In my opinion, so long as one is careful to pay due attention to what it was that a particular experimenter actually saw, one is not obliged to follow his interpretation or explanation. Indeed, it may well be that an alternative interpretation, when put together with fresh interpretations of other findings, can lead to a more satisfactory overall scheme. It is this principle that I have adopted in constructing the story presented in this book. I have not felt it appropriate to burden the text with refer-ences since many of the findings I refer to are also given, with their references, in standard textbooks. With the interpretations given by the original authors, these reports tend to give the impression of an array of unrelated facts, and for this reason the reader may be confused rather than enlightened by consulting the original papers. When the findings are freshly reinterpreted in the light of new data, including experiments of my own, they can now, I believe, be welded together into a coherent story.

T.D.M. Roberts
Fintry, April 1994

Acknowledgements

In developing the ideas presented in this book I have been greatly helped by discussions over the years with colleagues, collaborators and students. The late Professor Ian A. Boyd prepared for me the drawing of spindle structure (Figure 8.5) summarizing his histological findings, and has allowed me to use his schematic diagram of the actions of the intrafusal system (Figure 8.9). He also provided the drawing of a spray ending (Figure 8.1). Dr Neil C. Spurway prepared for me the sketch illustrating the interrelations of the many complex structures to be found within a skeletal muscle cell (Figure 4.1). Professor Milton Hildebrand, of the University of California at Davis, lent me the large set of measurements from his own cine films that provided the basis for my analysis of gait variants in the horse, as set out in Chapter 7. Some other figures are taken from the literature, as acknowledged briefly in the captions, the full bibliographical details being set out in the Sources of figures at the end of the book. I most gratefully acknowledge the absolutely invaluable support and encouragement provided, at all stages in the preparation of this text, by Mr John D. Christie, who has given most generously of his time and very considerable expertise. Discussions with him have guided my attempts to disentangle and simplify, and thus to clarify, the heavily convoluted ideas that form the core of the argument of the book. He has also helped with the index and with the proofs.

The problem

1

A curious thing about balance is that people usually expect to find that balancing is a fairly simple process, since nearly everyone can perform the routine balancing acts of everyday existence without having to think about what they are doing. In fact, the more one looks into it, the more complex and mysterious balancing behaviour becomes. The study of balancing behaviour leads one to examine deep problems of sensory perception normally treated under the heading of philosophy, and to reconsider those underlying principles of mechanics that are obscured by the simplifications of normal schoolroom teaching.

The primary aim of the scientist may be held to be that of trying to formulate explanatory descriptions that will have predictive value. In this endeavour it is clearly important, as a preliminary step, to ascertain just what it is that actually happens in any particular phenomenon that is to be explained. From this point of view the traditional accounts of how the body achieves and maintains its upright posture appear to leave a good deal to be desired.

In the account that follows it will be convenient to make use of a number of concepts developed in the field of physics. Some of these ideas are superficially quite familiar and, perhaps because of this very familiarity, many terms have come to be used even by professional physicists without a proper regard for the strict precision of their definitions. Accordingly, where the present argument depends on the interpretation of physical concepts, reminders of the definitions have been included in the text to make clear what usage is intended.

For many years neurophysiologists have sought to build an understanding of the operations of the nervous system in such activity as balancing behaviour using, as a basis, only straightforward engineering principles. They have regarded the sense organs as akin to the transducers of the engineer, generating signals to convey the physical parameters of environmental change. These signals were then supposed to be processed by the nervous system as command signals in a network of servomechanisms governing the forces developed by the individual muscles in much the same way as occurs in robots such as those used in the conveyor-belt manufacture of motor cars.

This attitude is a reflection of a common world view which, although it does not stand up to detailed scrutiny in terms of modern physics, is greatly influenced by the observable behaviour of resilient objects of such sizes as can be held in the hand. Collisions between billiard balls provide the basis for Newtonian mechanics, with its account of 'forces' associated with the changes in behaviour occurring at the interaction between objects. The 'force' of common experience is the stress force responsible for the cohesion and rigidity of solid objects. To this type of force, Newton added another, hypothetical, type of force which he called 'gravity' to account for the observed accelerations of unsupported objects such as his legendary falling apple. In contrast to stress forces, which depend on contiguity, gravity is a force that can act at a distance.

Our ideas on balance and equilibrium go back to very early times in the history of civilization, to the problems of the assessment and standardization of weights in commerce. A 'balance' is a device for comparing the weights of two scale pans (bi- = 'two', lanx = 'scale-pan'), as with a beam having three pivots and which is supported at the centre pivot. The scale pans are suspended from the two end pivots, which are equidistant from the centre pivot. 'Equilibrium' implies that the weights in the two scale pans are equal. The 'balance' then comes to rest with the beam horizontal.

An extension of the idea is to distinguish between 'stable' and 'unstable' equilibrium, where 'stable' means 'able to stand', or 'secure against being overthrown'. An equilibrium is stable if small casual perturbations are met by forces that tend to restore the system to the equilibrium state. In unstable equilibrium the effect of small perturbations is to generate forces that tend to increase the deviation from the equilibrium state.

The notion of equilibrium is extended to other systems besides those involving weighing. In the present context it is relevant to consider equilibrium in relation to the class of mechanisms known as 'servos'.

A 'servomechanism' is a system in which a strong 'slave' produces effects at the direction of a controlling 'master' whose exertion is limited to the issue of command signals. The effort applied by the slave is governed by the discrepancy (error) between the achieved state and that indicated as 'desired' in terms of the available interpretation of the command signal. Our modern world contains an increasing number of servomechanisms, familiar examples being those used in the braking and power-steering systems in motor cars. Thermostats and many other controlling mechanisms operate on similar principles.

The resting condition in a servomechanism is a condition of stable equilibrium, since any perturbation of the 'achieved state' will generate an error signal which in turn will call forth effort from the 'slave mechanism' to reduce the error.

We may take as a simple example of balancing behaviour the way a waking animal typically holds at least its head, and often its trunk also, clear of the supporting substrate. In some animals, such as the grazing herbivores, the plane of symmetry of the skull is often held vertical for a large part of the time, but this is not true of man. This behaviour allows one to speak of a 'normal' position, or attitude, of the head.

Sherrington and Magnus carried out experiments on the righting behaviour of decerebrated animals. The surgical operation of 'decerebration' involves the removal, under anaesthetic, of large parts of the brain. After the operation the animals can experience no sensations and are incapable of voluntary movement. They can then be allowed to recover from the anaesthetic without risk of inflicting pain. In this condition a number of automatic 'reflex' responses can be observed. The experimenters showed that certain of these animals keep their heads upright even when the trunk by which they are supported in the experimenter's hands is tilted out of the upright position. This righting of the animal's head does not occur if the balancing organs in the 'labyrinths' of the inner ears have been destroyed on each side at an earlier operation.

It is clear from these observations that the labyrinths have something to do with the maintenance of the upright posture.

The traditional view, based on these observations and still widely held, is that the upright posture is maintained by the operation of some sort of servomechanism in which the muscular activity in the limbs is controlled by deviations from an ideal upright position, presumed to be sensed by the labyrinth, in what are referred to as the 'postural' or 'righting' reflexes.

According to this view, the mechanism by which an animal maintains its 'upright posture' is a simple and obvious matter, not warranting the expenditure of the effort of detailed investigation. All that is required is a sensor of the gravitational vertical, supposedly located in the balancing organ in the inner ear, together with a reflex system of motor control.

However, that this is not the whole story is also clear from the fact that animals do not always hold their heads in the same position. If it were true that a set of reflexes operate to restore the 'normal' posture of the head whenever there is any deviation from this posture, then we should expect to see very little in the way of deviation in the absence of strong disturbing influences. But this is not what we do see. Animals characteristically move their heads about a good deal, turning from side to side and looking up and down at their surroundings.

Accordingly, we must reject the idea that the upright posture is maintained by some automatic regulating mechanism, and there will be little profit in searching for the components of such a mechanism. Nevertheless it is clearly true that animals and men do regulate their posture to the extent that we can readily recognize a 'normal' posture and distinguish it from an 'abnormal' one. Furthermore, overbalancing is a relatively rare occurrence.

The essence of balancing behaviour consists of the appropriate organization of the forces developed between the body and its supports. The traditional simple scheme has a great many things wrong with it. This book sets out to explore the situation in some detail.

In our search for explanatory descriptions that have predictive value, we start with a careful analysis of what actually happens during balancing behaviour before going on to consider the mechanisms by which the various observed effects are brought about. It is necessary at the outset to make clear what is to be understood by the concept of 'force'. Here the simplifications of high school physics need to be interpreted with caution.

The concept of 'force'   2

It is convenient to start with Newton whose First Law reads: 'Every body continues in its state of rest, or of uniform motion in a straight line, unless it is compelled to change that state by forces impressed upon it'. This formulation arose from consideration of the effects of applying muscular effort in setting objects into motion, and from the observed consequences of collisions and other interactions between bodies in contact with one another. Newton classified such instances together as involving what he called 'impressed force', but he also recognized that one body can influence another without actual contact. This action at a distance he called 'centripetal force', of which magnetism and gravity are examples. His First Law thus comes to serve as a definition of 'force' as that which causes bodies to change their state of motion.

Newton's Second Law tells us how forces are to be measured. It reads: 'Change of motion is proportional to the impressed force and takes place in the direction of the straight line in which the force acts'. The expression 'state of motion' is nowadays interpreted as the 'momentum', defined as the product of the mass multiplied by the velocity. In these terms, the magnitude of the force on a body is to be taken as equal to the rate-of-change of the momentum of that body. Thus when an unsupported object, such as a projectile, moves in a curved path, changing its momentum by the change in the direction of its motion, the curvature of the path is to be attributed to the action of a force at a distance. In setting out his Law of Gravitation, to cover the motions of the celestial bodies as well as those of projectiles and of objects in free fall, Newton departed from the previously held notion of *'gravitas'*, meaning 'heaviness', which had up to that time been taken to be an inherent property of massive objects. For Newton, gravity is a force acting at a distance. Any two objects exert an attractive force upon each other. The magnitude of the force is proportional to the product of the masses of the two bodies and is inversely proportional to the square of the distance between their centres of mass.

GRAVITY, WEIGHT AND STRESS

It is necessary to distinguish between gravitational force and weight. The notion of weight comes from the effort we have to exert to lift things, 'heaving' them up. The force involved here is an impressed force, depending on contact, not a force acting at a distance, like gravity. When objects are supported at rest relative to the earth's surface they exert a force against their supports. At the same time, the supports exert an upthrust against the objects resting upon them. When we lift an object we exert an upthrust on the object and at the same time we press downwards upon the ground. Forces of this kind are called 'stress forces'. They are associated with disturbances of the molecular architecture of the solid materials that are under load.

It is a characteristic of the solid state that the molecules which make up the material of the solid are each held in place by intermolecular forces. If a block of solid material is loaded by applying impressed forces on opposite faces, as when we squeeze a rubber eraser between finger and thumb, some of the molecules are displaced from their rest positions. The deformation is resisted by the intermolecular forces so that the compressed rubber pushes back against our fingers. All solid objects behave in this way, although some materials are more easily deformed than others. The relative deformation is called the 'strain' and we need to specify the direction in which the measurements have been taken. The force with which the strain is resisted depends upon the cross-sectional area of the block of material that is available. It is thus convenient to speak of the 'force per unit area'. This measure is called the 'stress' in the material, and again we have to specify the direction in which the forces are to be measured. The material under stress may be either in compression or in tension. It is usual for a compressive strain in one direction to be accompanied by tensile strain in directions at right angles. The converse is also true: when we stretch a piece of rubber, it gets thinner.

When we consider a hypothetical plane of section through a block of material that is under load, it is clear that the molecules that are on one side of this plane will exert forces on the molecules on the other side. These forces must be equal and opposite, otherwise the material would move. If we now shift the position of the hypothetical plane of section until it coincides with the area of contact between two bodies, such as the area of contact between our forefinger and the block of rubber in our earlier example, we see that the force with which the finger presses against the rubber is equal and opposite to the force exerted by the rubber against the finger. This is the basis of Newton's Third Law: 'The mutual actions of two bodies upon each other are always equal and in opposite directions'.

VECTORS

Early studies on the interactions of forces were carried out with strings, weights and pulleys. It is natural to represent the tension in a string by a simple line. Often we are concerned, not with the conditions within the material of the string itself, but only with the action of the string upon the body to which it is attached. This leads to the representation of forces as vectors, having directedness as well as orientation. In diagrams one puts arrowheads on the lines to indicate the effect of the string upon the object of interest. The analysis of the interaction of tensions in terms of vector diagrams leads to the paralellogram rule for the combination and resolution of vectors, and to the rules about 'couples' or pairs of non-coincident parallel vectors.

For many purposes vector diagrams are used to represent compressive thrusts as well as tensions. This convention works for the analysis of such structures as can be represented as a lattice of struts and ties connected together by pin joints. Each link between two joints is referred to as a 'member', where a strut is a member stressed in compression and a tie is a member stressed in tension. Lattice diagrams are generalized, by analogy, to cover solid structures, as in the development of beam theory in engineering.

The practice of representing the thrust in a strut as a simple vector with a geometrical point of application tends to conceal an important difficulty. It is easy to recognize the line of action of a string in tension because we can usually neglect the thickness of the string in comparison with its length. For material in compression the cross-sectional area cannot be neglected because it is an important factor in the resistance to buckling. Where one member presses against another the transmitted force is distributed as stress over the whole area of contact, this stress being accompanied inevitably by a corresponding strain. The representation of the area of contact as a pin joint is therefore unrealistic, though often convenient. Additional complications arise where the members are fastened together. The joint may resist a change in the angle between the members by developing torque, some parts of the material being under tension while other parts are compressed. In such a situation it may not be a simple matter to determine the 'point of application' of the transmitted force.

Because the development of stress forces is necessarily accompanied by the development of strain, all structures will become deformed to some extent when loaded by impressed external forces. Movement of the point of application of a force involves a transfer of energy in the form of work, and we can accordingly distinguish between 'load points', where the applied forces perform work against the structure, and 'supports' where the structure under consideration performs work against some other body. At a support, the force acting on the supported structure is called the 'reaction force'. If the structure is at rest, the combined effect of the imposed loads is in equilibrium with the combined effect of the reaction forces. If a sufficient number of the relevant forces are known, the others can all be calculated. The rules for such calculations constitute the science of statics.

D'ALEMBERT'S PRINCIPLE

The rules of statics are not directly applicable to situations in which there is movement. Problems in dynamics can, however, be treated by the rules of statics using a procedure devised by d'Alembert. If we know how each mass in the system is accelerating during the movement, we can calculate from Newton's Second Law what forces on each of the masses could produce the observed accelerations. D'Alembert called such forces the 'effective forces'. The Principle of d'Alembert states that the effective forces, if reversed, would be in equilibrium with the impressed forces. Thus, to solve a problem in dynamics we consider each mass in the system to be subject to an additional force of such a magnitude and direction as to oppose the observed acceleration of that mass. The combined system can then be analysed by the rules of statics as though it were in equilibrium.

It is important to remember that d'Alembertian reversed effective forces are not real forces, they are notional forces introduced merely for purposes of calculation. When we represent two forces as vectors and then use the parallelogram law to derive a third vector as the resultant, we are not creating a new force. Similarly, when we introduce a vector for the 'reversed effective force' in solving a problem in dynamics by the method of d'Alembert, we are not representing a force present in the real world.

As an example of the use of the method of d'Alembert, let us consider the action of gravity on an unsupported body. Each of the particles of which the body is composed will be attracted towards the earth by a force mg where m is the mass of the particle and g is the gravitational acceleration. The combined effect of all the gravitational forces on the individual particles produces an acceleration g of the total mass M of the body. The d'Alembertian reversed effective force thus has a magnitude Mg and it is directed upwards along a radius of the earth. We determine the point of application of this effective force by considering the equilibrium between this notional upward force and the combined effect of all the downward forces on the individual particles. The method of moments allows us to calculate where the upward force needs to be applied in order to avoid rotation and to preserve equilibrium. If we repeat the procedure with the body in a different orientation, we arrive at a new position for the line of effective force. The intersection of such lines is usually called the 'centre of gravity' of the body. (It would be more appropriate to call it the 'centre of inertia' since it is true of other forces beside gravity that no rotations are produced if the line of action of the resultant passes through this point. The expression 'centre of mass' is not appropriate since the proportions of the total mass lying on opposite sides of this point are not necessarily equal.) The reversed effective force for the acceleration of a body under gravity is a force Mg taken as acting upwards at the centre of gravity of the body.

There is a temptation to suppose the d'Alembertian upward force Mg to be the same as the reaction force developed against a support. The error in this supposition can be made clear by considering a hollow structure such as a picture frame. It is not possible to support a picture frame by a nail through its centre of gravity! The reaction force corresponding to the downward pull of the earth upon the body under consideration is another gravitational force, namely the attraction exerted by the body upon the earth.

When we push against a massive object to set it into motion, we set up stress forces that act in both directions. We push against the object to accelerate it, and it pushes back against us with a reaction force. In analysing the motion of the object we may introduce a d'Alembertian reversed effective force to facilitate calculation, but this must not be taken to imply that a 'force of inertia' is acting on the object to restrain its motion. The reaction force that leads to the sensation that our push is being resisted is a stress force acting on our body; it does not act on the object that is being accelerated.

The 'centrifugal force' of common speech is another example of a misunderstanding of reaction forces. When we stand in a vehicle that is moving in a curved path, we feel ourselves thrown outwards away from the centre of curvature of the path. To preserve our relative position within the vehicle we need to push against the outer wall. Our sensations correspond to the relative movement of our body within the vehicle whereas, in fact, it is the vehicle that is accelerating, towards the centre of curvature of the path, while the mass of our body is tending to preserve its state of motion in a straight line. If we are to be carried round with the vehicle, a centripetal force has to be transmitted from the vehicle to our body. The stress developed involves equal and opposite forces. One is the inward force that accelerates our body towards the centre of curvature of the path, the other is the outwardly directed reaction force with which we push against the vehicle. Correspondingly, if we hang a weight from a string and then swing the weight round in a circle, the force to accelerate the weight into the curved path of the circle is provided by the tension in the string. The tension pulls the weight towards the support. The string cannot apply centrifugal force on the weight because it cannot develop thrust in compression. The only truly 'centrifugal' force present is that transmitted to the support by the tension in the string. There is no centrifugal force on the weight itself.

THE RELATIONSHIP BETWEEN WEIGHT AND GRAVITY

We can now turn back to the relationship between weight and gravity. As already explained, the notion of weight is associated with the stress force developed between the body and its supports to prevent it from accelerating towards the centre of the earth under the influence of the earth's gravitational attraction. This stress force is indistinguishable in character from the stress developed against the wall of a vehicle that is moving in a curved path. Thus, in a human centrifuge, one feels an increase in weight, and in an orbiting spacecraft, after the rocket motors have been switched off and no further stress forces are acting to restrain the free fall of the vehicle, the astronauts experience the sensation of weightlessness. They no longer need to push against the floor. This does not mean that gravity has ceased to act. Indeed, the very fact that the spacecraft moves in an orbit round the earth is evidence for the continued action of gravity. Accordingly it appears quite perverse to adopt the practice that has grown up in recent years of using such expressions as 'zero gravity' or 'microgravity' in relation to orbital flight, because these suggest that conditions in an orbiting spacecraft in some way provide an escape from the influence of the earth's gravitational field. What such an environment does provide is a relief from the need to exert supporting stress forces.

In the elementary treatment of weight-bearing structures the effects of loading a structure with weights are dealt with by representing the loads as downwardly-directed vectors indicating forces of magnitudes such as Mg for a weight of mass M. This treatment corresponds to the procedure of hanging weights by strings attached to the appropriate points on the structure. The tension in a string is, however, a stress force, and it is not correct to suppose that the vectors so drawn indicate gravitational forces. The stress in such a string is accompanied by a strain in the structure, and complications arise if it is not acceptable to treat the load point as a pin joint exerting thrust on the adjacent members of the structure.

The analysis of the interaction between gravitational and stress forces calls for some care when we are dealing with structures whose mass cannot be neglected in comparison with the imposed loads, and in particular when dealing with the self mass of the structure itself. Because the stress forces involve strain and the gravitational forces do not, it is convenient to analyse the two force systems separately.

The effects of the gravitational forces are comparatively simple: each molecule accelerates with the same acceleration in a gravitational field of a particular strength, without in any way affecting the acceleration of neighbouring molecules. The relative positions, and the relative velocities, of any specific pair of molecules thus remain unaffected by the presence of the gravitational field. Consequently it is not possible to devise any material indicator of the presence or strength of the field, so long as it is uniform. Our knowledge of gravitational phenomena comes exclusively from inhomogeneities in the gravitational field. We observe the motions of objects relative to the earth, which, of course, does not accelerate under the influence of its own gravitational field, or we observe the movements of the celestial bodies relative to one another. Gravitational forces do not develop strain.

To clarify those effects of stress forces on a structure that arise because the material itself, of which the structure is composed, has its own mass, we consider a block of material that is being accelerated by a thrust F_1 applied from the left, as in Figure 2.1. We suppose the block to be arbitrarily divided into three portions by two parallel planes, AB and CD, at right angles to the direction of the acceleration. Let the masses of the three portions be m_1, m_2 and m_3 respectively, where the total mass is

$$M = m_1 + m_2 + m_3$$

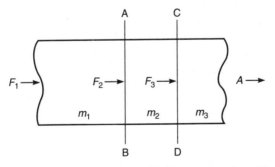

Figure 2.1 Stress distribution associated with acceleration. The stress force exerted across the section AB is greater than that exerted across CD because of the difference in the masses which they accelerate. A stress gradient is present throughout the material of the block.

Then we have

$$F_1 = MA$$

where A is the acceleration, which is the same for all parts of the block. Looking now at the slice of material between the two planes, we see that, at each of the planes, the force exerted has to accelerate the mass of material to the right of that plane. Thus, the stress force exerted from left to right across the plane AB is

$$F_2 = (m_2 + m_3)A$$

while that across the plane CD is

$$F_3 = m_3A$$

The stress at the left hand plane is greater than that at the right hand plane. The acceleration by stress forces of a block of material having distributed mass thus implies a gradient of stress in the direction of the imposed acceleration.

The stress gradient involved in accelerating distributed masses by imposed contact forces is illustrated in Figure 2.2(d). No gradient is present in free fall (Figure 2.2(a)) in spite of the acceleration due to gravity, since gravity itself does not involve strain. If the structure is restrained from falling freely, the supporting stress forces involve a stress gradient (Figure 2.2(b)). No stress gradients arise in directions at right angles to the supporting thrust in the absence of acceleration, either at rest (Figure 2.2(c)) or where the imposed stress forces balance one another (Figure 2.2(e)).

To separate the effects of stress from those attributable to gravity, we first resolve the accelerations of the parts into two components, respectively gravitational and stress-related. The gravitational acceleration is straightforward; it depends only on the local gravitational field strength. The stress-related component of acceleration is accordingly obtained by adding to the vector expressing the observed motion an additional acceleration vector equal in magnitude to the gravitational vector but directed in the opposite sense. The effects of the stress forces on the masses composing the structure under consideration are then determined by reference to the new combined stress–acceleration vector, taking account of the way the mass is distributed through the structure and of the stiffnesses of those parts of the structure that contribute to load bearing.

Because of the mass distribution and as a consequence of local variations in stiffness, the stresses and strains will be different in different parts of the structure. It is accordingly convenient, instead of specifying the accelerating stress forces in newtons, to refer to their effects in terms of the accelerations themselves, using as a unit the

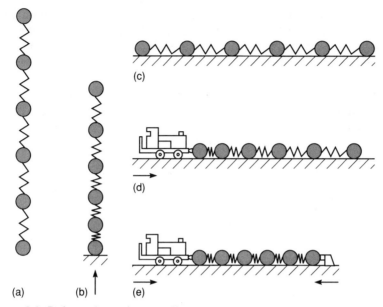

Figure 2.2 Deformations of a compliant structure with distributed mass. (a) Free fall: no deformation. (b) Supported on end: stress-gradient aligned with impressed force. (c) Supported on side: no horizontal deformation. (d) Accelerated by unbalanced stress forces: stress-gradient aligned with inpressed force. (e) Compressed by balanced stress forces: no stress-gradient.

standard value for the acceleration due to gravity at the earth's surface, namely 9.81 m/s^2, or g. Forces expressed in this way are sometimes referred to as 'g-forces'. This must not be taken to mean that they are in any sense gravitational. They remain stress forces in character, although the unit of measurement is derived from studies on gravity.

With these conventions, a body that is held at rest with respect to the earth's surface needs to be supported by stress forces amounting to 1g. If the support thrust exceeds this value the object will move away from the earth, as during a rocket launch. If the support thrust is less than 1g, the body will fall. Thrusts that act at an angle to the earth's radius will produce a horizontal component of motion relative to the earth's surface.

When a body is supported at rest on the earth's surface, the stress forces and the gravitational forces do not cancel out, although the combined acceleration is zero. The stress forces are always accompanied by the local deformations of strain. In orbit, on the other hand, the g-forces are absent, or very small, while the action of the gravitational field is unopposed. There is no question of the gravitational forces being 'neutralized' or 'compensated' in some way, as might be inferred from the publications of the Space Agencies, NASA and ESA, in relation to their so-called 'Microgravity Research Programmmes'. Instead of speaking of 'zero gravity', it would be preferable to use the expression 'zero-g', since it is the g-forces that are diminished in orbit, not the gravitational forces.

It may be that this confusion has arisen from thinking of force and acceleration in terms of cause and effect. It is preferable to regard these expressions as equivalent alternative ways of measuring a single type of event, namely a change in motion. If we are interested in forces, then we measure in newtons-per-kilogram, or as g-forces using the scale-factor g to relate to the standard conditions of field strength obtaining in the gravitational field at mean sea level on the surface of the earth. If we are interested in the acceleration aspect, we measure in metres-per-second per second. Here the unit g is specified as $9.81\,\text{m/s}^2$. The relationsip between these two measures is given by an algebraic rearrangement of Newton's Second Law to read: 'The acceleration of a body is equal to the ratio between the force on it and its mass'; i.e.

$$A = F/M$$

In an orbiting spacecraft there are no convenient reference points from which to measure the common accelerations of all the parts. It is a false conclusion to suppose that the absence of indications from accelerometers in the spacecraft may be taken as evidence that no gravitational force is acting. Indeed, without it there would be no orbital motion.

The conventional downwardly-directed arrow drawn through the centre of gravity (as in schoolbook representations of problems in dynamics) is to be taken, not as a vector indicating the pull of gravity, but as representing the d'Alembertian 'reversed effective force' required for resolution of the pattern of imposed stress forces considered on their own. When the imposed stress forces are in equilibrium, as they are in free fall, the 'effective force', in relation to these stress forces alone, is zero. But the gravitational force is still present, to account for the centripetal acceleration of the orbit.

Struts and springs 3

All the active forces developed by the muscles of the body are tensions. In contrast, the forces needed to support the body in an upright posture, with the feet below the centre of gravity, are compressive thrusts against the ground. We need, therefore, to consider the relationship between tensions and thrusts.

THE SOLID STATE

One of the properties that distinguishes the solid state is that the individual molecules are held together in a specific geometric arrangement by intermolecular cohesive forces. It is this property that gives solids their rigidity. Attempts to change the geometric arrangement, that is to say attempts to change the shape of the solid, are met by those intermolecular forces that resist the relative displacement of the molecules. In a particular region where two molecules interact, the force between them is dependent on the distance of separation in a complicated way. At very short distances the molecules repel one another; at somewhat larger distances they attract one another; at yet larger distances this attractive force decreases very rapidly with further increase in distance. Thus while the cohesive force that holds the molecules together depends on their being close enough to one another, any attempt to push them even closer will be resisted.

If we consider a pile of sand, the individual grains resist distortion but the pile as a whole does not, unless it is supported laterally. Dry sand appears to behave rather like a fluid. The reason is that the individual grains can move relative to one another. To give resistance to deformation we need to add a component capable of withstanding tensile stress, such as cement, to hold the individual grains together. Modern synthetic adhesives and cements rely for their tensile properties on the formation of long molecules which have their own intrinsic strength and which are attached to one another at various places along their length to form chains or networks that resist deformation in tension. The structure of bone includes mineral components to resist compression, together with organic components to resist local tensions and to hold the whole together in a rigid shape.

In general, a watery solution of long organic molecules will not support tensile stress, because the molecules do not come close enough together. They can be brought together by drying out the solution, as in the setting of carpenter's glue, or by the various biological processes that organize the linking up of long molecules, as in the fine structure of the muscle cell (described in detail in the next chapter).

The geometrical organization of the molecules of myosin and actin in muscle cells forms myofibrils capable of supporting tension. This tension is transmitted through tendons where the long molecules that support the tension include collagen, a protein which, when extracted with water, gives glue (*kolla* in Greek). The development of muscle tension is carried out wholly within the cells. At the ends of these cells it is necessary for the tension to be transmitted to extracellular structures. The Z-membranes in muscle cells contain collagen, and the last Z-membrane at the end of a muscle cell communicates its tension to the extracellular collagen of the tendon. At the attachment of a tendon to bone we find further organized collagen molecules linked to similar proteins forming the tensile matrix of the bone.

To understand the way the muscles interact with the bones we need to rely on a modelling procedure. The models may be physical structures or they can be purely conceptual in nature. In making a model we need to define the properties of the individual components and we need to specify the way these components are linked together and interact with one another. We suppose the model to be subjected to some treatment and we then compare the way the model responds to this treatment with the response observed when comparable treatments are applied to the system under study. Any discrepancies prompt us to modify our model. When the agreement is fairly good we can conclude that the principles on which our model is constructed bear a useful relationship of similarity to the principles of operation of the subject of study. It is often helpful to start with simple models even though it is obvious that they have certain defects.

Our consideration above of a pile of sand is an example of this kind of modelling procedure. To pursue this example further, we note that, although a pile of sand has no structural rigidity of itself, we can impart some rigidity to it by packing the sand into a number of sandbags. The bags can then be piled on top of one another to form a wall with sufficient rigidity to act as a defence against flooding or to form part of an air raid shelter. In this case the cohesion needed for rigidity is provided by the tension developed in the fibres of the sackcloth forming the bags.

The effect of a compressive stress can be considered in relation to a packed group of spheres. Let us look at a group of four spheres arranged as in Figure 3.1. A compressive thrust is applied along the line AB to push the spheres A and B towards one another. Relative movement in this direction is impeded by the spheres C and D which would have to be pushed apart to allow A and B to come closer together. We may suppose the compressive forces transmitted from one sphere to another to act along the normal to the surface at the point of contact. In a real case, the particles of a solid are not true spheres, so the angles between the forces at the points of interaction will not be precisely those that are applicable for the interaction of spheres. Nevertheless, the principles that emerge from our treatment of this simple model will prove instructive.

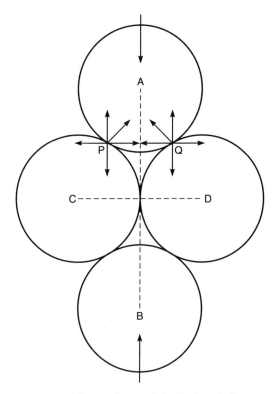

Figure 3.1 Arrangement of four spheres, labelled at their centres, to illustrate the effects of compressive forces. Compression between A and B produces stresses at P and Q with components, at right angles to AB, which push C and D apart.

If P is the point of contact between A and C the thrust normal to the surface of contact at P can be resolved into two components, one parallel to AB and the other at right angles to this direction. Similarly, at Q, the point of contact between A and D, we have two components one parallel to AB and the other at right angles to it. The forces acting on the sphere A at P and Q in a direction parallel to CD serve to compress the sphere A. The reaction forces to these components act on the spheres C and D to push them apart.

The compressive thrust applied along the line AB thus develops other thrusts radiating out in all directions in the plane at right angles to the direction AB. We can see the effect of such radial thrusts when the end of a rivet is struck with a hammer to form the swelling that gives the rivet its function.

The reason why a pile of sand offers little resistance to deformation is that, when a thrust is applied to it in any particular direction, the grains are pushed aside by the radial thrusts that develop at right angles to the line of the applied thrust. The fabric of the sandbag serves to restrain this radial flow.

The action of the tension in the fibres of the sackcloth of the sandbags can be worked out with the aid of Figure 3.2. This shows a portion of a fibre AB, curved downwards in the plane of the paper. The tensions at A and B each act at an angle to the line AB, and we can resolve these forces into components parallel to AB and components at right angles to this direction. The components parallel to AB are equal and opposite to one another but the components at right angles to AB combine to give a lateral thrust, downwards in the plane of the paper, towards the centre of curvature of the fibre. In the case of the sandbag, comparable lateral thrusts exerted by the fibres of the bag compress the sand inside the bag and prevent the particles from being pushed aside when the bags are piled on top of one another.

A somewhat similar action is exerted by the muscles of the walls of the hollow organs, such as the blood vessels, bladder and gut, and also of the abdomen. Tension in curved fibres develops inwardly-directed radial thrust to meet the hydrostatic pressure of the fluid contained in the cavity of the organ.

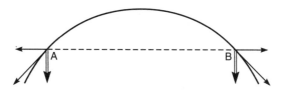

Figure 3.2 Tension in a curved fibre, as in the fabric of a sandbag, produces lateral compression.

When a solid is subjected to a compressive thrust, as in Figure 3.3, the line of this thrust is surrounded by other thrusts radiating outwards, together with tensile stresses arising from intermolecular cohesion and acting at right angles to these radial thrusts, as do the tensions in the fibres of the sandbag. The presence of these circumferentially-oriented tensile stresses can be appreciated by observing that, if a rod of metal is repeatedly struck on the end with a hammer, after the end has begun to splay out somewhat, it develops radial cracks at the outer edges of the swelling. These cracks arise when the tensile stresses exceed the cohesive strength of the metal.

The directions of action of the tensile cohesive forces between molecules are not, in general, lined up with the line of action of any tension that might be imposed upon the material as a whole. Such tensions will, accordingly, set up internal compressive thrusts.

We can see the effect of longitudinal tension in developing internal compression when a wetted rope is put under tension. When a slack rope is wetted, water is taken up into the spaces between the fibres. Then, when tension is applied, water is wrung out and drips from the tautened rope. Because the fibres from which the rope is formed are twisted together, the applied longitudinal tension has the effect of compressing the fibres laterally against one another, thus squeezing out the water previously trapped between the fibres.

The whole pattern of thrusts and tensions within a particular piece of material subjected to external forces, either in tension or in compression, will therefore vary from place to place within the material according to the details of the local molecular architecture.

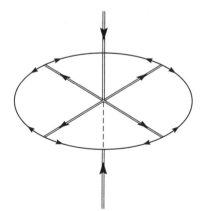

Figure 3.3 The spreading produced by a compressive stress generates circumferential tensile stresses.

LEVERS

Another way in which tension can be converted into thrust is by the action of a lever. In elementary treatments the lever is regarded as a straight beam subjected to three parallel external forces, where the points of application of these forces lie in a straight line and their direction of action lies at right angles to this line. In such an arrangement we may refer to the three points of application of the external forces as A, B and C, where B lies between A and C. The forces may be applied either as tensions or as thrusts, but the force at B must be in the opposite sense to the other two forces. It is often convenient to regard the lever as receiving 'effort' at one point and delivering it to a 'load' at another point, the third point being regarded as a passive support called the 'fulcrum'. Levers are classified in three 'orders' according to which of the three points, fulcrum, load or effort, lies between the other two.

Consider the lever shown in Figure 3.4, where the fulcrum is at B, supported by a thrust directed upwards in the plane of the paper. The forces at A and C are tensions, acting downwards. The magnitude of the thrust at B must, at equilibrium, be equal to the sum of the magnitudes of the tensions at A and C.

The action of the tension at A, in conjunction with the support at B, is to tend to rotate the lever anticlockwise about B. The magnitude of the turning effect, or 'turning moment' as it is called, is measured as the product of the force at A multiplied by the offset distance from B to the line of action of the tension at A. The tension at C also exerts a turning moment, this time clockwise about B. At equilibrium the two turning moments must be equal and opposite.

The combined action of the three forces at A, B and C is to tend to bend the beam. To support this 'bending stress' the material of which the beam is composed develops internal stresses. The material of the upper part of the beam in Figure 3.4 is in tension, while the lower part is in compression.

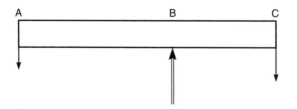

Figure 3.4 Bending effect of forces on a lever. The upper part of the material in the beam is in tension while the lower part is in compression.

In real cases, the beam of a lever is not necessarily straight, nor are the points of application of the external forces located in a single line. To analyse the behaviour of such a complex lever, for example that shown in Figure 3.5, we select one of the applied forces (acting at B in the figure) such that its line of action lies between the points of application of the other two (labelled A and C). We then produce the line of action of the force at B to intersect the line joining A and C. Let the point of intersection be P. If, for the moment, we consider only the external forces and ignore the internal stresses, the effect of the force at B will be just the same as that of an equal force applied at P. We now resolve each of the three forces, at A, P and C, into components parallel to and at right angles to AC.

The operation of a lever can be considered from another point of view. In Figure 3.6 a force P is shown as directed upwards at A together with an equal force P directed downwards at B, where the distance AB $= x$. The turning moment of the force at A about another point C, where BC $= y$, is $P(x + y)$ in a clockwise direction, while the turning moment of the force at B about the same axis is Py anticlockwise. The combined turning moment is

$$\{P(x + y) - Py\} = Px$$

clockwise, which is independent of y. It follows that the combined turning moment of a pair of equal and opposite parallel but non-coincident forces is independent of the position of the axis of rotation. Such a pair of forces is referred to as a 'couple'.

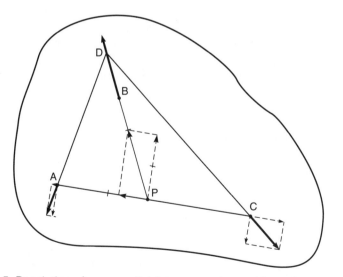

Figure 3.5 Resolution of non-parallel forces on a lever of irregular shape.

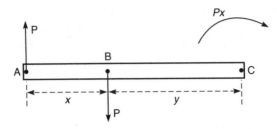

Figure 3.6 Parallel non-coincident forces. The turning moment, Px, about any point, C, is independent of y.

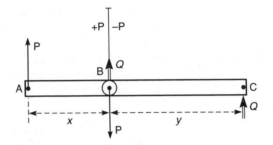

Figure 3.7 Lever working against a restraint, at B, under the influence of the combination of a couple with a thrust.

TORQUE

Since the same turning moment can be produced by different pairs of forces, each at the appropriate offset, so long as the product Px is the same, we may speak in terms of the product of force multiplied by offset as a 'torque', instead of speaking of the individual forces or of a couple.

The lever in Figure 3.7 is just like that in Figure 3.6 but with the addition of an upthrust Q applied at C. If we now suppose the point B to be restrained by an external support, the upward force exerted against the support must, at equilibrium, be equal to the sum of the two upthrust forces, P at A and Q at C, less the downward force P at B, i.e. $(P + Q) - P$, or Q. The turning moment produced by the couple consisting of P upwards at A together with P downwards at B is equivalent to a clockwise torque Px applied anywhere along the length of the lever. Thus the effect of adding the clockwise couple Px to the upthrust Q at C is to shift the point of application of the upthrust from C to B through the distance y, where $Qy = Px$ (Figure 3.8).

It is sometimes convenient to represent couples as vectors. The

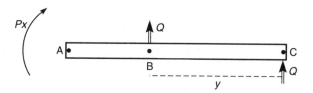

Figure 3.8 Action of an applied torque in shifting the line of action of a force. The application of the torque Px at any point on the lever has the effect of shifting the line of action of the thrust Q from C to B, where $Qy = Px$.

length of the vector is taken as indicating the magnitude of the turning moment; its line of action is along the axis about which the turning effect is to take place; and the direction of the arrowhead on the vector is selected to indicate that, if a rotation in the sense of the couple is accompanied by a movement in the direction of the arrow, this will produce a movement along a right-handed screw.

Using this convention, we can assess the effect of any combination of external forces upon a body by the following procedure. We first pick some arbitrary reference point as our origin and resolve each of the linear force vectors into components parallel to three mutually perpendicular axes. We then work out what couples are required to shift each of these linear components of force along the appropriate axis until it acts through the origin. We then recombine the resultants in the three reference planes to give a single force through the origin. Next we represent each of the couples as vectors through the origin and combine these into a single vector. We finish up with a single linear force and a single couple.

The conditions for equilibrium are that each of these two components must have zero magnitude. Another useful rule is that, at an equilibrium between three forces, the lines of action of the forces can be produced to meet in a single point.

When a torque is applied to a beam which is being used as a lever, the beam tends to bend. The stresses of bending are not uniformly distributed through the material of the beam. Figure 3.9 represents a longitudinal section through a beam subjected to a clockwise torque in its right-hand portion and to a balancing anticlockwise torque in its left-hand portion.

Consider the conditions in the material lying in a plane at right angles to the long axis of the beam, cutting the plane of the figure in the line AB. The material to the left of AB exerts an anticlockwise torque on the material to the right of that plane which, in turn, exerts a clockwise reaction torque on the material to the left. This means that the material near the upper surface of the beam will be stressed in tension while the stress in the lower parts of the beam will be in

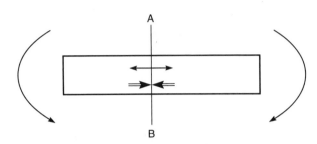

Figure 3.9 Effect of opposed torques on internal forces.

compression. The intensity of the stress varies continuously across the thickness of the beam, being greatest near the surface and falling to zero at some neutral position somewhere in the thickness of the beam, the precise location of the zero stress depending upon the fine structure of the beam.

A cross-section through a piece of bone reveals that the hard material responsible for the stiffness of the bone is not uniformly distributed through the cross-section. The bone is much denser near the surface, while the inner parts have a spongy appearance. The hard material is here restricted to relatively thin sheets and pillars, called 'trabeculae', with spaces in between containing blood vessels and other soft tissues.

This disposition of hard, 'compact', bone near the surface and the spongy, 'cancellous', structure of the inner parts reflects the distribution of the intensity of the stresses. The trabeculae form an intricate three-dimensional lattice and it is possible that the axes of the individual trabeculae lie along lines of stress-concentration. This is particularly apparent near the end regions of the long bones, where there is a concentration of the influences of the forces at the joints.

All the hard material of living bone is subject to continual demolition and reconstruction by the action of the soft tissues lying in the various spaces. This process permits the remodelling needed for growth and the more intense activity of healing and repair after fracture.

SHEAR

If the torques applied at the two ends of a beam are in the same sense, as in Figure 3.10, the stress distribution within the material of the beam is different from that in pure bending. We again consider the effects upon one another, across a hypothetical plane of section cutting the figure in the line AB, of the material forming the opposing faces. The material to the left of AB will tend to slide downwards, while that to the right will be forced upwards. Such a stress distribution is called **shear stress**. It can be shown to be made up, on the microscopic scale,

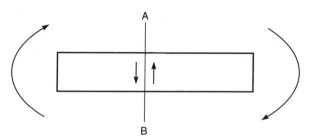

Figure 3.10 Torques applied in the same sense at the two ends of a beam involve shear stresses, the material to the left of the plane AB pulling down against the upward pull of the material to the right of the plane.

of a combination of compressive and tensile stresses at right angles to one another and at 45° to the plane of shear.

Up to this point, in relation to the effect of parallel non-coincident forces acting as a couple to apply torque to a beam, we have considered only cases where the axis of the beam lies in the same plane as that of the parallel forces. The external effects are those of a lever, while the internal effect is a bending of the beam. We now turn to the situation in which the axis of the beam lies at an angle to the plane of the couple.

In such a case, each of the imposed forces can be resolved into two components, one in a plane containing the long axis of the beam, and the other in a plane at right angles to this. We can then recombine the four resolved components to form one couple in the same plane as the axis of the beam together with a second couple in a plane at right angles to this. The first of these couples tends to bend the beam, while the second tends to twist it about its long axis. The twisting sets up torsional shear stresses in the material of the beam.

The relation between torsion and shear can be appreciated by thinking of what happens when we take the lid off a screw-top jar. The twistings applied in opposite directions to lid and jar together cause the lid to slide round relative to the jar. Sliding is what happens when shear forces exceed the strength of the material under stress.

The relationship between shear stresses and the combination of compressive and tensile stresses, referred to above, may be illustrated by twisting a stick of blackboard chalk. The fracture surfaces have a spiral shape, corresponding to the fact that chalk can resist compression better than tension. The chalk fractures along a plane at right angles to the tensile stress.

There are very few instances in which bones are called upon to resist torsional stresses. They nearly always act either as struts or as levers. In some animals, e.g. amphibians and reptiles, the vertical plane through the joints at the two ends of the proximal long bone of a limb (humerus or femur) does not always pass through the point of contact of the foot with the ground. In such cases this long bone is subjected to torsional stresses and the limb behaves as a crank (Figure 3.11).

We are now in a position to start analysing what goes on when a man stands on one leg with the knee slightly bent, as in Figure 3.12. The centre of gravity, C, of the body must be vertically over the point of application, F, of the upthrust at the foot. To find the position of F we resort to a specially designed force platform.

THE FORCE PLATFORM

Figure 3.13 shows some of the details of the principles on which such a force platform is constructed. Sets of strain gauges are fitted to the supports of the platform at the four corners of a rectangle, front left and right (FL and FR), and back left and right (BL and BR), respectively. Each set of gauges indicates the vertical and two horizontal components of force. The horizontal forces are lined up along the fore-and-aft and lateral directions.

The sum of all the vertical indications gives the magnitude of the vertical component of the resultant upthrust. Similarly the horizontal indications can be added in groups to give overall components in the fore-and-aft and lateral directions.

If we combine the upthrusts indicated at the two front supports, their sum will be independent of the lateral position of the resultant upthrust. Call this combined indication U. Combine the two upthrusts at the back edge of the platform similarly to get V. Now $(U + V)$ is the

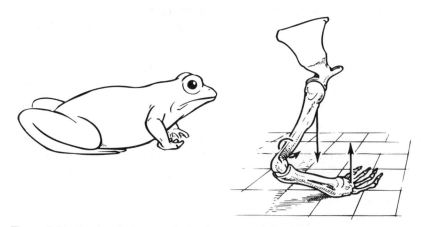

Figure 3.11 Torsional stresses in the humerus of the frog.

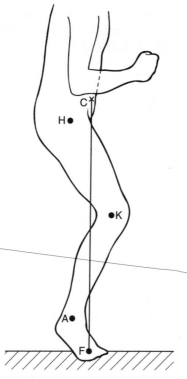

Figure 3.12 Side view of a man standing with knee bent. Upthrust exerted against the foot at F is transmitted to the centre of gravity, C, by a jointed framework in which torques are exerted at the pivot points; A, at the ankle; K, at the knee; H, at the hip.

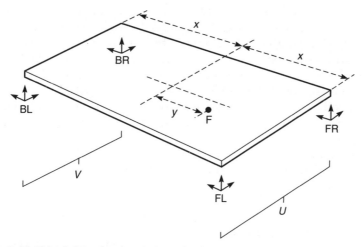

Figure 3.13 Principles of construction of a force platform with three-directional strain transducers at each corner.

magnitude of the combined vertical component of upthrust. Suppose U is greater than V. Then the point of application of the resultant will be nearer to the front of the platform than to the back. If the length of the platform is $2x$, and y is the distance between the midpoint and the point of application of the resultant upthrust (measured in the forward direction), then we can consider the tendency for the two components of upthrust to tilt the platform about the point of application of the resultant. These tendencies must be equal and we have

$$U(x - y) = V(x + y)$$

hence

$$y = x(U - V)/(U + V)$$

This gives us the position, in the fore-and-aft direction, of the point of application of the resultant upthrust. We can also derive a value for its position in the lateral direction.

If all the horizontal indications are taken together, with due regard to sign and to the dimensions of the rectangle, as well as to the position within this rectangle of the point of application of the resultant upthrust, we can derive an indication of the torque exerted against the ground about a vertical axis, as well as the direction and magnitude of the horizontal component of the upthrust. Since there are no tensions exerted between the feet and the platform, there can be no torques about horizontal axes.

STANDING WITH A BENT KNEE

We now return to Figure 3.12. In an inert structure, the centre of gravity is supported above the ground by rigid struts, as a table is supported by rigid legs. In contrast, the legs of a man are not simple rigid struts. The bones of the leg are loosely hinged together and, although each is rigid in itself, they are thus unable, on their own, to withstand the longitudinal compressive stress imposed by the weight of the body. The rigidity of the bones has to be combined with the action of muscular forces to convert the leg as a whole into a suitably rigid pillar.

The diagram of Figure 3.14 represents the human leg in a very much simplified manner. Attention is confined to a single fore-and-aft plane. No account is taken of the effects of muscles that act in directions that lie outside this plane, nor of the actions of muscles that span more than one joint. Even with these simplifications, there remain a number of complexities that display instructive features.

In this figure the pivots at the ankle, knee and hip do not lie vertically above the foot, so the weight of the body would collapse the

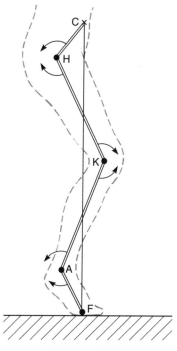

Figure 3.14 Simplified version of Figure 3.12.

leg were it not for the turning moments applied at each of these joints by muscular action. The effect of these torques is to shift the position of the upthrust so that it can be transmitted from one bone to another, eventually communicating the thrust from the ground right up to the centre of gravity.

Thus the couple acting on the foot at A, in Figure 3.14, shifts the line of the upthrust from F to A, while the reaction couple acting on the tibia shifts the upthrust back to the vertical over F. The couple acting on the tibia at K shifts the upthrust out to K, while the reaction couple on the femur shifts it back again. Similarly, at the hip the couple acting on the femur moves the upthrust out to H, while the reaction couple acting on the trunk moves it back to C.

The foot and ankle are shown in more detail in Figure 3.15. The position of the point F is derived from the indications of the gauges on the force platform. The line of action of the tension in the tendon, T, can be determined by inspection. The axis of rotation at the ankle is governed by the anatomy of the joint. The lower end of the tibia has a hollow, roughly cylindrical, cavity that slides over the convex cylindrical upper surface of the ankle bone (the talus). The centre of

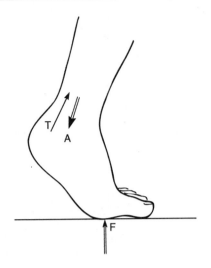

Figure 3.15 Forces on the foot.

rotation for flexion and extension of the foot is thus the centre of curvature of the surface of the talus.

The forces acting on the foot are: the upthrust from the ground, the pull of the Achilles tendon, and the thrust of the tibia against the ankle bone. At equilibrium, the lines of these three forces must meet in a point (labelled I in Figure 3.16, which shows the lines of action of these same forces on a different scale). It is of interest to observe that this point does not lie within the substance of the tibia since it must lie on the line of action of the muscles pulling on the Achilles tendon.

The line of action of the thrust from the tibia is given by the position of the intersection point, I, since the upthrust from the ground must be vertical and the line of action of the pull of the Achilles tendon must lie along the tendon, which cannot support a bending stress.

The tension in the Achilles tendon is provided by two muscle groups, one having its origin on the tibia and the other with its origin on the femur. The action of this second group crosses two joints and does not contribute to weight-bearing. The arrangement does, however, greatly complicate the overall picture.

We arrive at the magnitude of the contribution of the weight-bearing single-joint muscle to the tension in the tendon, from the magnitude of the upthrust at F (which is equal to the body weight), taking account of the two offsets, a, the horizontal distance from A to F, and t the offset from A to the tendon. If the force in the tendon is T, and the body weight is W, then $Wa = Tt$, so that $T = Wa/t$.

To get the magnitude of the thrust at the ankle, we adopt the

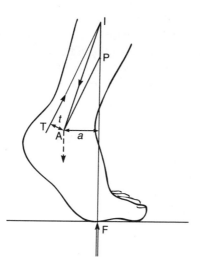

Figure 3.16 Graphical determination of forces acting at the foot, from Figure 3.15. Note that I does not lie within the tibial bone, implying that the bone supports bending stress as well as longitudinal compression.

following graphical construction. Draw a line from A parallel to the line of the tendon to meet FI at P. Then, if the length of PI is taken to represent the magnitude of the upthrust W, the magnitude of the tension in the tendon and that of the thrust from the tibia are given, on the same scale, by the lengths of the lines AP and IA respectively.

To convince ourselves that this construction gives the right answer, proceed as follows. Draw a perpendicular from A to IF. The length of this will be a. Draw another perpendicular from A to IT. The length of this is t. Now consider the triangle API. The area of a triangle is equal to half the base multiplied by the height. If we take PI as the base, the height will be a, and the area is $(PI)a/2$. If we take AP as the base, the height will be t, and the area is $(AP)t/2$. These two calculations must give the same area as we are dealing with the same triangle in each case. Hence

$$(PI)a = (AP)t$$

which is the relationship we require. This argument also provides the justification for the parallelogram rule for the resolution and combination of vectors.

It is clear from the figure that the thrust transmitted across the ankle joint is considerably greater than the body weight.

The interplay of the three external forces on the foot in Figure 3.15 would be just the same if the foot were to be replaced by a simple triangular structure made up of three straight members linked by pin joints, as in Figure 3.17. The two members AF and AT are under compression and are called 'struts', while FT is under tension and is called a 'tie'. The relative magnitudes of the forces in the three members can be obtained by using the parallelogram rule at each corner in turn. The operation of such a triangular structure as a lever may be analysed by the method of Figure 3.5.

TRIANGULATED LATTICE STRUCTURES

This type of model is an example of a very useful principle. It is always possible to design a theoretical triangulated lattice structure, made up of straight struts and ties linked by pin joints, to support any given set of external forces. Indeed, many modern engineering structures are constructed on this same principle. The triangulated lattice structures of cranes, roof trusses and bridges have become quite familiar features of our city skylines.

It is important to remember that, in the discussion of models consisting of triangulated lattice structures, we are dealing only with the **external** forces. The distribution of internal stresses in the material of a structure subjected to external forces, such as the effect of the force applied at B in Figure 3.5, is not at all the same as the effect of an equal force applied at P.

One way to find out about internal stresses is to make use of the fact that certain plastics, such as perspex or lucite, show differences in their optical properties when they are put under strain. If a model of the structure of interest is made out of one of these plastics, the distribution of internal strains can be made visible by examining the specimen

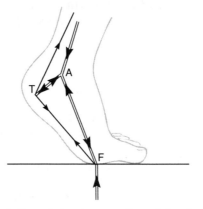

Figure 3.17 Representation of the lever action of the foot by a triangulated lattice. In this case each triangle consists of two struts and a tie.

with transmitted polarized light. The pattern of strains is often quite complicated.

This procedure with a plastic model is not applicable if the structure is not homogeneous. The foot is not a homogeneous structure. The stresses in the foot are distributed unequally among a number of bones, ligaments, tendons and muscles, and also through important fibrous pads, in a manner that is dependent on the nervous control of the various muscles involved, those in the leg as well as those in the foot itself. The intricate coordination of the activities of all these elements serves to alter the distribution of pressure against the ground and thus to shift the position of the resultant upthrust. One can feel the effect of these adjustments taking place when moving one's weight slowly over the feet. An indication of the separate contributions to weight-bearing made by the individual toes is given by the prints left by someone running barefoot on wet sand. Detailed analysis of the control of the foot is beyond the scope of the elementary treatment presented in this book.

There is little problem in assigning a position to the centre of rotation at the ankle joint because of the geometry of the articular surfaces.

At the hip, the anatomy of the joint also defines the centre of rotation, this being a ball-and-socket joint. One might suppose, therefore, that the conditions at the hip could, in principle, be analysed in a similar manner to that used for the ankle, since the torque required is given by the horizontal offset from H to C in Figure 3.12.

Problems arise in two ways. It is not always clear just where the centre of gravity is located anatomically, since it shifts when the limbs are moved relative to the trunk. On the other hand, we know that the centre of gravity of the body must always lie vertically over the point of application of the resultant upthrust from the ground, and the position of this point of application is given by the indications from the force platform.

Another difficulty arises in assigning a position to the line of action of the muscles spanning the hip joint, since there are several of these and they are arranged in three dimensions around the joint. The lateral position of the hip relative to the foot may vary from time to time since the weight is moved from side to side in the natural swaying action of quiet standing. The effect of this is that different amounts of lateral torque are required at the hip, this torque being supplied by the same set of muscles as are used for torque in the fore-and-aft plane. Furthermore it will, in general, not be known which of the muscles is active at any particular time.

These problems have proved a serious obstacle in working out what forces are likely to be imposed on an artificial replacement for the hip joint, such as is sometimes required in the treatment of joint disease.

THE KNEE JOINT

The articular surfaces at the knee joint do not define the axis of rotation, since the bones forming the joint do not fit snugly together (Figure 3.18). The lower end of the femur is formed into a pair of rounded rollers (the femoral condyles), with some resemblance to the paired wheels used on airliners and heavy lorries. These rollers bear against relatively flat surfaces on the upper end of the tibia. During a change in the angle at the knee there is a combination of rolling and sliding movements of the femur over the tibia. The amount of sliding is not the same for the two rollers, and this allows for some rotation of the tibia about its own axis. Lateral sliding is prevented by a promontory on the upper end of the tibia that engages in a groove between the two rollers of the femur.

There are four ligaments spanning the joint to limit relative movement of the bones. Two of these, the 'cruciate ligaments', are situated close together near to the promontory on the head of the tibia. The other two lie at the medial and lateral limits of the joint respectively, confining movement of the tibia to a single plane fixed relative to the femur, while permitting a small amount of axial rotation of the tibia itself.

If the knee is flexed, and an attempt is made to impose a sliding movement at the joint, either passively or by the action of muscles, the tibia cannot be made to move either backwards or forwards under the femur (in the absence of injury). Furthermore, it is not possible to pull the bones away from one another at any position of the joint. It follows

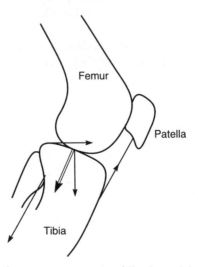

Figure 3.18 Profiles of some components of the knee joint, with indications of the forces (not to scale).

that neither of the cruciate ligaments has any slack in it in any position of the joint.

It has been demonstrated that the profile of the articular cartilages is such as just to keep the cruciate ligaments from going slack when the joint is moved. A possible mechanism for this might be that high points are rubbed off, while the cartilage is built up to fill the available space wherever it is not intermittently pressed upon.

One may conclude that the instantaneous centre of rotation for relative movement of the bones at the joint must lie at the intersection of the projection, onto the median plane of the joint, of the lines of action of the two cruciate ligaments.

There is a complication that affects this conclusion. Each of the cruciate ligaments has an appreciable thickness, and the points of attachment of the individual fibres forming a ligament are distributed over a considerable area of bone in each case. It is not immediately clear where the 'lines of action' of the ligaments should be drawn so there is some doubt about the true position of the centre of rotation at any particular angle of the joint. Whatever the actual position of the centre of rotation, some fibres must lie in front of and some behind it. This means that, when the joint is being flexed, fibres crossing from one bone to the other in front of the axis of rotation will be stretched while those lying behind the centre of rotation will be slackened.

There is presumably some tolerance on the change of length for a ligamentous fibre to survive without rupture, and some help may be available from the fact that the fibres are twisted round one another. Nevertheless, it is interesting to inquire about the possible uniqueness of locations on the two bones that can be linked by constant-length links at all positions of the joint, and whether the body uses all the possible locations for the attachment of ligaments, remembering that the lateral ligaments have to be accommodated as well as the cruciate ligaments.

The torque required at the knee is provided by the action of the quadriceps muscle, acting through its tendon, through the patella, and through the patellar tendon. The patella runs in a circular groove in the end of the femur, but the centre of curvature of this groove is some way away from the axis of rotation of the joint. All of these factors contribute to making the analysis of the forces at the knee a very complicated task.

In dealing with the foot, we regarded it as a single element acted upon by two thrusts and a single tension, where the lines of action of these three forces meet in a point. The patella is also acted on by three forces, two tensions and a single thrust. For the tibia, we have to consider two thrusts, one at each end, and three tensions, while for the femur we need three thrusts and three tensions.

At the knee we have to take account of tension in the ligaments spanning the joint as well as of the actions of muscles. This is because the direction of the thrust transmitted from femur to tibia must always be normal to the articular surface at the point of contact, otherwise the bones would slide over one another. Since the normal to the articular surface is not necessarily parallel to the line of the patellar tendon, and since it is usually not vertical either, there has to be another component of tension across the joint in a direction parallel to the surface of contact to combine with the normal thrust to give a resultant in the required direction.

The five forces on the tibia are represented in Figure 3.19. From our analysis of the forces on the foot we know that the upthrust from the ankle combines with the pull of the Achilles tendon to provide an

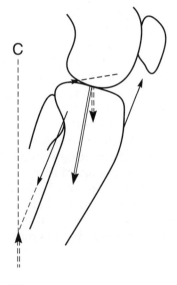

Figure 3.19 Relative magnitudes of the forces on the head of the tibia. At the lower end, the tension in the Achilles tendon converts the thrust exerted at the end of the tibia into a vertical upthrust in the line FC. At the upper end, the tension in the patellar tendon acts, in conjunction with that in the posterior cruciate ligament, to convert the stress at the point of contact with the femur (which necessarily acts at right angles to the articular surface) into a vertical upthrust exerted against the femur. In this configuration of the joint, the tension in the posterior cruciate ligament is too small to show up on the scale of this figure and the anterior ligament is not loaded at all. Forces exerted in paddle action, by muscles spanning more than one joint, would have to be added. Note that the compressive thrust acting across the articular surfaces between femur and tibia considerably exceeds bodyweight.

upthrust of magnitude W acting in the line FC. The lines of action of the other three forces are known so that, if we assign variables to the magnitudes of these forces, we can write an expression for the sum of their turning moments about the point of contact between the articular surfaces of the tibia and the femur. This total turning moment must be equal to Wk, where k is the offset from the point of contact between the bones to the vertical line FC. Each of the three forces can be resolved into vertical and horizontal components. The sum of the vertical components must be a downward thrust of magnitude W, and the sum of the horizontal components must be zero. We thus have three equations which may be solved to give the values of our three unknown magnitudes for the three forces acting between the femur and the tibia.

Once the tension in the patellar tendon is known, we can derive the magnitudes of the other two forces on the patella since the positions and directions of their lines of action are known.

We now have all the magnitudes and directions of the single-joint forces on the femur with the exception of the actions at the hip, where we encounter the difficulties mentioned earlier.

WEIGHT-BEARING BY THE LEG

In these discussions of the forces in the leg we have so far considered the leg as remaining at the same length throughout. In practice, there will be changes both in the length of the leg and in the load which it is called upon to bear. Changes in the overall load involve changes in the stresses on the individual parts, which will be deformed in different ways. In the analogy with a triangulated lattice structure, each of the members will behave like a spring, and indeed the leg as a whole can be expected to behave as a springy strut. For a particular leg to support the body in a specific posture it will be necessary to adjust the springiness of that leg so that the appropriate upthrust force is available at the right length of leg. Adjustments of this kind are made by adjusting the activity of the muscles in the leg carrying the load.

Let us consider the way the force developed in the single-joint portion of the quadriceps muscle has to be adjusted when the leg changes its length without changing the magnitude of the compressive thrust to be exerted between the hip and the ground. If the knee bends, the muscle will clearly be stretched, but the amount of stretch will depend on the way the patella moves in its groove in the femur. At the same time there will be an increase in the offset from the knee to the line of thrust through the hip to the point of contact with the ground. There will also be changes in all the leverages at the knee because of the rolling and sliding between the bones and the altered dispositions of the ligaments in relation to the instantaneous centre of rotation.

We can take all these factors into account to calculate the relationship between the stretching of the muscle and the increase in the tension that it must exert to remain in equilibrium with a given compressive load on the limb as a whole. It is not convenient to make all the necessary measurements from a real leg. As an alternative, we can make a working model using the best values we can find for the dimensions of the model and we can then make the measurements required for our calculations from the model instead of from the real leg.

In making one such model (Figure 3.20), profiles of the femur and tibia were obtained by projection and pivot points were fitted to correspond with the points of insertion of the cruciate ligaments. The ligaments themselves were represented by rigid struts, the compression of which simulated the action of the articular surfaces in transmitting thrust without incurring the complications of sliding friction. The model of the patella was supported by a rigid strut pivoted at a point corresponding to the centre of curvature of the groove in the end of the femur, again avoiding sliding friction. The lower end of the tibia was

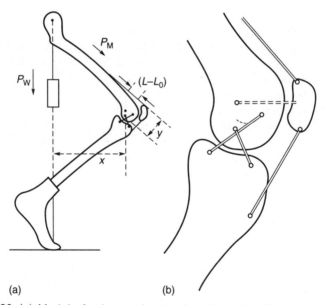

(a)   (b)

Figure 3.20 (a) Model of a human leg to show how the offsets x and y were measured. (b) Detail of the pivot points and linkages. The dotted line shows the profile of the bone round which the posterior cruciate ligament becomes wrapped in full flexion of the knee. (From Roberts, 1971, by courtesy of *Nature*.)

continued into a fixed profile of a foot with dorsiflexed toes. Offsets x and y were measured from the point of intersection of the cruciate ligaments to the line of action of the muscle and to the line from hip to foot, as in Figure 3.20(a). The change in length that would be imposed on the muscle was also measured. From these measurements we derive a curve (Figure 3.21) that indicates the shape of the relationship between muscle tension and muscle length that is required to balance the effect of a constant compressive thrust in the line of the leg.

Rather surprisingly, this relationship between tension and length for the single-joint portion of the quadriceps muscle to support a constant load turns out to be very near to a straight line over a large range of positions of the knee (Figure 3.21). This means that if we were to replace the muscle by a steel spring with a linear tension–extension

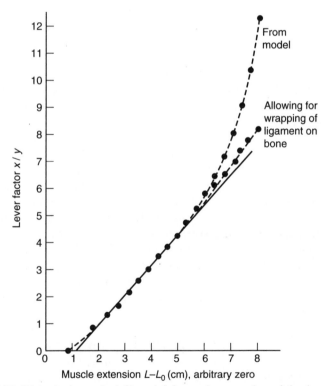

Figure 3.21 Plot of x/y against $(L - L_0)$ for various angles of the knee joint in the model shown in Figure 3.20. Note that, because $P_M/P_w = x/y$, this graph gives the shape of the tension–length diagram which a single-joint extensor of the knee would need to have if it were to be in equilibrium with a constant compressive load. For a linear spring, $P_M = S(L - L_0)$, as shown by the full line, where S is the stiffness. (From Roberts, 1971, by courtesy of *Nature*.)

relation, the leg as a whole would act as a constant-force strut. When we do this and measure the thrust developed by the model leg at different angles of the knee we find very little variation in thrust over quite a large range of knee angles.

These results confirm that the geometry of the knee has the effect of converting the linear tension–extension relationship of the spring into a constant-thrust characteristic for the leg as a whole.

Now the force developed by an active muscle cell varies with its length, and the total force in the tendon attached to a number of muscle cells will depend on how many of these cells are active at a particular time. The tension–extension relationship of a whole muscle will therefore depend on a number of factors, and particularly on the motor command signals that the muscle receives from the central nervous system.

It is perhaps unreasonable to expect an exact match between the tension–extension relationship for a particular muscle and the curve representing the effects of changing leverages under a constant load, but we can consider four possibilities.

1. The slope of the muscle curve is correct but the muscle curve lies to the right of the load curve in Figure 3.21. In this case, whatever the starting position, the muscle develops insufficient force to support the load, and the limb collapses.
2. The slope is correct but the muscle curve lies to the left of the load curve. The muscle now develops excess force at all positions and the limb springs into full extension.
3. The slope of the muscle curve is less than that of the load curve. This means that, at joint angles greater than that corresponding to the intersection of the two curves, the limb collapses. From smaller starting angles the limb springs into full extension.
4. The slope of the muscle curve is greater than that of the load curve. The intersection of the curves now defines a position of stable equilibrium that can be shifted in either direction by adjustment of the activity of the muscle. Clearly this latter condition is the most useful.

In this analysis of our simplified model we have not yet taken account of the effect of the weights of the individual segments of the leg. The magnitude of the upthrust measured at the foot differs from that of the upthrust required at the hip by the weight of the leg, so that adjustments have to be added into our calculations at each of the joints of the leg to take account of which segments are above and which are below the joint.

MULTIJOINT MUSCLES

Further complications arise when we start to take account of the actions of the muscles that span more than one joint. For example, the hamstrings and biceps femoris cross both the hip joint and the knee. When they are active they must put the femur under compressive stress. They are, however, not well placed to resist collapse of the leg under the weight of the body since the stretching that would occur at the hip when the body sinks down is offset by a movement in the opposite direction at the knee. The function of these two-joint muscles is to convey torque across two joints. Thus the leverage of the lower leg is made available in addition to that of the upper leg in providing the torque necessary to prevent the trunk from tipping forward over the hip. Paddle action of this kind is very important in rapid locomotion where large short-lasting thrusts have to be transmitted to the trunk without the hip being lined up between the foot and the centre of gravity.

The two heads of the gastrocnemius muscle run from the distal end of the femur, just behind the condyles, to the Achilles tendon. Their action spans both knee and ankle. They serve to convey torque from the femur to the foot, lengthening the lever by which torque is applied to the hip by forces exerted between the foot and the ground.

The analogy between the actions of muscles on bones and the diagrammatic representation as a triangulated lattice structure is not precise. The attachments of muscles and tendons to bones do not run to single points. They are distributed over an area of bone surface, often not very near to the points of articulation between the bones. Furthermore, each 'triangular' arrangement of bones and muscles is actually a three-dimensional structure. The bones carry torsional and bending stresses as well as simple compressions. In spite of these detailed differences, the 'triangulation principle' gives useful insights into the way in which forces are communicated between one part of the body and another.

In most cases the individual bones do not themselves come into direct contact. Where they do do so, they tend to become fused, so that relative movement is thereafter no longer possible. Where a compressive thrust has to be transmitted from one bone to another across a movable joint, the separation of the bones is maintained by cushions of cartilage or by fibrous pads, each of which serves to distribute the stresses. Tendencies for the bones to be pulled apart are resisted by ligaments. Relative movement in other directions involves the sliding of one bone over the other. There is usually also a certain amount of rolling as well as the sliding. Special lubrication mechanisms reduce friction and facilitate sliding. The most obvious forms of relative movement are changes in the angle between the axes of the bones forming the joint together with rotations about these axes.

The bones, muscles and tendons of the body together form a resilient lattice structure from which the soft tissues are suspended. A consequence of the distributed mass is that stress forces exerted at the areas of contact with the external supports, during normal standing and in the course of locomotion, produce a complex pattern of stresses in the various parts of the lattice. The resulting changes in the configuration of the body parts depend on the pattern of resistances to extension developed in the individual muscles. Each of these individual resistances depends in turn on the moment-to-moment pattern of motor-nerve impulses received from the central nervous system. This topic is discussed in detail in the next chapter. As a consequence of the 'give' in the muscles, the resilience of the whole structure involves movement at many joints.

JOINT LUBRICATION

In view of this inevitable continual movement, it is important that there should not be too much friction at the joints. In fact, the magnitude of the frictional resistance in normal animal joints turns out to be very small indeed. This is brought about by rather complicated means. The bones forming a synovial joint are kept apart by two layers of specialized cartilage, one attached to each of the two bones that are linked at the joint.

The articular cartilages play an important role in distributing the stresses at the point of contact, acting as a shock absorber to reduce the risk of shattering the bones on sudden impact. They also contribute to the lubrication of the joint.

In the hydrodynamic lubrication of engineering bearings, the designer seeks to achieve smooth surfaces that can be kept apart by an oil film. When there is relative movement of the surfaces, the separating fluid layer is commonly not of uniform thickness. Because the lubricating fluid is viscous, it gets dragged into the regions where the bearing surfaces are closer together. This leads to the development of localized small regions of high hydrostatic pressure which together provide enough force to support the external load on the bearing. In another mechanism, called boundary lubrication, the molecules of the lubricant react chemically with the bearing surfaces to form strong slippery films.

Where the bearing surfaces are not perfectly smooth, the effect of the irregularities is to produce small areas of high local stress where the opposing bumps may actually plough into one another, producing small temporary welds. The subsequent shearing of these welds accounts for much of the energy lost in friction.

With soft bearing materials the opposing bumps deform one another and greatly increase the effective area of contact over which the lubricating fluid can exert hydrostatic separation.

The joints in the body are anatomically specialized structures that link together the relatively more rigid bones of the skeleton. Apart from such replications as the interphalangeal and intervertebral joints, there are almost as many types of joint as there are joints themselves. The action of one bone upon another under the influence of the associated muscles resembles the action against the ground of the pole of a bell tent, the free end of which is pulled upon in many different directions. At any specific joint between two bones there exist, in principle, six degrees of freedom for the relative movement of the bones, namely linear displacements about three mutually perpendicular axes, together with rotations about each of these three axes.

Because the ligaments linking the bones at a joint are necessarily somewhat springy, it is possible for unusually large forces to produce a temporary separation of the bones forming certain joints. This can result in a dislocation if the bones do not thereafter spring back correctly to their proper relative positions.

In addition to the ligaments, the bones at a joint are also linked by a loose connective-tissue capsule which encloses a quantity of the special 'synovial fluid' that bathes the moving parts. In the knee joint, the rounded surfaces of the condyles of the femur work against the relatively much flatter surfaces of the tibia, to leave spaces around the area of contact. These spaces are neatly filled by crescent-shaped blocks of cartilage, triangular in section, one surrounding each of the two condyles of the femur. These 'menisci', or 'semi-lunar cartilages', are tethered by a complex set of ligaments which allow sliding in and out of the joint space when the condyles of the femur roll over those of the tibia. At the same time, the ligaments prevent the incomplete rings of the menisci from opening out to allow the wedges to escape completely. As a result, the menisci contribute substantially to supporting the compressive load across the joint. In certain conditions of exceptional or sudden loading, the menisci fail to move appropriately and may become split, as happens in certain sports injuries.

Synovial fluid consists, essentially, of a watery solution of hyaluronic acid. Water is itself an excellent lubricant in certain conditions. It is responsible for the notorious slipperiness of ice. The ice melts locally where it is pressed upon and the resulting water layer presents only fluid friction in place of the static friction expected at a direct contact between solids. At low relative speeds, fluid friction presents only neglible resistance to movement. The presence of hyaluronic acid greatly enhances the lubricating properties of the watery fluid in the synovial space.

Hyaluronic acid is one of a group of substances called proteoglycans in which long unbranched chains of disaccharides, called glycosaminoglycans, are linked to proteins. The resulting very long molecules increase the viscosity and the slipperiness of the water in much the same way as do the synthetic detergents used in washing. In other situations in the body a similar function is performed by mucin.

Another component of the synovial fluid, called 'lubricating glycoprotein', adsorbs onto the cartilage surfaces and functions as a 'boundary lubricant'. The synovial fluid provides sufficient lubrication for the contact surfaces that are not under heavy stress, but an additional mechanism is required at the load-bearing surfaces themselves. This additional mechanism depends on the specialized structure of the cartilage forming the joint surfaces.

A complication is that the cartilage forming the bearing surfaces is porous as well as being deformable and not perfectly smooth. This means that when a joint is subjected to a compressive load, the stressed areas of cartilage will be deformed. The contained fluid is relatively incompressible, so it gets squeezed away from the area of high stress, travelling through the matrix of the cartilage as well as being expelled into the space between the opposed bearing surfaces. The resistance to flow through the narrow channels in the cartilage matrix allows a local build-up of hydrostatic pressure at the 'high spots' of the bearing to provide short-term support for the external load, while the fluid layer provides lubrication. In the everyday use of the joints in the body there is commonly some rolling motion as well as sliding. The position of the high spots is thus continually changing, allowing previously compressed regions of cartilage to become resoaked with fluid that can now enter directly through short low-resistance channels from the free surface.

Articular cartilage consists mainly of collagen fibres embedded in a proteoglycan gel. Collagen is a fibrous protein whose principal components are made up of two types of subunit each of which has the form of a left-handed helix. Two subunits of one type and one subunit of the other are wound and bonded together in a right-handed helix to form a strong rod-like unit. A large number of these units are packed side by side in echelon to form very long fibres capable of supporting tensile stress.

The molecules of the gel consist of long hyaluronic acid molecules linked by protein to two other different glycosaminoglycans to form large, complicated, proteoglycans. In turn, these proteoglycan molecules are linked at intervals to the collagen fibres so that they are not free to move through the tissue. The proteoglycan molecules carry a number of fixed negatively charged subunits so that the whole is strongly osmotically active. In consequence of the osmotic activity a considerable swelling pressure develops, which is resisted by tensile stresses in the collagen fibres.

The mechanism by which cartilage resists compression resembles that responsible for the resistance offered by a pile of sandbags. The sand particles cannot escape through the fabric of the sandbag and are restrained by the tension in that fabric; the proteoglycan molecules, drawing in water by osmotic forces, are restrained from swelling by the network of collagen fibres to which they are attached. The water molecules can pass freely in either direction.

When a block of articular cartilage is subjected to an external deforming force, the balance between the osmotic swelling pressure and the restraining tensile stress is disturbed. There is relative deformation of all the components. The deformation of short-term loading is rapidly recovered, but sustained loading leads to movement of fluid through the matrix. This leads, in turn, to a local increase in osmotic pressure, which then supports the load. As fluid continues to move, the block of cartilage undergoes 'creep'. When the imposed load is eventually removed, the cartilage gradually returns to its former configuration by re-imbibition of fluid.

In summary: much of the compressive thrust across a joint is carried by hydrostatic pressure in the trapped fluid. A fluid layer between opposing surfaces provides purely viscous friction like that involved in sliding on ice. Some contact between the protuberances of opposing surfaces (which are far from smooth) is to be expected. Here boundary lubrication is provided by the lubricating glycoprotein of the synovial fluid. Local deformations produce local increases in osmotic pressure, leading to local increases in hydrostatic pressure to carry the local loads. Fluid moves through the matrix of the cartilage away from the stressed region to allow local deformation. Fluid is also squeezed out locally from the space between the opposing surfaces, to flow back in again as soon as the local stress is relieved by a movement of the joint. The resoaking of the matrix restores the profile more rapidly than the deformation on the initial loading.

We have now seen that the maintenance of the normal upright posture depends on coordinating the stress forces with which we push against the ground. These stress forces are applied through a lattice structure of struts (bones) and ties (muscles and tendons) with low-friction joints between the struts. We now turn to the processes by which the necessary forces are generated and controlled.

The generation and deployment of muscle force

4

The forces with which the limbs support the body all arise from the action of muscles pulling upon bones. In the generation of these forces a number of factors come into play which interact with one another in complicated ways. In what follows, these factors will be discussed in relation to skeletal or 'striated' muscle only. (Smooth muscle and cardiac muscle differ in certain particulars from skeletal muscle, but these differences will not be dealt with in this book.)

The anatomical naming of the skeletal muscles depends on the fact that different parts of the whole muscle mass are attached to, and pull upon, different tendons. As a consequence, natural cleavage planes occur and these can be revealed by gross dissection. Each separable block of muscular tissue can accordingly be named either by its characteristic shape or in terms of the bones to which it is attached through the tendons at its ends.

MOTOR UNITS

Microscopic examination reveals that each anatomically-named muscle consists of a large number of separate elements, the muscle cells, bound together by connective tissue. Each muscle cell has its own controlling nerve supply and consequently operates as a functional unit which is, in general, independent in its activity from the activity of neighbouring muscle cells. The detailed organization of muscle activity is not arranged on the basis of the anatomically separable muscle masses but rather on a basis of individual muscle cells. There is some grouping, however, imposed by the anatomy of the nerves controlling the muscle cells. Each motor nerve-fibre commonly serves a number of muscle cells, each of which will be made active whenever the nerve-fibre is active. Accordingly, the unit of organization consists of a single motor nerve-fibre together with all the muscle-fibres with which it is connected. This unit is referred to as a 'motor unit'.

The separation into strands sometimes seen in cooked meat is a consequence of the arrangement of the connective tissue holding the muscle-fibres together and of the way this connective tissue breaks up on cooking. Each resulting strand contains a few dozen muscle-fibres. The way the muscle mass is bound into strands that can be separated by cooking does not correspond to the functional subdivision into motor units.

The number of muscle cells in a motor unit usually lies somewhere in the range from about 40 to about 400, but varies widely between different muscles and in different species. The different muscle cells forming a single motor unit do not all lie side by side. They are scattered through the muscle mass with the muscle cells of other motor units lying in between, an arrangement which has important consequences in relation to the liability of the muscle to fatigue.

ELECTRICAL ACTIVITY

The cycles of activity in muscle cells, just as in nerve cells, are dependent on the properties of the cell membrane and on the concentrations of certain ions in the fluids inside and outside these membranes. In each case there is a resting 'membrane potential', i.e. a voltage difference between the inside and the outside of the cell. This voltage changes rapidly when the cell is made active and it is thereafter rapidly restored again to the resting level, the whole cycle, or 'action-potential', lasting only about one thousandth of a second.

Because of the short time-course of the action-potential, and of the fact that nerve cells and muscle cells are long narrow structures (often spoken of as 'fibres'), it is possible for one part of a cell to be active while other parts are resting. The different electrical conditions at the active and inactive regions lead to the passage of electric currents (called 'local circuit currents') which can have the effect of making inactive regions active in their turn. In this way the activity-cycle 'propagates' along the length of the fibre. Nerve cells are commonly made active only at one end, and accordingly the propagated action-potential passes always in the same direction in a particular nerve-fibre, from one end to the other.

The role of the nerve-fibres in the body is to carry messages from one place to another. The passage of such a message is accompanied by the sequence of electrical events that manifest themselves as an action-potential. When such a message arrives at the junction between a motor nerve-fibre and a muscle cell, this leads to the development of mechanical activity in the muscle cell. Usually this activity shows itself as the sudden development of force. In physics a 'force suddenly communicated' is referred to as an 'impulse'. By an extension of this idea, the nervous message itself has come to be called an 'impulse' also, though the sense here is somewhat different.

NEUROMUSCULAR TRANSMISSION

The region where a motor nerve-fibre makes functional connection with a muscle-fibre is the site of considerable anatomical specialization of the cell membranes of both cells. The resulting complex is called an 'end-plate', from its histological appearance. The two cell membranes come very close together but do not fuse.

When an impulse in a motor nerve-fibre reaches the specialized end-plate region where the nerve-fibre comes into functional relation with a muscle cell, the electrical mechanism that was effective for the propagation of an action-potential along the length of a single cell turns out to be inadequate to produce activation of the muscle cell directly, because of the very great disparity between the areas of cell membrane involved.

The transmission of the activating message from nerve to muscle is achieved by a cycle of chemical events triggered off by the arrival of the nerve impulse. A 'chemical messenger' (acetylcholine) is liberated from the nerve-fibre into the small space between the nerve and the muscle. This substance has the effect of changing the electrical properties of the muscle-cell membrane, depolarizing the membrane for a brief period. The muscle-cell membrane at the end-plate region then undergoes a sequence of localized voltage fluctuations referred to as an 'end-plate potential'.

When the end-plate region of the muscle cell is depolarized during the end-plate potential, local circuit currents are generated. These make the neighbouring parts of the muscle-cell membrane active in turn so that a cycle of electrical activity then propagates over the whole length of the muscle cell.

The generation and propagation of action-potentials in nerve-fibres by local circuit currents, and the similar processes in muscle-fibres, together with the activation of the muscle-cell membrane by the currents arising from the depolarization of the end-plate region, all appear to be purely passive processes involving only the voltage-dependent permeability of the cell membrane to various ions and the presence of the resting membrane potential. The number of ions transferred across the cell membrane during a single impulse is trivial compared to the total number present in a cell, so that a comparatively slow process of ion pumping is quite adequate to maintain the membrane potential.

The pumping requires energy which is ultimately derived from oxidative metabolic processes, but even in the absence of oxygen a cell can sustain something like a million impulses before the membrane potential runs down. In contrast, the tension-generating mechanisms in a muscle cell are much more dependent on a steady supply of oxygen and on the availability of the necessary fuel, as well as on the removal of the products of metabolism, including heat. Accordingly, the adequacy of the blood supply is an important feature in governing what force a muscle can develop at any particular time. The way the individual cells of a motor unit are distributed through the mass of a muscle ensures that the effects of cumulative local changes in concentration, such as might arise from repetitive activation, are kept to a minimum.

INTERNAL STRUCTURE OF A MUSCLE CELL

The internal structure of a muscle cell contains a number of elements, each with a different role to play in the linkage between the electrical activation of the cell membrane and the development of tension (Figure 4.1). The bulk of the protein content of a muscle cell is made up of actin and myosin whose long molecules are packed together in a very orderly pattern to form rod-like filaments. These filaments are all oriented parallel to the long axis of the muscle-fibre, with similar filaments lying side by side in accurate register. Layers of actin filaments alternate with layers of myosin filaments to form fibrils that run the whole length of the cell. It is the regular alternation of the constituents of the fibrils that gives to the whole muscle a cross-banded appearance in histological preparations.

One of the bands, called the Z-line, corresponds to a structure that links together, by their central regions, all the actin filaments of a single layer running right across one fibril. The part of a fibril lying between adjacent Z-lines is called a 'sarcomere', which thus consists of one half of a layer of actin filaments, a layer of myosin filaments, and one half of the next layer of actin filaments. The layers of actin and myosin filaments interdigitate, like the bristles of a pair of hairbrushes when they are put together.

Each muscle cell contains a good number of separate fibrils with many other structures packed into the spaces between them. These structures include nuclei, mitochondria, glycogen granules and a complex system of tubules referred to as the 'sarcoplasmic reticulum' in which two components can be distinguished, a longitudinal system

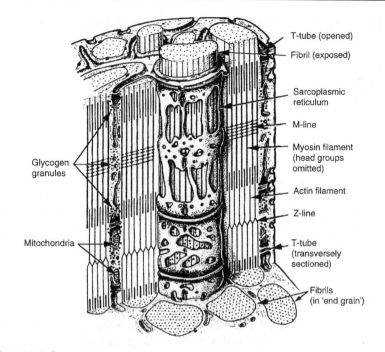

T-tube (opened)

Fibril (exposed)

Sarcoplasmic
reticulum

M-line

Myosin filament
(head groups
omitted)

Actin filament

Z-line

T-tube
(transversely
sectioned)

Fibrils
(in 'end grain')

Glycogen
granules

Mitochondria

Figure 4.1 Semi-diagrammatic representation of some features of muscle structure. The filaments of myosin (thick) and actin (thin) are shown grouped into fibrils, separated by the sarcoplasmic reticulum (s.r.) and other cell inclusions. The upper transverse section cuts only the thin filaments and shows the transverse tubule system laid open. The lower section cuts both thin and thick filaments, together with parts of the longitudinal tubule system formed by the fenestration of the curtain of s.r. lying between the fibrils. At their regions of apposition the T-tubules are sandwiched between densely granular cisternae of the longitudinal tubule system, to form the 'triads'. Three sets of triads are shown (the upper one halved). The T-tubules open to the extracellular space (at the top of the figure). Numerous caveoli occur in the cell membrane. (It is not clear how many of these communicate with the T-tubule system.) The thin filaments are shown attached to the Z-membrane (schematic). A second cross-linkage system forms the M-line connecting the midpoints of the thick filaments. Mitochondria and glycogen granules are to be found scattered in the spaces between the fibrils. Different muscles in different species show variations in the detailed relationships between the individual components illustrated here. (Sketch by N. C. Spurway.)

and a transverse system, with specialized regions of intercommunication called 'triads'.

The system of transverse tubules communicates with the cell membrane and also with the longitudinal tubules. The sarcoplasmic reticulum thus forms a link between the surface of the cell, which is the site of the electrical activity, and the tension-generating fibrils which lie deep inside the cytoplasm.

The electrical changes at the cell membrane during the action-potential lead to the release of calcium ions from the longitudinal tubule system into the fluid surrounding the fibrils. These calcium ions catalyse a chemical reaction between actin and myosin and thus activate the tension-generating mechanism. After a very short interval the calcium ions are withdrawn again into the tubule system. The mechanical response to activation is accordingly of very short duration and the muscle cell needs to be reactivated repeatedly if the tension is to be maintained.

TENSION GENERATION

It is the fibrils that are responsible for the generation of tension. Each molecule of myosin bears a reactive group at one end. During the association to form a filament, some of the myosin molecules come to lie with their reactive groups towards one end of the filament and some with the reactive groups towards the other end. The reactive groups form small projections on the sides of the myosin filaments. These projections are capable of becoming attached to the neighbouring actin filaments in the region of overlap to form a set of 'cross-bridges' of a size near the limit of resolution of present-day electron microscopes.

If a number of such cross-bridges are present in each of its sarcomeres, a fibril can withstand longitudinal tension. When a muscle cell is made active, the number of cross-bridges is increased in a chemical reaction between the actin and the myosin. The orientation of the cross-bridges is such that the filaments of actin linked to the opposite ends of a myosin filament are drawn towards one another. Lateral movement is prevented by the packing and by the fact that the bridges are formed on all sides of the myosin filaments. If the ends of the muscle are not restrained, longitudinal movement is possible and this results in a change in the spacing of the bands.

When a muscle is made active, it will do one or more of three things, depending on the conditions:

1. it will shorten if it can;
2. it will develop a tension against a resistance;
3. it will show an increased resistance to extension.

The amount of the tension developed in a particular muscle fibril is dependent on the number of cross-bridges that are available in each sarcomere. Thus the tension developed by a whole muscle is very much dependent on the length of the muscle in relation to the resting value.

ENERGY SUPPLY

The energy for the work done in shortening against a load comes from oxidative metabolism through a sequence of chemical reactions that involves both a short-term and a long-term system of energy storage. The long-term energy store inside the muscle cell consists of glycogen granules that are built up from the glucose circulating in the blood. The short-term store consists of the energy-rich phosphate bonds in adenosine triphosphate (ATP), which is one of the components in the chemical reaction involved in the formation of the cross-bridges between the actin and the myosin filaments. This is the energy source first drawn on in the development of tension.

The energy stored in ATP is sufficient for only a very few activations, say about ten, corresponding to rather less than a second of tension generation at the frequencies of activation used in the maintenance of posture. The glycogen store, on the other hand, will support over an hour of fairly heavy mechanical work. Beyond this point the muscles are entirely dependent on the continued supply of glucose from the blood stream.

The ATP broken down to provide the energy for tension generation is rapidly reformed using another small back-up store of energy in the form of creatine phosphate. This in turn is then recharged by a series of chemical reactions that obtain their energy from glucose molecules. The normal process of mobilizing energy from glucose requires a supply of oxygen and there are severe limits on the amount of mechanical work that a muscle can perform if its oxygen supply is restricted.

Some energy can be made available from stored glucose in the absence of oxygen, using a different chain of chemical reactions from those used in oxidative metabolism. This system of 'anaerobic metabolism' is employed to provide energy for sudden emergencies, such as in sprinting, where the rate of supply of oxygen through the respiratory system is not fast enough to meet the demands of the mechanical work that has to be performed. A disadvantage of the anaerobic system is that it entails the accumulation of lactic acid as a by-product. The sprint can therefore be maintained for only a short time, after which the rate of working has to be slowed down to a pace that can be matched by the oxygen uptake. The lactic acid accumulated during a sprint is metabolized later in a phase in which the oxygen uptake is continued at a rate exceeding that then needed to sustain the mechanical work. Anaerobic metabolism during sprinting thus involves incurring an 'oxygen debt' which has to be repaid when the emergency is over.

The amount of shortening that a sarcomere can undergo is clearly very much greater than the length-change to be expected from a single cross-bridge. This means that, as well as cross-bridges being formed during activity, they must also become detached again after they have shortened as far as they can. One has to imagine that the individual cross-bridges cooperate in pulling on the actin filaments rather as a group of men might haul in a rope hand over hand, each hand releasing the rope after pulling in as far as it can and then shifting its grip ready for another pull.

The detachment of the cross-bridges involves the ATP molecules. If the mechanism for regenerating ATP is not available, as for example in the period of rigor mortis following the death of the animal, the cross-bridges remain permanently attached and the muscles are very resistant to extension. In these conditions the ATP concentration in the muscle cytoplasm falls to very low levels. At the same time, the calcium ions accumulate in the cytoplasmic fluid because the mechanism for pumping these ions into the longitudinal tubule system is put out of action by the failure of the oxygen supply. These observations lead to the following conceptual model of the way the system operates.

The chemical energy from the breakdown of ATP is used in a process which detaches those cross-bridges that have already shortened and then extends all the unattached side branches of the myosin filaments and develops strain energy in them, shortening being restrained by a catch involving the adenosine monophosphate molecules derived from the splitting of ATP. The strained side branches of the myosin molecules constitute a store of mechanical energy, in the same way as one stores strain energy in the spring of a break-back mousetrap when setting it. When the concentration of calcium ions in the cytoplasm rises, in response to the message communicated from the cell membrane by the sarcoplasmic reticulum, the myosin side-branches become attached to the actin filaments to form the cross-bridges, and the catch holding back the strain energy is released. In this model, the cross-bridges are already under strain before they become attached to the actin filaments. The strain energy becomes available immediately the bridges have been formed. Tension develops rapidly in the muscle fibrils and can at once start to perform the mechanical work of shortening, provided that the ends of the muscle are free to move.

The role assigned to the calcium ions in this scheme has been confirmed in experiments with the jellyfish protein aequorin. This protein has the property of luminescing in the presence of calcium ions. A solution of the protein is injected into a muscle cell and the intensity of the light emission is measured with a sensitive photomultiplier. No light is emitted when the muscle is resting, but immediately after the muscle cell has been activated by an electric shock there is a sudden flash. The peak intensity of the emitted light occurs just at the moment when the rate-of-increase in tension in the muscle is at its maximum. Thereafter the light output falls off during the next few tens of milliseconds. The decline in tension follows a different time-course from the decay of light-emission, in accord with the idea that separate processes are involved in the detachment of the cross-bridges from those involved in their formation.

In considering the time-course of the development of tension in a tendon there are several factors that have to be taken into account. Tension is a stress force inevitably accompanied by strain. Thus when tension is developed in a structure that is composed of several elements in series, each of the elements will be strained by an amount dependent on its compliance. The passive parts need to be stretched to develop tension and this implies that the parts that generate the tension will have to shorten unless the whole structure is being stretched at the same time as it is being made active.

FUNCTIONAL COMPONENTS IN MUSCLE

It is convenient to consider the structure of a muscle, together with the tendons to which it is attached, as made up of three components (Figure 4.2):

1. the contractile mechanism that develops the tension when the muscle is made active;
2. a passive series elastic element that transmits the tension from the contractile element to the supports;
3. a passive elastic element that is in parallel with the other two elements and which can be held responsible for the tension that a muscle can support when it is not being activated.

The tension-generating apparatus, or 'contractile mechanism', thus lies entirely within the cell membrane of the muscle-fibre. For most of the length of the cell the majority of the myofibrils are separated from the cell membrane by a cytoplasmic fluid space containing the tubules of the reticulum, the nuclei, the mitochondria and other cell inclusions.

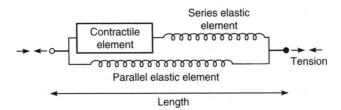

Figure 4.2 Conceptual model of tension-bearing elements in muscle. The changes which occur in the mechanical properties of the muscle during activity are confined to changes in the contractile element. The mechanical properties of the elastic elements are not altered.

The collagen fibres of the tendons, to which the muscle tension must eventually be transmitted, are extracellular structures. This means that the tension has to be passed at some point through the cell membrane. Collagen fibres, continuous with the fibres of the tendon, extend into pouches of cell membrane invaginated into the ends of the spaces between the myofibrils. Each myofibril thus comes to be surrounded near the end of the muscle cell by cell membrane, which forms a cap over the end of the myofibril. The Z-membrane formed from the actin filaments of the last half-sarcomere of the myofibril is closely apposed to the cell membrane of this cap region. On its 'morphologically outer' side, the cell membrane is closely covered by collagen to form the sarcolemma, which in turn is continuous with the collagen fibres of the fingers of tendon. Thus the tension, generated by the interaction between filaments of actin and filaments of myosin, is transferred from actin filaments to Z-membranes, thence to the cell membrane, and thereafter, through the collagenous outer coating of the cell membrane, to the collagen fibres of the tendon itself.

ELASTIN

In addition to collagen fibres, tendons contain other fibrous proteins, including 'elastin' which has important special properties. Different tendons contain different proportions of these various constituents according to the degree of extensibility appropriate to the location of each tendon. While collagen fibres present considerable resistance to extension, fibres of elastin can be extended to twice or even to two-and-a-half times their resting length. The force developed obeys Hooke's Law over a large range, tension being proportional to relative extension. When released, elastin fibres spring back to their resting length, delivering up most of the strain energy stored during the initial stretching. Elastin does not show 'creep' during sustained loading. The behaviour of elastin thus closely resembles that of lightly vulcanized rubber, whereas that of collagen fibres is responsible for the relative inextensibility of leather. The molecular configuration responsible for the behaviour of rubbers involves an open-meshed network of convoluted long thread-like molecules with cross-links between them at intervals. The unsupported threads between the cross-links are slack in the unstressed condition and are pulled out when the material is stressed.

In elastin, which has a very different chemical composition from that of collagen, the constituent aminoacids in the fibrous proteins forming the network have non-polar side-chains. These side-chains tend to aggregate into hydrophobic globules from which water is excluded. It is this tendency that is responsible for the resting configuration of the unsupported threads and thus for the mean distance between nodes in the unstressed condition. In watery solution, the water molecules surround the hydrophobic non-polar material with hydrogen-bonded cage structures. When elastin is stressed, either in tension or in compression, some of the non-polar side-chains are displaced from inside their hydrophobic globules. The consequent organization of the water molecules involves a large positive free energy change. Thus the unfolding of the protein by the applied stress requires an input of energy. This energy can be recovered by allowing the hydrophobic side-chains to relax back into their hydrophobic 'homes'. This mechanism, which has some resemblances to the mechanism of the development of surface tension, accounts for the elastic extensibility of elastin in its normal watery environment.

The extensibility of rubber depends on a different mechanism. The component molecules of rubbers also consist of convoluted flexible threads linked together only here and there. Heat energy keeps the long threads in continual motion, resulting in a particular mean distance between links in the unstressed condition. Under tensile stress the threads are pulled out while the Brownian motion tends to restore them to the entropy level of their unstressed mean configuration. This 'entropy' mechanism of extensibility is also shown by samples of elastin placed in a 30% solution of ethylene glycol in water, where the glycol interferes with the 'surface tension' mechanism described above. The two mechanisms are distinguishable by thermodynamic measurements involving stretching elastin samples in a microcalorimeter.

ISOLATED MUSCLE

The traditional method for studying the development of muscle tension involves the use of an isolated muscle together with its motor nerve supply. One end of the muscle is firmly anchored while the other end is connected to a device that controls and monitors both the length and the tension (Figure 4.3). The muscle is made active by applying an electric shock to the motor nerve, using a sufficient intensity of stimulation to be sure of activating all the motor nerve-fibres. The muscle responds by developing a sudden increase in tension, or by a sudden shortening, both types of response being referred to as a 'twitch'.

Various routines are employed. In 'isometric' recording the intention is to measure the tension developed by the muscle at a known constant length. This intention cannot be achieved in practice because of the need to stretch the passive series elastic element before it can carry any tension. The contractile element inevitably shortens, so that so far as that element is concerned, the conditions are not truly isometric. To get over this difficulty, the muscle may be suddenly stretched by a cal-

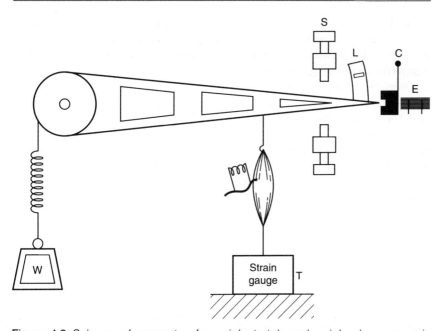

Figure 4.3 Scheme of apparatus for quick-stretch and quick-release experiments. W = weight, adjusted to provide the desired tension (small for quick release, large for quick stretch, intermediate for study of the force−velocity relationship); T = strain-gauge tension recorder; S = adjustable stops set to desired final length of the muscle; L = photoelectric length transducer; C = catch to restrain the muscle support during initial development of tension; E = electromagnet to release the catch at a predetermined interval after the onset of stimulation.After setting the stops and the weight to the conditions required, the lever is moved to engage the catch. The muscle is set into tetanic contraction by a series of electric shocks and, at a predetermined moment, the catch is released. The lever jumps to the appropriate stop according as the muscle tension is greater or less than that preset by the weight. By using a light lever and a soft spring the inertia that has to be accelerated during the length-change is kept to a minimum. By winding back the stops and choosing a suitable intermediate value for the weight, the apparatus may be used to collect data for the force−velocity curve.

culated amount just after it has been made active. If the length-change has not been selected correctly, the tension record will show either a rise, during which the elastic elements are being stretched, or a fall, during which the excess tension in the elastic element is extending the contractile element.

In another routine, called 'isotonic' recording, the muscle is called upon to support a constant force while attention is concentrated on the length-changes. Difficulties arise here from the forces needed to accelerate the unavoidable inertia of the recording device, and also from the fact that inactive muscle cannot support as much tension as active muscle. One solution is to arrange for the muscle length to be restrained by a catch until the desired tension has been developed in isometric conditions, and then to release the catch and allow the muscle to shorten or lengthen as appropriate.

The tensions developed by a muscle are dependent upon activation, and the magnitudes of the tensions vary with the time since the most recent activation. The onset of tension-development occurs rapidly in response to the sudden increase of calcium concentration at activation. The rate at which the tension subsequently falls off depends on the concentration of ATP. In repetitive activation a new increase in calcium concentration may be initiated before all the bridges formed by the earlier activation have been detached. The next mechanical response then starts from a 'contraction remainder' left over from the previous activation (Figure 4.4). With a suitable frequency of repeated activation,

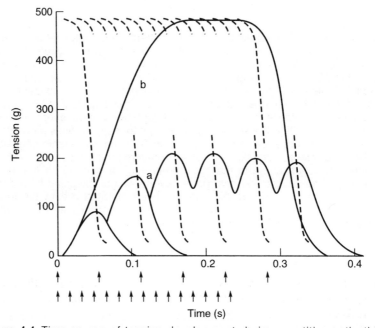

Figure 4.4 Time-course of tension-development during repetitive activation at the moments indicated by the arrows. 'a' Responses to one, two, and six shocks at 18 shocks per second; 'b' response to 15 shocks at 60 shocks per second. The traces have been brought into coincidence at the moment of the first shock in each series. The broken lines indicate portions of the relevant 'active-state curves'. (Frog gastrocnemius muscle stimulated by way of the sciatic nerve, 20°C.)

the successive mechanical responses become fused into a sustained tension called the 'tetanic tension'.

The results from experiments with isometric and isotonic recording, together with those from quick stretches and quick releases, lead to the following generalizations.

TENSION–LENGTH RELATIONSHIP

Inactive muscle resists stretch with a stiffness that increases with increasing length (lower broken curve in Figure 4.5). In an ideal spring, i.e. one that obeys Hooke's Law, the stiffness is independent of length and the tension T at different lengths L can be expressed by the equation

$$T = S(L - L_0)$$

where S is the stiffness and L_0 is the maximum length at which no tension is exerted. L_0 may be referred to as the 'slack length'. Consider

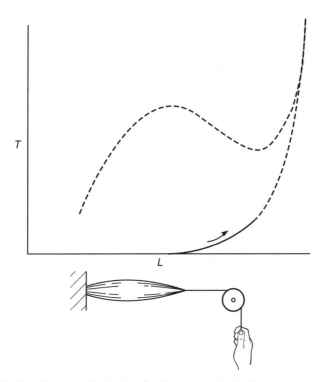

Figure 4.5 Inactive muscle being forcibly extended. The tension rises along curve 'a' in Figure 4.8, which is reproduced here by broken lines.

now a system made up of a number of ideal springs arranged in parallel and each having a different slack length (Figure 4.6). If this system is stretched, the different springs will begin to contribute tension one by one as their slack lengths are exceeded. The overall stiffness of the system will then increase, in a series of steps, as the length increases, and it is easy to imagine how a smooth curve may be made up of the contributions of a large number of such elements arranged in parallel. The curved tension–length relation found in many inert biological tissues, such as tendons and connective tissue, can thus be regarded as a quite straightforward property of a complex arrangement of simple elements. Similar curved tension–length relations are, in fact, found in textiles and particularly in knitted fabrics.

If a muscle is held at a set of fixed lengths in a series of experiments, and is maximally stimulated at each length, using repetitive stimuli to produce fused tetanic contraction and with adequate rest periods between the trials, a plot of the resulting peak tensions gives a curve like the upper broken curve in Figure 4.7. In Figure 4.8, the results of Figures 4.5 and 4.7 are presented together. Curve 'a' is the inactive tension from Figure 4.5 and curve 'b' shows the tension when the muscle is fully active at various fixed lengths. Curve 'c' is obtained by subtracting curve 'a' from curve 'b'. The resulting, roughly parabolic, curve represents the tension contributed by the contractile mechanism at the various lengths indicated.

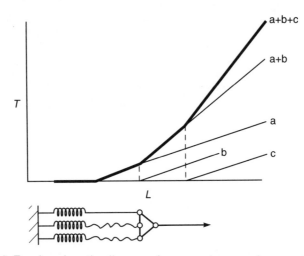

Figure 4.6 Tension–length diagram for a system made up of a parallel assembly of three simple springs, each with a different slack length. As the system is progressively extended, the tension contributions of the individual springs are brought into play one by one. Because the springs are in parallel, the tensions add. Compare with curve 'a' in Figure 4.8.

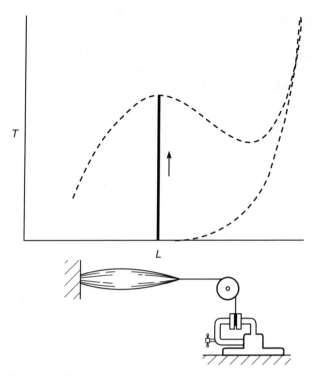

Figure 4.7 Muscle pulling against a rigid device. Tension rises vertically, with no change in length, to the appropriate point on the isometric tension–length diagram of Figure 4.8.

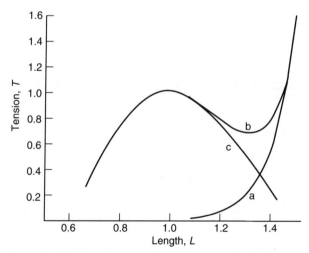

Figure 4.8 Characteristic tension–length diagram for skeletal muscle: curve 'a' for inactive muscle, as in Figure 4.5; 'b' tetanic tensions obtained at various lengths in isometric recording conditions with repetitive activation, as in Figure 4.7; 'c' tension contributed by the contractile element, obtained by subtracting 'a' from 'b'. (After Hill, 1953.)

The shape of this curve can be accounted for in terms of differences, at the various lengths, in the degree of overlap between the actin and myosin filaments (Figure 4.9). For a single sarcomere, there is a plateau in the tension–length curve corresponding ,to the range of sarcomere lengths at which all possible cross-bridges are effective ('c' in Figure 4.9). At larger sarcomere lengths ('d' in Figure 4.9), there is less overlap and some of the cross-bridges cannot be brought into play. The tension thus falls off with increasing length. During progressive shortening, the actin filaments of the two ends of the sarcomere begin to overlap with one another and may engage with cross-bridges pulling in opposite directions ('b' in Figure 4.9). With further shortening, the myosin

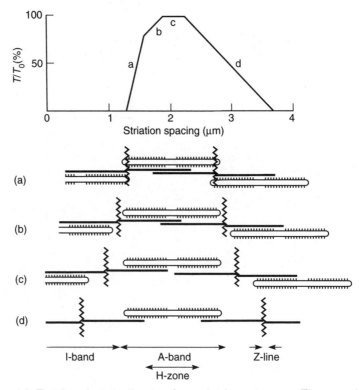

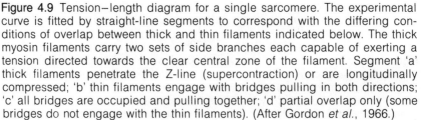

Figure 4.9 Tension–length diagram for a single sarcomere. The experimental curve is fitted by straight-line segments to correspond with the differing conditions of overlap between thick and thin filaments indicated below. The thick myosin filaments carry two sets of side branches each capable of exerting a tension directed towards the clear central zone of the filament. Segment 'a' thick filaments penetrate the Z-line (supercontraction) or are longitudinally compressed; 'b' thin filaments engage with bridges pulling in both directions; 'c' all bridges are occupied and pulling together; 'd' partial overlap only (some bridges do not engage with the thin filaments). (After Gordon et al., 1966.)

filaments come up against, and may have to penetrate, the Z-membranes, with further reduction in the overall tension developed by the sarcomere. The corners in the tension–length relations for different sarcomeres occur at slightly different lengths. With a large number of sarcomeres in series, as in any whole muscle, the corners are not seen, the overall effect having the rounded appearance of curve 'c' in Figure 4.8.

The maximum active tension developed by the contractile element at constant length occurs at a length near to the normal resting length of the muscle in the body. The total tension exerted against the recording device (curve 'b') is the sum of those shown in curves 'a' and 'c'. The general shape of these two curves for different muscles is usually similar to those shown in the figure, but there are individual differences in the relative positions of these curves on the length axis. The shape of curve 'b' for different muscles may accordingly differ from that shown here in the extent of the dip appearing to the right of the peak of active tension.

If a muscle is allowed to shorten it does not develop as much tension as it can at constant length. The shortfall in tension is dependent on the speed of shortening, with a relation that resembles the rectangular hyperbola

$$(T + a)(V + b) = \text{constant}$$

where T is the tension and V is the speed of shortening, and a and b are constants. This relation is illustrated by the part of the curve in Figure 4.10 that lies to the left of the line for zero velocity.

The equation can be rearranged to give

$$TV + aV = b(T_0 - T)$$

a form which tells us something about the way a muscle may be expected to behave. The product TV is the rate at which the contractile element does work against the load. The term aV can be interpreted as the rate at which energy is dissipated within the contractile mechanism itself when it shortens. This is akin to the energy 'lost' in overcoming friction in a machine. The sum of the two terms on the left is thus the rate at which energy is set free by the muscle. The equation tells us that this rate is proportional to the amount by which the tension currently exerted on the load falls short of the maximum tension of which the contractile mechanism is capable.

If it were not for the presence of the aV term, which represents internal damping within the contractile mechanism, we would expect a muscle to be able to do more work by moving faster against a smaller load. The effect of the internal damping is to make very rapid movements wasteful. In consequence, as the speed of movement is gradually increased, the rate of doing external work at first rises and then falls, and there is, for each muscle, a particular optimum speed of working against external loads.

If an active muscle is stretched slowly it can develop more tension than at constant length, but if the rate of stretching is increased beyond a certain point there comes a stage at which the rate of formation of cross-bridges cannot keep pace with the rate at which the bridges are being broken by the stretching. The tension accordingly falls off and slippage occurs. This is illustrated by the right-hand portion of the curve in Figure 4.10.

The speeds of shortening and of lengthening for a particular muscle are greatly influenced by the way the muscles are connected to the bones of the skeleton and by the way these bones move on one another. The triangulation of muscles and bones is used to generate the torques needed at the various joints of the overall lattice structure of the body. The same torque can be produced either by a small force operating at a large offset, or by a larger force operating at a smaller offset. In the design of each triangle there is a conflict betwen the degree of extension of which a muscle is capable and the magnitude of the total force that it will be called upon to exert, since a larger offset

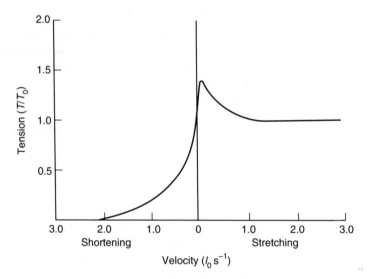

Figure 4.10 Force–velocity curve for tetanized muscle. For shortening only, the curve resembles the rectangular hyperbola $(T + a)(V + b) = (T_0 + a)b = $ constant. The curve for lengthening shows that the muscle is able to develop a force greater than the isometric tension if it is forcibly extended at a moderate speed. (After Curtin and Davies, 1972.)

implies a greater length-change of the muscle for the same change in the angle at the joint.

Each sarcomere can accommodate only a very restricted range of changes in length. A muscle that needs to operate over a large range of extensions consequently needs to have many sarcomeres in series. This is achieved in long muscles with parallel fibres. If less extension can be tolerated, the required extra force can be provided by packing short muscle-fibres in herring-bone pattern on either side of a sheet of tendon. Such 'pinnate' muscles can develop large tensions but can operate over only a small range of extensions.

The curves given for the relations between tension and length (Figure 4.8) and between tension and the speeds of shortening or lengthening (Figure 4.10) are intended to illustrate the general shape of such relations. In different muscles, different calibrations of the scales are appropriate. There may also be differences in the relative positions in Figure 4.8 of curves 'a' and 'c', with consequent changes in the appearance of curve 'b' for overall tension. These characteristic curves represent results either at constant length or at constant tension. In any practical use of a muscle in the body, tension and length will be changing at the same time. In such conditions predictions from the characteristic curves turn out not to be borne out precisely.

The nature of the problem may be illustrated by Figures 4.11–4.14.

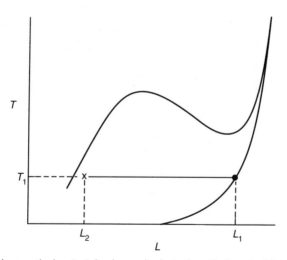

Figure 4.11 A muscle is stretched passively to length L_1, at which it develops tension T_1. It is then made active and allowed to shorten isotonically. Shortening proceeds to L_2, stopping before reaching the tension–length curve for isometric tensions.

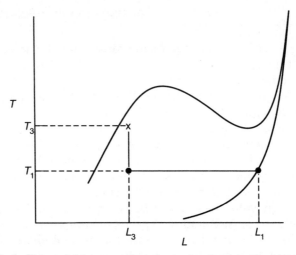

Figure 4.12 As Figure 4.11 except that shortening is restrained by interposing a stop at L_3.

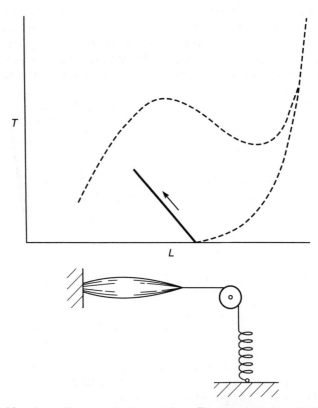

Figure 4.13 Muscle pulling against a spring. The tension–length diagram reflects the stiffness of the spring.

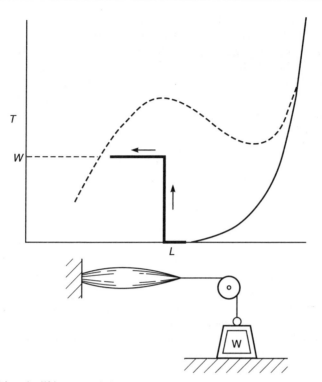

Figure 4.14 Muscle lifting a weight.

In Figure 4.11, a muscle is forcibly extended to length L_1 while it is inactive. It is then made active and allowed to shorten at constant load T_1. The shortening does not proceed as far as the length at which this tension can be developed without shortening.

In Figure 4.12, the muscle is extended to L_1, and is then activated and allowed to shorten at constant load T_1, just as in Figure 4.11, but shortening is restrained by a stop at L_3. Tension now rises isometrically to T_3, a tension which is less than that which could have been obtained isometrically at that length without the earlier shortening phase.

Figure 4.13 shows what happens when the muscle develops tension against a spring. As the force increases, the spring is pulled out, so the muscle has to shorten. The tension does not continue to rise as far as curve 'b', but stops short.

Figure 4.14 illustrates what happens when lifting a weight. If there is any slack in the connection to the weight, the muscle will at first shorten to take up the slack. During this unrestrained shortening, no tension is developed. The muscle then builds up tension at constant length until sufficient force has been developed to lift the weight. Once the weight is clear of its support, the muscle shortens at constant tension, but not as far as to reach the curve 'b'.

This curve 'b' indicates the maximum tension that the muscle can develop when fully activated at constant length. In practice, muscles are not usually fully activated. The various factors influencing tension development all interact in ways that make prediction difficult. We may record the muscle length, the way the length is changing, and the history of previous activations, but although, in principle, these are the main factors to be taken into account, in practice we do not know enough detail about the effectiveness of each of the factors in the same muscle at the same time to be able to make useful predictions as to just how much tension will be generated in any particular circumstances.

The influence of previous activations is particularly difficult to assess. Both the rate of uptake of calcium by the longitudinal tubule system and the rate of regeneration of ATP are dependent on the oxygen supply. The efficacy of the circulation also affects the removal of the products of metabolism and in intense exercise there may be cumulative effects on the acidity and on other factors that can then play a part in influencing the tension-generating mechanism. In the normal course, the regulation of muscular activity is carried out in terms of the regulation of the motor impulses transmitted to the muscles from the nervous system, but clearly the relationship between motoneuron firing-frequency and muscle tension is a very remote one. Nevertheless, the only control available to the nervous system is to select which motoneurons shall be active and at what times and repetition-frequencies.

TYPES OF MUSCLE-FIBRE

Further complications arise because muscle-fibres are not all identical in their behaviour. They also differ in the relative proportions of the various cell inclusions. For example, some fibres are large in cross-section, with many fibrils. Others are smaller, with fewer fibrils and relatively more of the constituents involved in oxidative metabolism. Of these, both myoglobin and the cytochromes are coloured. Fibres may thus be classified as 'white' or 'red'. These differences reflect specializations for anaerobic or for oxidative energy usage respectively, the smallness of the red fibres favouring the diffusion exchange with the capillaries. A consequence of this specialization in relation to energy usage is that white muscle is more susceptible to fatigue, while red muscle can continue to perform useful work for extended periods.

Another type of specialization concerns the rate at which tension builds up after the moment of activation, and also the rate at which the tension falls off during subsequent relaxation. We come, on this basis, to speak of 'fast' and 'slow' muscle. Fast muscle-fibres are appropriate to tasks involving small loads and rapid movements, such as the movements of the eyeballs or of the digits. Slow muscle-fibres are appropriate when the load has substantial inertia and for the sustained support of the weight of the body.

VARYING LOADS

In many physiological situations, muscles are called upon to support varying loads. In general, if the load first increases and then decreases, the relation between tension and length in the muscle does not follow the same path in both directions. This is because the muscle, at a particular intensity of activation, can develop more tension while being forcibly stretched than it does when shortening to move the load. There is hysteresis. Practical cases are complicated by the fact that, when working against fluctuating loads, the degree of activation of the muscle is altered during the stretching and again during the subsequent relaxation.

To get some idea of what may be happening in a particular case, we may proceed as follows. Figure 4.15 shows the curve for full activation (curve 'c' from Figure 4.8) together with two other curves in which the ordinates are respectively 60% and 30% of the values for full activation. In Figure 4.16 the curve for inactive tension (curve 'a' from Figure 4.8) has been added to each of the curves of Figure 4.15. We now suppose

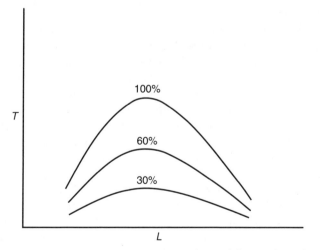

Figure 4.15 Active tensions for various proportions of the total number of motor units.

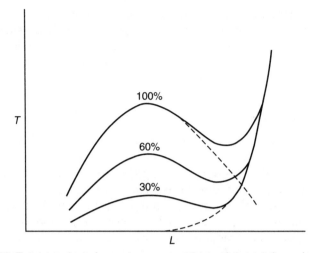

Figure 4.16 Total tensions for various proportions of the total number of motor units.

that the degree of activation increases when the muscle is stretched by a movement of the load (Figure 4.17). This increase in activation may correspond to an increase in the number of motor units contributing to the development of force, each of the active motor units behaving in an all-or-none manner and developing all the force of which it is capable. During stretching, the working point moves through positions like those marked 1, 2, 3 and 4, each corresponding to a different position of the tension–length curve according to the progressive increase in the proportion of the total number of motor units that have been recruited into activity. The muscle behaves like a spring.

The rate of recruitment of motor units during stretching depends on the conditions, so the path of the working point on the tension–length diagram may vary in different situations. Figure 4.18 is from an actual experiment with a muscle which was in functional connection with the nervous system (soleus muscle in a decerebrate cat). A fluctuating tension was applied to the tendon of the muscle by a special device which permitted the muscle to take up its own length without constraint. Tension and length were recorded, to produce the display shown in the figure. The resulting tension–length diagram shows that tension is not linearly related to extension, and that there is noticeable hysteresis, the tension at a particular length being greater during stretching than it is during shortening. The hysteresis appears to be a quite general aspect of the development of tension by muscle in physiological conditions and it has important consequences in the

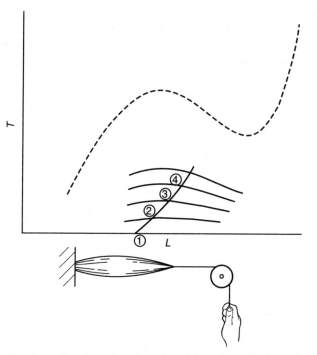

Figure 4.17 Tensions developed during stretching of a reflexly active muscle.

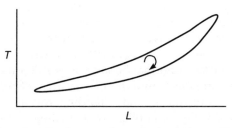

Figure 4.18 Tension–length diagram for reflexly active soleus muscle of the decerebrate cat during harmonic changes in applied tension. The curve is traced in a clockwise direction. (From Roberts, 1963, by courtesy of *Quart. J. Exp. Physiol.*)

avoidance of oscillation in supporting forces. Its effect is akin to that of the shock-absorbers used in motor vehicle suspensions.

In most circumstances, the repetition-frequencies used by the nervous system for postural purposes are lower than those which might produce fused tetanic contractions. The consequent fluctuations in tension permit the blood to flow through the muscle, albeit intermittently, and this avoids the adverse effects that would follow from the complete occlusion of the blood supply that occurs during fused tetanus. The option to use higher frequencies of activation is retained for special occasions when a large tension is required for a short time, as for example in operating a pair of wire-cutters.

At the normal subtetanic frequencies of activation of individual motor units, the resulting fluctuations in tension are smoothed, in the process of transmission from the muscle-fibres to the attached tendon, by the activity of other motor units. Because the activations of the individual motor nerve-fibres are not normally synchronized with one another, the peaks and troughs in tension in different units occur at different times. When one unit is relaxing after its peak tension, another unit will be starting its cycle of activity with an increasing tension. Most of the fluctuations in tension are thus ironed out. There is an advantage in restricting the rate of firing to a small range, since slowly-repeated activations are less easily smoothed, and more rapidly-repeated activations lead to fused tetanus so that no advantage is gained by further increasing the firing rate.

In the special conditions of the laboratory, when one wishes to study the mechanical behaviour during a muscle activation, it is convenient to arrange for simultaneous activation of the motor units. This is readily achieved by applying electric shocks to the motor nerve so that all the relevant motor nerve-fibres are activated simultaneously. In some other conditions also the motor units in a particular muscle are, for some reason, activated almost synchronously at a low frequency. When this happens, the result is a perceptible tremor.

Just how the muscle activity is regulated by the nervous system to produce the necessary fine adjustments in resistance to extension for all the different tasks in normal behaviour is still a matter of considerable doubt. An immense amount of research effort has been, and continues to be, directed at understanding this process. The neuro-anatomy involved is very complicated, as is the relationship, described in this chapter, between motor-nerve impulses and the mechanical activity of the muscle cells. Many different schemes have been put forward, each based on simplifying assumptions that later studies have shown to be unwarranted. The topic will be discussed in more detail in a later part of this book.

We have now seen that the maintenance of the normal upright posture depends on coordinating the stress forces with which we push against the ground. These stress forces are applied through a lattice structure of struts (bones) and ties (muscles and tendons) with low-friction joints between the struts. We now turn to the processes by which the necessary forces are generated and controlled.

Active balance   5

In considering the balancing behaviour of animals and men it is not sufficient to confine attention to such stress forces as might just be in static equilibrium with the gravitational forces. The support forces have to be generated by muscles and, in consequence, the amount of force available is necessarily changing all the time. We have, therefore, to take account of the effects of fluctuating forces. For this we shall need to use the concepts of momentum, work and energy. These concepts are usually introduced rather summarily in the early stages of the teaching of elementary physics and they tend thereafter to be taken for granted without further analysis. Because the body is a flexible structure with distributed mass, the simplifications of conventional schoolbook mechanics are not appropriate. They can indeed be actually misleading. Readers who are not in the habit of dealing daily with these concepts may accordingly find the following reminder useful.

MOMENTUM, WORK AND ENERGY

Let us start by considering two masses, M and m, and let us suppose them to be at rest close beside one another. We then consider what happens when they become separated by the action of a force F that is active for a time T (Figure 5.1). Suppose that M moves to the right and m to the left and that the final velocities are respectively V and U. M attains a momentum MV to the right while m attains a momentum mU to the left, where 'momentum' is the product of the mass multiplied by the velocity. The velocities are in opposite directions and, with the usual convention, V will be positive and U negative. According to Newton's Second Law, 'force' is the rate-of-change of momentum, and according to the Third Law the forces on the two bodies are equal in magnitude but opposite in direction. Thus we have

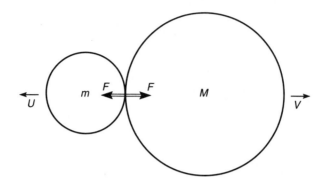

Figure 5.1 Force and momentum. A force, *F*, acts to separate two masses, *M* and *m*, which move away with different velocities, *V* and *U*. Note that *MV* = −*mU*.

$$F = M\frac{dV}{dt} \quad \text{and} \quad -F = m\frac{dU}{dt}$$

In each case the velocity starts at zero and increases steadily over the time *T*. The effect of the force can be expressed as the 'impulse', which is the product of the force multiplied by the time for which it acts. The impulse is then the same as the change in momentum. As a general formulation, we have that the impulse on *M* is

$$\int_0^T F dt = \int_0^T M\frac{dV}{dt} dt = MV$$

Similarly, the impulse on *m* is

$$\int_0^T m\frac{dU}{dt} dt = mU$$

The total momentum at the outset is zero, because the masses are at rest. At the end of time *T* the total momentum is *MV* + *mU*. Because the magnitudes of the two impulses are equal although they act in opposite directions, the momentum gained to the right by *M* is equal and opposite to the momentum gained to the left by *m*. The total momentum is accordingly still zero. That is to say, momentum is conserved, and *MV* = −*mU* (remember that *U* is negative).

We now consider the work done by the forces. This is measured as the product of the force multiplied by the distance over which it acts. The distance travelled to the right by *M* in the time *T* is

$$\int_0^T V dt$$

or

$$\int_0^T At\,dt$$

where A is the acceleration, which is constant under constant force. Evaluating the integral, the distance travelled by M under the action of the force is

$$\frac{1}{2}AT^2 = S \text{ (say)}$$

The work done on M is then

$$\int_0^S F\,ds \quad \text{or} \quad \int_0^S M\frac{dV}{dt}\,ds$$

which, since $ds/dt = V$, can be rearranged as

$$\int_0^V MV\,dV = \frac{1}{2}MV^2$$

This expression, in terms of V, is referred to as the 'energy' of the body M by virtue of its motion, designated as 'kinetic energy' to distinguish it from other forms of energy. We may now say that the work done to accelerate a mass is converted into the resulting kinetic energy of that mass.

If $M = km$, then $U = -kV$, and the acceleration of m is $-kA$, so that the distance travelled by m is $-\frac{1}{2}kAT^2$, and more work is done on the lighter mass.

Although momentum is conserved, energy has to be supplied to effect the separation of the masses. We have to supply $\frac{1}{2}MV^2$ to M and $\frac{1}{2}mk^2V^2$ to m, i.e. more energy has to be supplied to the lighter mass.

Let us now consider the case where a mass M, moving with velocity V towards the right, is brought to rest by compressing a spring the other end of which is anchored to some large mass, such as the earth (Figure 5.2). The moving mass gives up its momentum of MV. Because the mass of the earth is relatively so large, the change in its velocity is very small. Although this change in velocity can usually be neglected, we ought not to forget that the earth does, in fact, acquire momentum from the impact.

For simplicity let us suppose that the spring obeys Hooke's Law so that the force developed when it is compressed is proportional to the displacement. Correspondingly, the deceleration of the mass will vary, rising from zero at the moment of impact to a maximum when the mass has been brought to rest at the point of maximum compression of the spring. At intermediate times we have

$$F = -ks$$

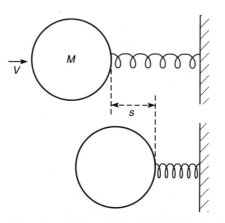

Figure 5.2 A mass, *M*, moving to the right with initial velocity, *V*, is brought to rest in a distance, *s*, by compressing a spring, the other end of which is tethered to a large mass.

where *k* is the stiffness of the spring and *s* is the distance travelled by the mass at time *t* after the initial impact. The minus sign is required because the force acts in a direction to reduce the displacement.

Now

$$F = M\frac{dv}{dt} \quad \text{and} \quad V = \frac{ds}{dt}$$

This means that the time-course of the change in *s* is governed by the differential equation

$$M\frac{d^2s}{dt^2} = -ks$$

The general solution of equations of this type is

$$s = A\sin Bt + C\cos Dt$$

and we find the values of the parameters *A*, *B*, *C*, and *D* by considering the initial conditions.

At *t* = 0, *s* = 0 and sin *Bt* = 0. Therefore *C* = 0 and our solution reduces to the form

$$s = A\sin Bt$$

Differentiating, we have

$$\frac{ds}{dt} = A\frac{d}{dt}(\sin BT) = AB\cos Bt$$

At $t = 0$, $ds/dt = V$ and $\cos Bt = 1$, therefore $AB = V$. The left-hand side of the original equation then becomes

$$M\frac{d^2s}{dt^2} = M\frac{d^2}{dt^2}(A \sin Bt)$$

$$= -MAB^2 \sin Bt$$

$$= -MVB \sin Bt$$

while the right-hand side yields

$$-ks = -k\frac{V}{B}\sin Bt$$

i.e.

$$-MVB \sin Bt = -k\frac{V}{B}\sin Bt$$

hence

$$B^2 = \frac{k}{M}$$

so that

$$s = \frac{V}{B}\sin Bt$$

That is to say, the displacement follows a sinusoidal time-course. The parameter B, (whose value is $\sqrt{(k/M)}$) controls the period of the sinusoid, which repeats when $Bt = 2\pi$. The maximum value of s, arrived at when the mass has just been brought to rest, is given by the ratio of V to B.

At the moment at which the mass has just been brought to rest, the work done in bringing the mass to rest is $\int F ds$ and the whole of the kinetic energy previously associated with the mass in its movement before the impact, $\frac{1}{2}MV^2$, has become converted into the strain energy stored in the compressed spring.

REBOUND

The events of the collision are not completed when the mass has been brought to rest, because the compressed spring is still exerting a force on the mass. This force accelerates the mass to the left, the displacement of the spring, s, continuing to follow the time-course indicated by the equation $s = (V/B)\sin Bt$ until the mass loses contact with the spring at $s = 0$. By this time the mass has acquired momentum $-MV$ and it thereafter proceeds to the left with a velocity whose magnitude is equal to the original V, but which is now in the opposite direction.

At this point the whole of the energy stored in the spring during the collision has been returned to the moving mass. The momentum of the mass has changed by $2MV$ towards the left, so that the earth must have acquired momentum of $2MV$ to the right.

A recoil in which the whole of the original kinetic energy is recovered after a temporary change into strain energy, is referred to as perfectly 'elastic'. In treating the collision of masses for the purposes of elementary physics, elastic recoil is usually taken for granted and the details of what happens during the collision are passed over, as though the change in momentum could take place instantaneously. However, the exchange of momentum implies the action of an impulse whose magnitude is $\int Fdt$. If the time occupied by this impulse is very short, then the magnitude of the force has to be proportionally large, becoming infinite if the impulse is supposed to be instantaneous. Clearly this is not a realistic situation.

Another complication arises from the fact that real bodies have distributed mass, and the structure connecting the individual mass elements has a finite stiffness.

DISTRIBUTED MASS

As a first stage in attempting to deal with the problem of distributed mass let us consider a pair of equal masses linked by a spring and suppose these masses to be moving from left to right with velocity V, the line of the linking spring being at right angles to the direction of motion. We then suppose the masses to come into collision with a large mass attached to the earth, the impact being cushioned by a pair of springs, one for each of the masses, where the lines of action of these cushioning springs are symmetrically inclined to the direction of motion of the masses and act in directions tending to separate the masses (Figure 5.3).

The effect of the inclination of the cushioning springs is that when they begin to develop force, in the course of arresting the motion of the masses, they push these masses apart and stretch the spring that links the masses together. Then, at the point where the masses have been brought to rest, there is some strain energy stored in the linking spring as well as the strain energy stored in the cushioning springs.

During the recoil phase, the masses are accelerated to the left by the cushioning springs, and they are accelerated towards one another by the tension in the linking spring. If the linking spring is capable of exerting compressive thrust as well as tension, the masses will go into simple harmonic oscillation, moving towards and away from one another along the line joining their centres. The energy for this oscillation has come from the kinetic energy of the original motion of the

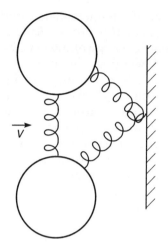

Figure 5.3 Effect of impact on distributed mass. See text.

masses. Accordingly there is not so much energy available for the recoil along the path from right to left, and the leftward velocity after the collision is less than the velocity of approach. If we were not aware of the oscillation occurring at right angles to the line of flight, we might suppose some energy to be 'lost' in the collision.

The situation inside a body having distributed mass is related to the conditions in this example. We may suppose the mass of the body to be concentrated in the individual molecules, which act as 'mass elements'. Each molecule is restrained in a network of intermolecular forces which act like springs capable of both compressive thrust and tension. When one body comes into collision with another, the lines of action of the intermolecular forces are, in general, inclined to the direction of motion of the bodies. In consequence, local oscillations of the molecules are produced by the impact. The energy for these oscillations has to come from the kinetic energy with which the bodies approach one another.

The molecular vibrations generated by impact are of two kinds. In one, the oscillations of the individual molecules are largely un-coordinated. Energy stored in such oscillations is classed as 'heat'. In another, there is sufficient order in the oscillations of neighbouring molecules for local changes in pressure to be produced. Energy in this form is classed as 'sound'. In both cases, the local disturbances arising from the effects of an impact influence neighbouring molecules so that these in turn are set into oscillations of their own. The disturbance propagates through the material of the bodies involved in the collision and may even spread to the surrounding medium. Thus some of the energy delivered to the collision is radiated from the point of impact, both as heat and as sound. It is not normally possible to recover this energy directly into kinetic energy of the mass as a whole. For practical purposes such radiated energy is truly lost.

If sufficient energy is delivered to the molecular oscillations, some of the molecules may become so separated from one another that the intermolecular attractive forces, instead of increasing with separation, begin to diminish. When this happens, the material begins to tear apart. Cracks begin to appear across which the intermolecular attractive forces are relatively weak. In consequence, the load carried by the material as a whole has to be distributed over a smaller cross-sectional area, and regions of stress-concentration arise in the neighbourhood of the cracks.

When a crack starts, some of the material in the immediate neigh-bourhood of the crack ceases to contribute to load-bearing. As the intermolecular linkages are relieved of imposed stress they release their stored energy and this energy becomes available to increase the oscil-lations of the stressed material close to the crack. Accordingly, once a crack has started, it tends to spread. Thus, if a collision is sufficiently violent, that is to say, if sufficient energy is delivered at impact, then not only does the collision generate heat and sound, but the material of the bodies in collision may be fractured.

We now consider what happens when a mass, falling freely towards the earth under the action of gravity, is arrested by impact with the ground. In many situations the mass will rebound upwards. Its upward movement after leaving the ground will be again subject to the unrestrained action of gravity. The upward velocity is gradually decelerated to zero, after which the mass falls back again towards the earth at increasing velocity, bouncing up again after another impact.

Bouncing occurs in different ways according to the conditions. The simple bouncing of an elastic ball, as in many ball games, involves two phases in each cycle: a free-fall phase of constant downward acceler-ation under gravity, and a phase of upward acceleration under the elastic forces of deformation developed partly by the structure of the ball and partly by the nature of the surface on which the ball bounces. For many instances, a fair account of the motion is given by supposing the deformation-stiffness to be representable by a straight-line relation between the deformation-displacement and the restoring force, without hysteresis, as in an idealized spring. The action of a linear spring upon a rigid mass results in simple harmonic motion. The time-course of bouncing in this idealized system then consists of a parabolic phase of downward acceleration, alternating with a sinusoidal 'half-cycle' of upward acceleration corresponding to the contact time. The durations of the two 'halves' of the cycle are unlikely to be equal. Such a system would continue to bounce indefinitely, which is not what is observed in practice.

In any real system, deformation is accompanied by internal friction in the material deformed, so that some of the energy of the motion is converted to heat. The stiffness of deformation cannot therefore be accurately represented as a linear relation. Some hysteresis has to be taken into account. Furthermore, many materials show curved relations between deformation-displacement and restoring force. Another complication of the real case is that practical objects are made up of distributed masses held together by deformable intermolecular bonds. Forces applied at the surface of contact between two objects are transmitted through the material of the objects by these intermolecular bonds, the mass to be accelerated by each such bond depending on the site of that bond within the structure of the object and on the distribution of mass through the whole structure.

If an object with distributed mass suffers a short-lasting vertical impulse, similar to that arising at the impact after a fall, some vertical oscillations may occur without the object actually leaving the ground. This is what happens when a moving vehicle encounters a hump in the road. Where such oscillations are undesirable, they may be minimized by the incorporation of suitable damping. This is the function of the shock-absorbers of a vehicle.

The body of an animal is a springy structure with distributed mass and it is inevitable that there will be some fluctuation in the magnitude of the supporting forces, because they are generated by muscles. The fact that the body does not usually show marked continuous bouncing oscillations is due to the presence of the inherent damping within the muscles themselves.

One consequence of the fluctuating nature of the supporting forces is that the centre of gravity of the body is liable to be moved relative to the position of the supports at the feet. This possibility raises the question of stability. The organization of the muscular forces needed to prevent overbalancing is the essence of balancing behaviour. Let us look again at what we mean by balancing.

STABILITY

Balance is a fairly familiar idea but, like many English words, it is used in several different senses, often without a clear understanding of the distinctions between them. The word itself comes from the Latin name for a device used for comparing weights. In a beam-balance, the beam pivots about a point just above its centre of gravity. When the weights in the two scale-pans are equal, the beam see-saws slowly before coming to rest in the 'balanced' position. The weights in the two scale-pans tend to tilt the beam in opposite directions. In the 'balanced' condition, with the beam at rest, the two opposing tendencies to tilt are equal in magnitude (Figure 5.4). This leads to the basic meaning of 'balance' to indicate the equality of opposing tendencies.

When the beam of the balance is swinging, the movements of the beam itself have to be taken into account. If the left-hand scale-pan moves downwards, this moves the centre of gravity of the beam towards the right of the pivot. The support force exerted by the pivot then tends to tilt the beam towards the right and this counteracts the displacement from the rest position. This is just what happens to anything that is hung from a support that is above its centre of gravity, such as a coat hanging on a peg.

Any situation in which a displacement from a particular condition generates forces that tend to reduce the displacement is referred to as a state of 'stable equilibrium'. (The word 'equilibrium' ('equal weight') is just another word for balance.) The contrast here is with an 'unstable equilibrium', such as that of a pencil stood up on its point where, even though the pencil may be in balance for a moment in the rest position, any displacement, however small, generates forces that tend to increase the displacement further so that the pencil falls. An intermediate condition, that might be referred to as one of 'precarious balance', arises where an object stands on a support that is below the centre of gravity and where the available area of support is relatively restricted. An example is the case of a coin stood up on its edge. So long as the centre of gravity of the coin remains vertically above the area of contact, the coin is in stable equilibrium and will stay upright. But as soon as the coin is displaced beyond the vertical projection of the edge of the area of support, the condition becomes unstable and the coin falls. The same is true of a man standing on one foot.

It is more usual for objects to be supported on multiple contacts distributed over an area that is at least comparable with the height of

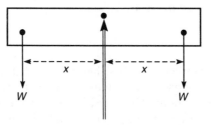

Figure 5.4 Principle of operation of a beam balance. Note that the central supporting pivot is offset slightly above the line joining the two load pivots at opposite ends of the beam.

the centre of gravity of the object above the supports. We may take as an example the case of a symmetrical rectangular table supported by four legs placed at the corners. Figure 5.5 represents an end view of such a table. Only two legs are shown, the other two being obscured. The position of the centre of gravity of the table is represented by a solid circle. As the feet of the table legs are equidistant from the vertical through the centre of gravity, the upthrust forces on the legs on the two sides of the centre of gravity are equal in magnitude.

If the table is loaded by placing a large weight on it to one side of the centre, the table does not fall over (Figure 5.6). The centre of gravity of the combination of table plus load now lies at O. The upthrusts at the feet are no longer equal on the two sides because the vertical through the new centre of gravity is not equidistant from the feet. The upthrust in the legs to the right of the centre of gravity, P_r, tends to tip the table to the left, while that of the legs to the left, P_l, tends to tip it to the right. The magnitudes of these two turning moments are respectively $P_r a$ and $P_l b$, where a and b are the offset distances. Since the table does

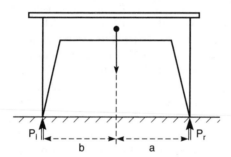

Figure 5.5 End view of a symmetrical table (schematic) at rest with its centre of gravity midway between equal upthrust forces.

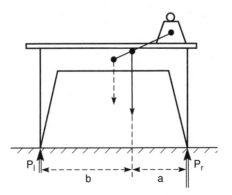

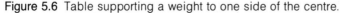

Figure 5.6 Table supporting a weight to one side of the centre.

not, in practice, tip over, these two turning moments must be equal in magnitude and opposite in direction, i.e. $P_r a = P_1 b$

A similar inequality in the upthrusts arises if the table is set on a sloping surface, as in Figure 5.7. There is clearly a limit to the degree of tilting that can be tolerated without the table toppling over. This limit is reached when the vertical projection of the centre of gravity passes through the edge of the area of contact of the feet with the supporting surface.

We may define an 'area of support' as that polygon, with no re-entrant angles, that just encloses the vertical projections of all the available points of support. This leads to a statement of general principle, that the equilibrium of a supported object is stable so long as the vertical projection of the centre of gravity falls within the area of support.

Figure 5.7 draws attention to the fact that the legs have to be firmly attached to the table. When the area of contact with the ground is not vertically below the attachment of the leg to the tabletop, the upthrust combines with the downward pressure of the tabletop to form a couple tending to tip the leg over to the left. This tendency has to be met by a torque exerted by the stiffness of the attachment of the leg to the tabletop. If this joint comes loose, the table will fail to stand up.

The definition of stable equilibrium given earlier refers to the effect of perturbations. Figure 5.8 illustrates the situation in which a horizontal perturbing force is applied to the tabletop. If the table is to remain stationary, it is necessary that this perturbing force be opposed by a horizontal component of force developed at the contact with the supports. This horizontal force combines with the resultant upthrust needed to support the weight of the table to form an inclined thrust. If the table is not to topple, the line of this combined thrust must pass

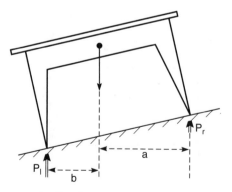

Figure 5.7 Table on an inclined support.

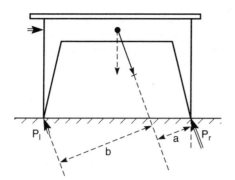
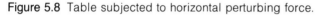

Figure 5.8 Table subjected to horizontal perturbing force.

through the centre of gravity of the table. From this we conclude that each of the forces at the individual feet of the table legs must also be inclined, and we can use a graphic method to work out the relative magnitudes of the vertical and horizontal components of force at each of the feet.

FRICTION

The horizontal force is provided by friction. The mechanics of dry friction are quite complicated. The frictional force that opposes sliding is very dependent on the nature of the materials in contact. The surfaces of most materials are usually contaminated in various ways and the nature of this contamination is also important, as we have already seen in the earlier consideration of lubrication. Surfaces that may appear smooth to the naked eye are invariably rough on the molecular scale. We can get some idea of what happens by supposing the opposing surfaces to be like irregular sandpaper. When two surfaces are pressed together, the various prominences in one surface engage with depressions in the other. When a shearing force is applied, projections from the two surfaces are brought up against one another and develop stress. The aggregate of minute stresses of this kind provides the force which prevents slipping. This force is sometimes referred to as 'stiction', in distinction from the force opposing sliding during actual relative motion of the two surfaces.

If the shearing force is large enough, the strain on the microprojections exceeds the limit for intermolecular cohesive forces and the projections are broken off. This is the process that produces wear at sliding surfaces. At the point of fracture, the molecular bonds previously strained rebound into oscillation. Sliding thus generates heat. A supply of energy is required to maintain the sliding motion. This energy comes from the work done against the force of the frictional resistance to motion. In many practical situations the force opposing sliding is proportional to the force pressing the surfaces together. The friction for a particular load is not dependent on the area of contact because an increase in area decreases the load per unit area while at the same time providing more contact sites at which frictional force can be developed.

An exception to this principle applies if a hard object presses against a large surface which is relatively soft. A small area of contact may then involve a gross deformation of the softer surface, with the formation of a depression, the walls of which can obstruct sliding movements. In such a case, an increase in surface area may make sliding easier because the depression is shallower and its edges present a smaller barrier. A further increase in ease of sliding may be achieved by rounding off the edges of the contact area. These principles are applied in the design of skis which, as well as spreading the skier's weight over a larger area, are turned up at the front end to assist the ski in climbing over the edge of the depression it makes in the snow. At the sides of the ski, the walls of the depression prevent lateral sliding.

THE 'POINT OF BALANCE'

The mechanics of the stability of a table apply also to the case of a person seated on a chair. Movements of the centre of gravity of the body, produced by leaning over, either to one side or in the fore-and-aft direction, are met by rearrangement of the distribution of pressure against the chair without overbalancing.

The expression 'balancing' is used for the process of setting one object on top of another where the available area of support is small compared with the height of the centre of gravity above the support. The result is not necessarily a condition of precarious balance. Consider the example of a pole balanced on an oil-drum laid on its side (Figure 5.9). It is necessary, first, to experiment by trying the pole in various positions in order to determine the 'point of balance' of the pole. Thereafter, the pole will stay in place even though the area of contact is very small. If you now give one end of the pole a little downward push, it will rock up and down like the beam-balance. The mechanics of the two oscillations are, however, quite different.

The beam of the balance is supported at a point **above** its centre of gravity, so it behaves like a pendulum. In contrast, the support for the pole in Figure 5.9 is the area of contact with the drum, which is necessarily **below** the centre of gravity of the pole. The pole is stable because of what happens at the support point. When the pole tilts, it rolls over the surface of the drum. The point of application of the

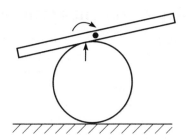

Figure 5.9 Stable equilibrium: pole balanced on a cylindrical drum. Note that the displacement of the point of contact, when the pole is disturbed, exceeds the horizontal excursion of the centre of gravity of the pole.

supporting thrust provided by the drum thus changes. The condition is stable so long as, for any displacement, the movement of the point of application of the support thrust is greater than the movement of the centre of gravity of the supported body. When this condition is satisfied, the support thrust always tends to tilt the supported object towards a rest position with its centre of gravity vertically over the point of support.

This is, in fact, a general statement of the condition that obtains also with any object whose centre of gravity is above the support, even where the supporting surface is not relatively restricted. We do not usually observe any rocking, unless parts of the supported structure are relatively springy. Nevertheless, the centre of pressure of the supporting force does move when any attempt is made to displace the supported object. The principle applies to living things, such as our own bodies and the bodies of animals, as well as to inert objects. It applies, as we have already seen, to a person seated on a chair.

In Figure 5.6, we considered the effect on the upthrusts exerted by the legs of a table when the centre of gravity of the whole is shifted by the addition of a weight. In an animal, in addition to those changes in the upthrusts by the legs that are occasioned purely as a passive reaction to such external perturbations, the animal can actively alter the thrusts in its legs. If the total of the combined upthrusts of the legs is less than that just needed to prevent the body from falling under the action of gravity, then the body will sink. Similarly, if the total upthrust exceeds what is needed, the body will be thrown upwards with an acceleration dependent on the magnitude of the excess thrust. Adjustment of the thrusts exerted by individual legs can actively alter the point of application of the resultant upthrust, and adjustment of the torques exerted at the proximal joints can alter the inclination of the resultant. The effect of these changes can be a toppling, a horizontal movement, or a combination of these. Any such movement involves a redistribution of momentum.

ANGULAR MOMENTUM AND THE MOMENT OF INERTIA

The momentum of toppling has to be treated differently from the momentum of linear movement. Whereas the resistance of an object to linear acceleration is a fixed property of that object, the resistance to angular acceleration depends on the distribution of the mass of the object through its structure and also on the relationship between the centre of gravity of the object and the axis about which it is to rotate. We need a separate measure of this resistance to angular acceleration. It is called the 'moment of inertia' of the object about the relevant axis. It is defined, by analogy with the definition of mass, as the ratio between applied torque and the resultant angular acceleration.

This leads to a definition of 'angular momentum' as the product of moment-of-inertia multiplied by angular-velocity, in the same way as linear momentum is the product of mass multiplied by linear velocity. The relations between these measures of angular motion are not mere analogies to the corresponding relations for linear motion; they are true alternative formulations of those same relations.

To show that this is so, we consider first a mass M constrained to move around an axis at a distance r from its centre of gravity (Figure 5.10), and set into motion by a torque, T, applied around that same axis. When the mass moves through a small distance dx, the line joining its centre of gravity to the axis of rotation moves through a small angle $d\theta$, where $\theta = x/r$.

The effective force accelerating the mass is T/r, so that

$$\frac{T}{r} = m\frac{d^2x}{dt^2} = mr\frac{d^2\theta}{dt^2}$$

hence

$$T = mr^2\frac{d^2\theta}{dt^2}$$

i.e. the ratio between applied torque and angular acceleration (the ratio that is to be called 'the moment of inertia') is, in this case, mr^2. This formula indicates how to calculate the magnitude of the moment of inertia.

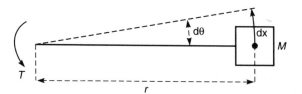

Figure 5.10 Torque and moment of inertia. See text.

For objects that have regular geometric shapes and which are of homogeneous density, we can evaluate the moment of inertia from this formula by the use of the calculus. The magnitude arrived at is dependent on the position and orientation of the axis of rotation in relation to the shape of the object. Objects that are not spherically symmetrical have different moments of inertia about different axes. For inhomogeneous or irregularly shaped objects it is necessary to resort to direct measurement. It is not necessary, however, to remeasure for each specific axis of rotation.

Consider an object constructed of two masses m and m' linked together by a straight, weightless, rigid rod (Figure 5.11). The moment of inertia of this object about an axis through its centre of gravity is $ma^2 + m'b^2$ where O, the centre of gravity of the object, lies at a distance a from m and b from m'. We require the moment of inertia of the object about another axis, parallel to the first, and passing through P, which is at a distance d from the centre of gravity, with the angle $POm' = \theta$. Suppose the distance of m from P to be x and that from m' to P to be y. The required value of the moment of inertia about P is

$$mx^2 + m'y^2$$

which we may call I'. Now

$$x^2 = a^2 + d^2 + 2ad \cos \theta$$

and

$$y^2 = b^2 + d^2 - 2bd \cos \theta$$

Therefore

$$I' = (ma^2 + m'b^2) + 2d \cos \theta(ma - m'b) + d^2(m + m')$$

Now

$$ma - m'b = 0$$

from the definition of centre of gravity, and $(ma^2 + m'b^2)$ is the moment of inertia of the object about its centre of gravity. Call this I and

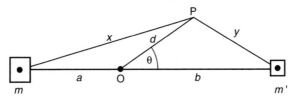

Figure 5.11 Moment of inertia about an axis not passing through the centre of gravity.

suppose it to be equal to Mr^2, where M is the total mass $(m + m')$. The value r is called the 'radius of gyration' of the object and

$$I' = M(r^2 + d^2)$$

The moment of inertia about any axis is thus dependent only on the moment of inertia about a parallel axis through the centre of gravity and on the offset distance between the axes. Clearly the moment of inertia of any object is at a minimum when the axis of rotation passes through the centre of gravity.

Expressing the moment of inertia in terms of a radius of gyration implies that the moment of inertia of a real object is the same as it would be if all the mass of the object was concentrated at a single point located at a specified distance from the centre of gravity. This simplification is convenient for certain calculations. It is open to the same objections as the treatment of an object, in relation to linear motion, as though all its mass was concentrated at its centre of gravity.

So long as we recognize that it is a possibly treacherous simplification, we may find the notion of the radius of gyration useful in helping to visualize what to expect in certain situations. Elongated objects have a larger moment of inertia about transverse axes than about their longitudinal axes, and the moment of inertia of any object is increased when the axis of rotation is remote from the object's centre of gravity. We need these ideas if we are to develop an understanding of what is going on during movements of the body parts.

TOPPLING

As we have seen, a shift in the position of the centre of gravity in relation to the upthrust currently being exerted will result in swaying, with a liability to toppling. There is always a certain amount of movement in the body, arising from the activity of the heart and from breathing. The resulting sway needs to be opposed if the body is to avoid falling over. If you stand on one foot you will be able to feel the process in operation. Pay attention to the sensations from your foot. You will be able to feel the way the body makes automatic adjustments to the pressure between the foot and the ground. You will feel the pressure moving between heel and toe, and from side to side of the foot. If you make a deliberate swaying movement, to take your centre of gravity outside the area of the foot, you will start to fall over. When this happens, you will find that your other leg is automatically swung out in the direction of the impending fall and stiffened to catch your weight on the other foot. It is by sequences of movements of this kind that we walk about, run, jump and so on. These reactions are so commonplace that we are usually quite unaware of what is going on.

To get some idea of the nature of this process, consider the task of balancing a broom upside down on your hand. Suppose you have the end of the handle resting on the palm of your hand and the broom-handle upright with the broomhead in the air (Figure 5.12). When the broom starts to topple in a particular direction you quickly move your hand in that same direction. Try to move far enough and fast enough to arrest the tilt. The broomhandle will start to tilt in a new direction, calling for a new corrective movement of the hand, and so on. Skill is needed, but this comes with practice. Some people are better at it than others. Eventually, you will be able to manage with quite small movements.

When the broom is tilting over, three things are happening: the falling towards the ground, the horizontal movement, and the tilting over. Each of these movements is affected by a different aspect of the support thrust that you are applying with your hand. The falling is produced by the gravitational attraction of the earth, directed along a radius of the planet, a direction that we can call the 'gravitational vertical'. When the thrust line is at an angle to this direction, we can regard the thrust as made up of two components, an upward one directed along the gravitational vertical, and another at right angles to this. The relative magnitudes of these two components depend on the angle between the thrust line and the gravitational vertical. The vertical component of the support thrust to a greater or lesser extent opposes the tendency of the broom to fall under gravity, and the horizontal component of thrust influences the horizontal movement of the broom. The tilting movement depends on the relationship between the thrust line and the centre of gravity of the broom. The movements of your hand alter the force with which you press up on the handle of the

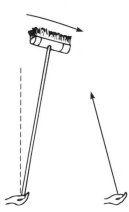

Figure 5.12 Active balancing.

broom. Your strategy for keeping the broom from falling is to keep changing the direction, magnitude, and point of application of the supporting thrust. The vertical and rotational movements occurring in various directions at different times then ·all eventually cancel one another, leaving only such desired horizontal movement as you decide upon.

ACTIVE BALANCING

Ordinary standing and walking about involve precisely similar adjustments of the direction and point of application of the support thrust provided from the ground. Instead of sliding our feet about, in the way we have to move the hand that supports the broom, we just use the two legs in turn, repositioning one leg while the other is supporting the weight. If, for some reason, we have only one leg available, the body has another trick for avoiding falling over. Suppose you are standing on one leg and have lifted the other foot to do something to your shoe. If your raised foot is still trapped when you start to tilt over, you will hop. Your supporting leg suddenly relaxes a little and then straightens strongly. This throws your body up in the air for a moment. The supporting foot is then lifted and moved smartly to a new position, where the leg stiffens again to catch the weight of the body and avoid the imminent fall.

A corresponding sequence of tossings and catchings, but using the two legs in turn, forms the basis of what we are doing when we run, where the extra thrust just before take-off in each stride is sufficient to allow both feet to be off the ground at the same time. The horse, with four legs available, uses his legs in different combinations for the different gaits, but the principle is the same: he applies a sequence of thrusts against the ground in different directions and at different places for each step.

Many of the component actions involved in our maintenance of uprightness and in locomotion appear automatic, or semi-automatic. We are not usually aware of the details of what we are doing during these complex actions. We can usually distinguish 'voluntary' from 'involuntary' actions when we are performing them ourselves, but it is less easy to make a similar distinction for the actions of others. Some of these component actions can be elicited in animals that have been prepared, by preliminary surgery under anaesthetic, in such a way as to preclude any possibility of conscious sensation or of spontaneous movement. We may then refer to the responses of such 'reduced preparations' as 'reflexes'.

REFLEXES AND HABITS

The word 'reflex' is often used rather loosely in common speech to indicate merely a certain promptness in reacting. In the strict neuro-physiological sense, however, a reflex is definable as 'a characterizable pattern of involuntary response that can be elicited with some regularity from an organism on presentation of the appropriate specific stimulus provided that the connections to the central nervous system are intact'. The underlying notion is that, when a stimulus is applied to some peripheral part of the body (as in striking the patellar tendon with a neurologist's hammer) a 'message' of some kind is sent to the central nervous system where it is 'reflected back' to the muscles, or other effectors, to produce the observed response (such as the knee-jerk). The elaborate wording of the definition quoted above is necessary to give the concept practical utility in diagnostic neurology. If a specific reflex can, or cannot, be elicited in a specific patient, conclusions can be drawn about the integrity or otherwise of definite nervous pathways and mechanisms of signal transmission.

At one time it was possible to believe that postural activity and most of locomotor activity consisted of a complexly interacting network of reflexes. Recent work has thrown doubt on this belief. It is not the reality of the reflex mechanisms that is in question. The problems lie in accounting for the central nervous processes involved in achieving the observed coordination of muscular activity. A complicating factor is that there are many apparently automatic actions that must depend, for their initial development, on some process of learning. Such behaviour patterns are to be classed as 'habits' rather than as 'reflexes'. The nature of the responses in the 'true reflexes', on the other hand, appears to depend entirely on the detailed anatomical structure and layout of neural connections within the central nervous system. Similarities between the reflexes found in different animals suggest that much of the relevant neural layout has a genetic basis, and is not dependent on learning.

Reflex responses and habits both depend on the mysterious process of 'recognition' by which conditions that are to generate a specfic response are distinguished from conditions that do not. Even reduced preparations, and indeed individual neurons also, are capable of some forms of recognition. This topic will be dealt with in detail in a later part of this book. Meanwhile we will confine our attention to the observable responses in the various reflexes of standing and of balance without attempting at this stage to account for the neural processing involved.

Staying upright

6

WHICH DIRECTION IS 'UP'?

The word 'vertical', when used in the context of balancing, is usually understood to mean the 'gravitational vertical'. In the neighbourhood of the earth's surface, this can be taken as the direction of a radius of the planet. (We disregard small-scale local variations associated with the proximity of high mountains and with other departures from the geometry of a homogeneous sphere.) It can be shown, however, that it is not the gravitational vertical itself that is relevant in the avoidance of falling.

If a long prism is balanced, on one end, on a small platform supported by strings, as in Figure 6.1, the whole assembly can be swung in a circle. It then becomes clear that the prism remains in place on the platform although tilted over, even so far that a gravitational vertical line through the centre of gravity of the prism does not then pass through the area of support provided by the end face of the prism. What is happening here is that the thrust exerted by the platform against the prism includes a horizontal component, directed towards the centre of curvature of the path, as well as a vertical component to prevent the prism from falling. The prism does not fall so long as the line of action of the resultant upthrust passes through the area of support. The direction of thrust is thus more important for stability than the direction of the gravitational vertical.

In the case of an animal, whose body is in continual motion, the upthrust vector also moves, both passively as a result of changes in the position of the centre of gravity relative to the area of support, and actively as a result of changes in muscular activity initiated by the animal. The animal does not necessarily wish to remain in the same place; he moves about by manipulating the thrusts exerted against the supports. He must, however, at all times have regard to the need to avoid falling over and hitting his head against the ground. This

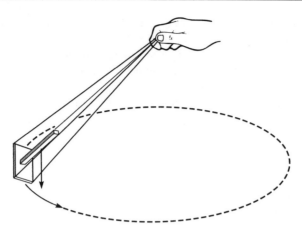

Figure 6.1 A narrow prism, supported on end on a platform swung in a circle, does not overbalance although its centre of gravity is not vertically above its area of support.

requirement involves a decision as to the best direction in which to push against the supports. This direction can be referred to as the 'behavioural vertical'. Uprightness is maintained by reference to the behavioural vertical, rather than to the gravitational vertical. The process of arriving at a decision as to which direction, in relation to the animal's body, is to be taken as the behavioural vertical involves a number of factors, and we need to consider each of these in turn.

WEIGHT-BEARING

The essence of standing in an animal is that the body is **actively** supported in an attitude that differs from that which would be taken up by the body parts in the absence of any of the 'activity' characteristic of the waking animal. Each of the bones of the skeleton is capable of withstanding compressive loading but, because the individual bones are linked together by flexible joints, an animal's skeleton is not able to support the weight of the body without the bracing provided by active tension in the muscles.

The bones and muscles of an animal's body support the weight by forming a triangulated lattice structure which distributes the necessary forces as required by the distribution of the masses of the parts. From one point of view, one might consider such a structure to be built up, triangle by triangle, from the foundations provided by firm contact with the ground. This is the way buildings and other engineering structures are constructed.

An alternative approach is to start from what may be taken to be the overriding objective of the organization of muscular activity in the body, namely the desirability of avoiding impact between the skull and the ground. This standpoint corresponds to the observable development of standing in the newborn. For a prey animal, such as a wildebeest living on the open plains, there is a survival advantage in establishing adequate behaviour patterns for standing and locomotion very early in the infant's life, so that he can run with the herd and escape from predators.

LEARNING TO STAND UP

The first visible action of a newborn infant wildebeest, after only a few panting breaths, is that the animal lifts its head clear of the ground, using its neck muscles. The head then lurches about from side to side and up and down. The momentum developed during these lurches has to be absorbed by intermittent muscular activity. The coordinated timing of this activity in the relevant muscle groups improves rapidly. Trunk muscles and limb muscles are soon brought into play. In place of the initial accidental lurchings of the head, the animal starts to make apparently deliberate lurchings which affect the trunk as well as the head. Lurchings of the trunk affect the legs and then these in turn are brought into coordinated action, until the whole of the forequarters, and eventually the hindquarters also, come clear of the ground. At this stage the infant's feet are widely spread, giving a very large area of support. With further lurchings, confidence improves, and the feet are brought gradually closer together. The infant is standing up within about three minutes from the moment of birth.

It is the lurching movements of the head, passing the momentum to the trunk when each lunge is arrested, that makes it possible for the infant to lift one or other of its feet momentarily and to reposition it. The infant now staggers about, rapidly acquiring increasing skill in controlling both the aiming of the legs and the magnitude of their thrusts. In only about 20 minutes, the infant wildebeest is ready to move off with its mother to join the herd. In other species, where the young are born in the protected environment of a nest or den of some kind, the various stages of development of the techniques of standing and locomotion are very much more spread out in time.

THE 'NORMAL' POSTURE

In general appearance, each of the bony structures of the axial skeleton, including the skull, may be classified as bilaterally symmetrical, though minor departures from precise symmetry can usually be detected by careful measurement. In many animals, other than man, a characteristic 'normal' attitude of the head can be distinguished. In this attitude the plane of symmetry of the skull is held in or near the vertical, with the direction of forward gaze nearly horizontal. It is into this attitude that the infant prey animal first lifts its head. Thereafter the head is supported on the occipital condyles of the skull.

SUPPORTING THE HEAD

The centre of gravity of the skull lies well forward of the condyles, so a considerable torque has to be exerted to shift the line of action of the upthrust available at the condyles forward until it passes through the centre of gravity of the skull. Otherwise the head would topple forward. Some of the initial lurching of the head arises from inaccurate early attempts to control the neck muscles to provide appropriate torque.

The upthrust against the occipital condyles is provided by the spine, or backbone, of the body. This consists of a number of separate bones, the vertebrae, firmly linked together by deformable intervertebral discs to form a column. This structural arrangement combines a very stiff resistance to longitudinal compression with a certain degree of flexibility in other directions.

THE VERTEBRAL COLUMN

In each disc, a tough fibrous ring, the annulus fibrosus, surrounds a deformable soft centre, the nucleus pulposus. The fibres of the annulus link the opposing faces of adjacent vertebral bodies in concentric sheets where the constituent fibres form left-handed and right-handed spirals in alternate sheets, with gradually changing pitch. In the outer layers the fibres run almost parallel to the axis of the disc, while the fibres in the innermost layers are more nearly circumferential. The nucleus pulposus is a watery gel of proteoglycans like that of articular cartilage but without the stiffening meshwork of collagen fibres. It is in contact with the cartilage covering the faces of the vertebral bodies. The swelling pressure of the strongly hydrophilic gel stretches the fibres of the annulus and builds up the considerable hydrostatic pressure with which the disc resists short-term compression. Under sustained compressive loading, water is slowly driven out of the gel, through the cartilage covering the vertebral bodies and into the cancellous spaces within them, and thence into the bloodstream. On release of the stress, water is slowly drawn back to reinflate the disc. It is this mechanism that is responsible for the fact that a man is usually slightly taller in the morning, on rising, than he is at the end of the day.

Relative movement of one vertebra against the next is restrained by paired sets of articular processes. These can make a contribution to load-bearing as a supplement to that provided by the disc in the midline. In principle, a three-point contact should be stable in resistance to compression, provided that the line of thrust passes within the triangular area of support. However, each of the joints between adjacent vertebrae is capable of a certain amount of movement. The articular facets can slide over one another and, although the discs bind adjacent vertebrae together very strongly and can support strong compression, the vertebral bodies are still able to slide, tilt, and rotate against one another to some extent. The amount of relative movement between adjacent vertebrae is severely limited by a complex array of ligaments.

In addition to the annulus fibrosus of the disc, adjacent vertebrae are linked by ligaments associated with the capsules of the articular joints, by the interspinous ligament, and by paired intertransverse ligaments. There are also four strong ligaments that run the full length of the vertebral column with connections, in passing, to each of the individual vertebrae.

Such relative movement between adjacent vertebrae as is allowed by the ligaments is regulated by an elaborate system of muscles, among which we may distinguish those linking each vertebra with a small number of its immediate neighbours and other muscles which span a larger number of intervertebral joints. For each vertebra, the vertebral body and the neural spine are each linked, on each side of the midline, by muscles running obliquely to the transverse processes of the nearest two or three vertebrae, both above and below (Figure 6.2). Similarly, the transverse processes of each vertebra are pulled upon by muscles from the vertebral bodies and neural spines of neighbouring vertebrae, both above and below. Adjacent transverse processes are also linked together by muscles (Figure 6.2). These sets of short-range muscles stiffen the column as well as producing changes in the curvature of its axis. The longer muscles of the backbone rely on the stiffening action of the short-range muscles in order to use the column as a continuous strut in the triangulated lattice that transfers supporting forces from the limbs to the other parts of the body. The balancing of the head on the neck is particularly dependent on long-range muscles. In addition to the short-range muscles linking the occiput to the atlas and axis and neighbouring vertebrae of the neck, longer muscles link the skull to thoracic vertebrae and to the bones of the shoulder girdle.

NECK MUSCLES

The task of balancing the head on the neck is not the same in man in the erect position as it is in the all-fours position of the quadrupeds.

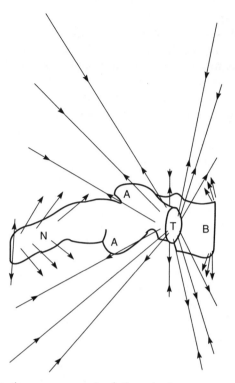

Figure 6.2 Schematic arrangement of the short-range muscles linking the vertebrae in the neck. N = neural spine; A = articular process; T = transverse process; B = vertebral body. In addition, long-range muscles (not shown) link the vertebrae to the skull above and to the thoracic vertebrae and limb girdles below. Of these long-range muscles, some attach to the neural spines, some to the transverse processes, and some to the vertebral bodies.

The available repertoire of axial muscles is, however, more or less identical among all the various mammalian species, with only comparatively minor variations in certain special cases, as called for by particular specializations in life-style. In describing the layout of the musculature, a minor problem of nomenclature arises. The terms 'dorsal' and 'ventral' that are appropriate to quadrupeds are replaced, in human anatomy, by 'posterior' and 'anterior' respectively. In the general treatment that follows it will be convenient, in relation to the backbone, to use 'dorsal' to indicate either 'dorsal' or 'posterior' as the case may be, and 'ventral' to indicate either 'ventral' or 'anterior'.

The loading of the long muscles on the dorsal aspect of the neck is clearly much greater in the quadrupeds, where the centre of gravity of the head is a long way in front of the support available from the forelegs, than it is in the usual upright posture of man. To provide the required upthrust at the skull, the neck vertebrae are each supported by the pull of muscles attached to the neural spines of the vertebrae of the thorax, these spines being especially elongated in the neighbourhood of the forelimb, to provide additional leverage (Figure 6.3).

In the ungulates, with their grazing habit and relatively heavy heads (which contain large masses of ivory in the form of the grinding teeth), the range of supporting tensions required rarely falls to the low value provided by inactive muscle. There is thus an advantage in providing the necessary tension by two mechanisms in parallel: an inert system (tendon), with constant mechanical properties, to provide some of the tension, supplemented by an active system (muscle), whose mechanical properties can be varied by nervous control to supply a variable amount of additional tension. The dorsal neck ligaments of the ungulates function in this fashion and they are correspondingly massive.

It is sometimes supposed, from the massiveness of the ligamentum nuchae in the ungulates, that this structure 'carries the weight of the head'. This cannot be strictly true, for a variety of reasons. The ligament may be functionally divided into two parts (Figure 6.3). The most dorsal part is a strong band running from the nuchal crest of the

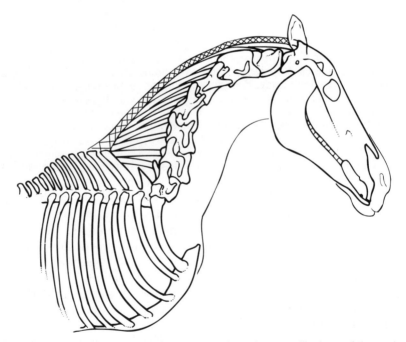

Figure 6.3 Detail of the neck of a horse to show the contributions of the various parts of the nuchal ligament in providing support to the skull. The dorsal band running to the skull is shown hatched. (See also Figure 6.4.)

occipital bone in the skull all the way down the neck to the tops of the long neural spines of the mid-thoracic vertebae. Below this band there are a number of strands which run from the neural spines of each of the neck vertebrae and which are collected together to join the dorsal band at its attachment to the thoracic neural spines. The weight of the head is carried by the occipital condyles bearing against the atlas vertebra, which is supported in turn by the other neck vertebrae. When the head is in the erect posture, the neck vertebrae are held in place by triangles of forces each made up of two struts and a tie. The vertebral column of the neck and the neural spines of the thoracic vertebrae act as struts, and the structures, both muscular and tendinous, connecting the neural spines act together as a tie. If the ligaments alone were to provide sufficient tension to support the neck in the erect position, the animal would have a problem in lowering its head to graze.

So far as concerns the dorsal band of the ligamentum nuchae, i.e. that part that runs directly to the skull, it forms part of a four-bar linkage (Figure 6.4), the other three components being the occipital bone, the vertebral column, and the thoracic neural spines. It is a property of four-bar linkages that they provide no resistance to shear forces. This system thus can play no part in 'carrying the weight of the head'.

A clue to the true function of the nuchal ligament is provided by its

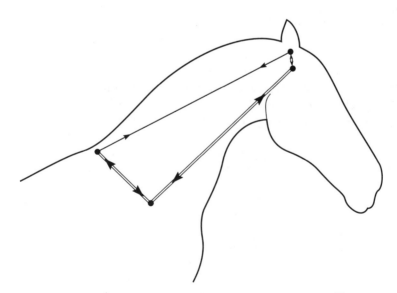

Figure 6.4 Four-bar linkage formed of three struts and a tie. (Compare with Figure 6.3.)

composition. It is made up almost entirely of elastin. This is a very springy material with comparatively little hysteresis in its tension–length relation. During locomotion, the limb thrusts are intermittent and there is, consequently, a tendency for the head to bounce up and down. Such nodding is particularly noticeable at the brisk walk. During this nodding, the momentum of the head changes continually. The kinetic energy acquired during downward movement has to be absorbed at each nod and further energy is then required to initiate the next upward movement. The downward movement of the head stretches the nuchal ligament, converting the kinetic energy of the downward movement into strain energy stored in the ligament. Much of this energy is recovered during the upward movement of the head, with a consequent saving of some of the energy that would otherwise have to be supplied by the muscles.

The contribution of the neck musculature to the support of the head in the quadruped can be considered as provided by three systems: one supporting the neck and the other two controlling the tendency for the skull to topple forward over the occipital condyles. In addition to the short-range muscles which stiffen the vertebral column in the neck, one set of long muscles runs from the transverse processes of the neck vertebrae to the neural spines of the thoracic vertebrae, and also to their transverse processes. This set, which supports the neck, includes a substantial component attached to the transverse processes of the atlas. In quadrupeds, these processes are sufficiently prominent to be called the 'wings of the atlas'. The second set of long muscles in the neck runs from the nuchal crest of the occipital bone of the skull to the transverse processes of the neck vertebrae. The third set runs from the nuchal crest of the skull to the neural spines of the thoracic vertebrae and of the posterior cervical vertebrae. This third set thus acts in parallel with the dorsal band of the nuchal ligament.

The neck muscles are all paired so that lateral bending of the neck can be produced by unequal activity in the muscles of the two sides.

In man the task of supporting the head is less severe since the neck vertebrae are more nearly vertical. The muscles on the posterior aspect of the vertebral column are correspondingly less well developed in man than in the quadrupeds, while those muscles on the anterior aspect are relatively more prominent. Anatomists distinguish some 14 pairs of muscles attached to the skull and contributing to this task. The masses of the paired sterno-cleido-mastoid muscles, lying on each side of the larynx, are a prominent feature of the anterior aspect of the neck. This muscle can be subdivided into parts, each with a different function, according to the locations of their attachments.

In addition to the attachments to the mastoid process, which give the muscle its name, other attachments are distributed over a considerable area of the occipital bone. At the lower end, some fibres run to the sternum and some to the clavicle. The two mastoid processes on the skull lie fairly close to a transverse line through the centre of rotation at the atlanto-occipital joint. The mastoid portions of this muscle can thus make no significant contribution to controlling tipping movements of the skull in the median plane. Their function is to pull the head and neck forwards together without tipping, and to control lateral movements of the head. The occipital fibres of this muscle form a crossed four-bar linkage (Figure 6.5) with the skull, the vertebral column, and the ribcage. The action of this linkage at any one time is very much dependent on what other muscles are doing at that time. If the vertebral column of the neck is stiffened by the short-range muscles, the occipital fibres of the sterno-mastoid will either pull the head and neck forwards without tipping, or will tip the head backwards over the occipital condyles, according to whether or not the neck is permitted, by other muscles, to bend forwards relative to the thorax. Unequal activity of these muscles on the two sides produces a rotation of the skull about the long axis of the neck, as in shaking the head.

Forward, nose-down, tipping of the skull over the occipital condyles is produced by long muscles on the ventral aspect of the neck, running from the base of the skull to the transverse processes of the neck vertebrae. Another two sets of long neck muscles run from the bodies

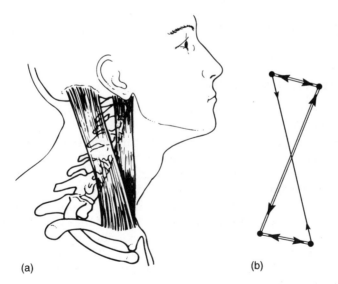

(a)   (b)

Figure 6.5 (a) Layout of the occipital and mastoid portions of the 'sternomastoid' muscle in relation to their contributions to head movement. (b) Crossed four-bar linkage to show the action of the occipital part of the muscle.

of the first few thoracic vertebrae; one set runs to the transverse processes, and the other to the vertebral bodies, of the neck vertebrae. These muscles serve to oppose backward curvature of the neck in the median plane, thus straightening the neck.

Mention should be made in this context of another system of muscles that can, in certain circumstances, influence the attitude of the head. The hyoid bone, lying in the neck just above the larynx, functions primarily as an anchorage for the tongue musculature. It is itself held in place by muscles running to the skull, to the lower jaw, to the sternum, and to the clavicle. The sternum is thus linked to the skull through a chain of muscles, by way of the hyoid and the lower jaw. If the muscles stabilizing the hyoid are made active at the same time as the masticatory muscles that close the jaw, the combined effect can be to tend to tip the head forward.

It may be questioned, however, whether this system acting by way of the hyoid should be taken as having a significant role to play in rotating the skull forward over the occipital condyles in man. The horse has a substantial muscle running directly from the sternum to the angle of the lower jaw, and this can have an effect comparable to that just described for muscles attached to the hyoid. It can thus provide assistance to the action of those deep muscles that run between the base of the skull and the upper neck vertebrae and which are the prime movers in tipping the head forward over the condyles. The presence of this special muscle in the horse reflects the importance of this movement in grazing. After the lips and teeth have taken a grip on a bunch of grass, the head is jerked briskly to pull the mouth towards the forefeet, thus tearing off the portion of grass that is to be eaten.

MOVEMENTS OF THE HEAD

The first two neck vertebrae, the atlas and the axis, differ markedly in shape from the other vertebrae. During embryonic development, part of what might otherwise be expected to turn into the vertebral body of the atlas becomes detached from that vertebra and fuses with the body of the adjacent vertebra. The resulting odontoid process on the axis then forms a synovial joint with the remains of the atlas, working in a socket formed by a strong transverse ligament completing the ring of bone representing the remainder of the body of the atlas. The pin joint between the atlas and the axis makes it possible for the head to rotate about an axis through the upper vertebrae of the neck.

The two articulations of the atlas with the occipital condyles of the skull provide a hinge joint permitting nodding movements of the head in the median plane. The articular surfaces are spherically curved, the occipital condyles on each side nestling within the hollow of the corresponding facet on the atlas. The facets are inclined towards one another so that each forms part of the surface of a single sphere, whose centre lies in the midline, within the cranium, and a little way above the foramen magnum. This geometric arrangement suggests that the atlanto-occipital joint is really a partial ball-and-socket joint with several degrees of freedom, rather than a simple hinge. However, movements of axial rotation and of lateral flexion at this joint are limited by ligaments to a very few degrees, compared with about 15° of possible movement in the median plane when the joint acts as a hinge.

Of the various movements that the head can make, relative to the trunk, axial rotation takes place primarily at the atlanto-axial joint, flexion and extension in the median plane involves the hinge action of the atlanto-occipital joint, combined with curving of the neck produced by small movements at each of the intervertebral joints, while lateral flexion, ear to shoulder, depends almost entirely on lateral curving of the column of neck vertebrae.

It may be seen from this brief summary that the muscular control of the attitude of the head on the neck, involving as it does the coordinated activity of a large number of muscles, calls for a quite complex process of organization.

THE SUPPORTING FRAMEWORK OF THE TRUNK

The pattern of short-range muscles linking each vertebra to its immediate neighbours, together with long-range muscles spanning several intervertebral joints, as described for the neck vertebrae, is continued throughout the length of the vertebral column. The set of individual vertebrae is thus welded together to form a fairly rigid beam from which the soft tissues of the viscera are suspended as it were in a bag, the abdominal cavity, held in place by tension in the muscles of the abdominal wall. A separate compartment is required for the lungs since tension in the curved walls of the abdomen increases the hydrostatic pressure within it, and the operation of the lung calls for a lower pressure in the thoracic cavity than that of the outside air. The reduced pressure needed for ventilation of the lungs is achieved by the reinforcement of the chest walls provided by the stiffness of the ribs, in conjunction with tension in the diaphragm, which forms a dome concave towards the abdomen.

The backbone, as the main weight-bearing structure, is itself supported in turn by the limbs, so long as the feet are on the ground. The weight-bearing action of the hindlimbs is transmitted to the vertebral column through the sacral articulation with the pelvis. The forelimb, in contrast, has no direct bony articulation with the vertebral column.

The bones of the pelvic girdle, together wih the fused vertebrae of the sacrum, form a rigid structure, parts of which act sometimes as struts and sometimes as ties (Figures 6.6 and 6.7) according to the attitude of the hindlegs. This structure receives the thrust of the femur at the hip and provides anchorages for the muscles spanning the hip joint to enable both propping thrust and paddle torque to be transmitted from the hindlimb to the pelvis. Onward transmission of supporting forces to the vertebral column is achieved partly by short intervertebral muscles in the pattern already described for other parts of the column, partly by additional long muscles linking the lumbar vertebrae and the ribs to the ilium of the pelvis, and partly by the muscles of the abdominal wall.

THE ABDOMEN AS A HYDRAULIC STRUT

If any foot is to be raised, the whole weight of the corresponding limb has to be added to the burden carried by the backbone. If both forelegs

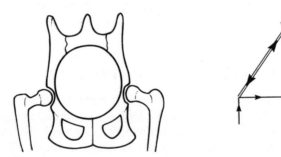

Figure 6.6 Projection, onto the transverse plane, of the pelvic girdle of the cat to show the disposition of struts and ties when the weight is symmetrically supported on the two hindlimbs.

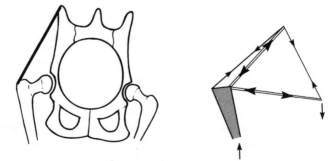

Figure 6.7 As Figure 6.6 but with the weight supported on the left hindleg alone.

are to be lifted at the same time, considerable torque has to be developed between the pelvis and the rest of the trunk, to carry the weight of the forequarters and the head. If this torque were to be developed by the tension of the back muscles in combination only with the compressive stress along the axis of the vertebral column, the tensile force required would be very great, since the offset distance between the forces is comparatively small. The task is made easier by bringing in the action of the abdominal muscles. At first sight, this might look like applying a tension in the wrong direction, since the abdominal muscles tend to pull the ribcage and forequarters downwards. However, activity in abdominal muscles in combination with activity in the diaphragm increases the hydrostatic pressure in the abdomen so that the abdominal contents can be used as a hydraulic strut to take some of the compressive load. This eases the stress on the vertebral column and, at the same time, by increasing the offset between the forces, greatly reduces the tension called for from the back muscles in the development of adequate torque. The hydraulic strut is not suitable for prolonged use because it interferes both with the pumping activity of the heart and with the ventilatory movements of respiration.

In the erect posture of man, the mass of the upper body is usually held more or less vertically over the pelvis so that the torque required for support is fairly small. The situation changes if the shoulders are moved forward of the hips, and especially so if a weight is to be lifted in the hands. Weight-lifters rely heavily on the abdominal hydraulic strut, often reinforcing the action of their abdominal muscles with a tight belt. There is some doubt, however, as to whether the belt actually confers any significant mechanical advantage, and many believe that the beneficial effect is mainly psychological. The belt is said to 'support the back' but, if the lower back is hollowed, as it should be for this type of task, the effect of the compressive stress on the column of vertebrae is likely to tend to move the vertebral bodies forwards rather than backwards. So the pressure of the belt on the small of the back appears to be in the wrong direction for support.

An alternative hypothesis, attempting to account for a possible advantage in the use of a tight belt, depends on the relation between wall tension and the hydrostatic pressure of the contained fluid. The pressure developed by a particular tension is greater for greater curvatures of the tensile fibres. The tight belt may serve to separate the abdominal wall into upper and lower regions, in each of which the curvature of the wall in the longitudinal direction is greater than it would be in the absence of a belt. The effect of the belt would then be to enable more pressure to be exerted for the same muscular effort. The question remains to be resolved by measurement.

It is, of course, very necessary, when lifting anything heavy, to adopt a posture in which the lower back is slightly hollowed. Injuries to the back can occur if the curvature is either too great or too small. If the back is too hollow, the compressive stress on the articular facets is increased at the expense of that on the intervertebral discs. This may lead to fracture of the articular processes, which are less suited to such large stress than the discs.

At the other extreme, if the lower back is too flat, or if it is at all arched, the angulation of the opposing faces of the vertebral bodies tends to squeeze the discs out backwards and the posterior part of the annulus may develop fissures and fail to contain the central gel. The resulting protruding masses then compress the spinal nerves to interfere with their function and produce the 'slipped disc' syndrome. At the same time, the articular facets tend to separate and may even slide over one another and become locked in dislocation.

LIMB DESIGN

The differences in life-style between species lead to greater differences in the structure of their limbs than in that of their vertebral columns. Both the musculature and the skeleton of the limbs and limb girdles show considerable variety, though all are derived from the same basic repertoire. Since the growth of bone, in certain circumstances, accommodates itself to the local intensity of mechanical stress, the variation between species in the forces called for from specific muscle groups results in characteristic differences in the shapes of the bones to which these muscles are attached. It thus comes about that, in the course of the evolution of particular animal groups, some bones are lost altogether along with their associated muscles.

It is characteristic of amphibians and reptiles that between bouts of activity they adopt a posture with the abdomen and thorax resting directly on the ground, with the limbs out to the side. Then, to lift the thorax for locomotion, paddle action has to be exerted with the humerus, to push downwards against the ground. The necessary force is provided by the pectoral muscles acting in conjunction with a bony strut between shoulder and sternum (Figure 6.8(a)). This strut also plays a part in supporting the weight of a forelimb when its foot is to be lifted from the ground (Figure 6.8(b)).

In contrast, many groups of mammals have become specialized for running. The feet are positioned close under the body, not far from the midline plane of symmetry. In this attitude the humerus is more nearly vertical than in the broad-shouldered animals, so that the trunk can be supported by propping, with little need for paddle action in the transverse plane (Figures 6.9 and 6.10). In association with this life-style, the clavicle has become much reduced; indeed in the ungulates it is absent altogether, the upthrust of the forelegs being conveyed from

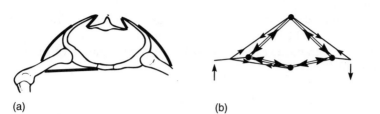

(a)   (b)

Figure 6.8 Projection, onto the transverse plane, of the pectoral girdle of a broad-shouldered animal (frog) to show the disposition of struts and ties when one foreleg is lifted from the ground. When the weight is supported symmetrically on the two forelimbs, the pattern on each side corresponds to that shown here on the left side.

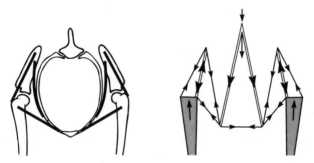

Figure 6.9 Projection, onto the transverse plane, of the pectoral girdle of a narrow-shouldered animal (cat) to show the disposition of struts and ties when the weight is symmetrically supported on the two forelimbs.

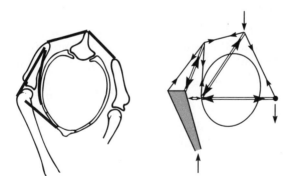

Figure 6.10 As Figure 6.9 but with one foreleg lifted.

the scapula to the ribs through a sling-like fan of muscles. This arrangement allows considerable freedom of movement between the scapula and the ribcage so that the shoulder can participate in the striding action of the forelimb.

The arboreal life-style of the primates calls for a different line of specialization. The clavicle has been retained to provide a stable platform from which the arm can be extended in a wide range of directions to reach out for food.

The limbs themselves consist of several bony segments articulated in zig-zag fashion so that the limb as a whole is not rigid either in compression, to act as a prop, or in resisting bending when the limb acts as a lever, in paddle action. To provide the necessary stiffness, each joint is spanned by sets of muscles which act either to flex or to extend. These muscles can also be distinguished according as they span a single joint or span more than one joint.

MUSCLES SPANNING MORE THAN ONE JOINT

The action of a single-joint muscle has been discussed in an earlier chapter, where it was pointed out that the two-joint muscles are not well placed to resist longitudinal compression of the limb if they are the only muscles acting. The interaction between single-joint muscles and two-joint muscles can be illustrated with a model of the hindleg of a horse (Figure 6.11). In this model the actions of two sets of two-joint muscles are represented by wire links of fixed length, one (representing biceps femoris and semimembranosus) running from ischium to tibia, and one (representing the two heads of gastrocnemius) running from femur to the point of the hock. The attitude of the pelvis is restrained by its attachment to the rest of the body of the model. It is quite clear that this model limb folds readily and is unable to support the rest of the model. However, the addition of just one single-joint wire link, between the greater trochanter of the femur and the iliac crest of the pelvis (to represent the action of the single-joint gluteal muscles), converts the limb into a pillar that resists longitudinal compression and supports the weight of the model.

This model is unrealistic in that a wire link of fixed length is not a fair representation of a muscle. Even tendons and ligaments are extensible, acting like springs, and muscles act like adjustable springs. In each case, the length taken up depends on the tensile load that the structure happens to be carrying and this may vary at different times either passively, as a consequence of what is happening elsewhere in the body, or actively under nervous control. For a limb as a whole to perform its functions as prop and paddle it is necessary to coordinate the activities of all the muscles in the limb with one another and with the activities of those muscles transmitting force to the backbone. A number of automatic and semi-automatic mechanisms contribute to this task of coordination.

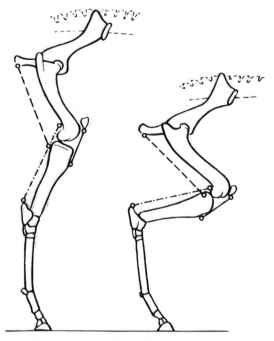

Figure 6.11 Lateral view of the hindleg of a horse to show that the two-joint muscles, biceps femoris O———O and gastrocnemius O—·—·O, undergo little change in length when the trunk is lowered by flexing the knee. They are therefore not well placed to provide the resistance to compression of the limb along its axis that is needed to support the weight of the animal. They do, however, serve to maintain the force preventing the pelvis from tipping forward over the hip in spite of the change in disposition of the limb bones.

'REFLEX' RESPONSES

It is convenient, at this point, to introduce the topic of automatic mechanisms by discussing a well-known example, the knee-jerk re-action. In principle, what happens in this reaction is that, when a person's patella tendon is struck with a physician's tendon hammer, the lower leg jerks forward. It can be shown that the effect is not due to a direct action on the tendon itself because a similar jerk response can be elicited by striking the patella downwards. What is common to these two different stimuli is the sudden stretch of the quadriceps muscle. A similar reaction can be elicited in animals, where it can be established that the response depends on the integrity of the spinal cord, together with the sensory and motor nerves connecting it to the muscle. This leads to the conclusion that a message is sent, from the peripheral site where the stimulus is detected, into the central nervous system where, after suitable processing, another message is formulated and sent out to the muscle to produce the observed response. It is the notion of messages being sent to and being 'reflected back from' the central nervous system that gives rise to the name 'reflex' for this type of behaviour.

Many other 'reflexes' beside the knee-jerk have been described, and several are routinely used in diagnostic neurology to test for defective function in various parts of the nervous system. It turns out that these reflexes are not as simple as might at first appear. For example, in testing for the knee-jerk response, some care has to be taken to see that the subject is in a suitably relaxed posture, with the lower leg hanging free. The tap has to be applied in the right place and with the right kind of force. The response is not elicited by every kind of muscle-stretch. For instance, it does not follow the sudden stretch of the same muscle that inevitably happens when the subject lands on that leg after a running step.

Electrical recording reveals that the blow of the tendon hammer sets up a synchronized volley of impulses in many sensory nerve-fibres. The cell bodies of a group of motoneurons in the spinal cord receive this sudden influx of synchronized excitatory activity and all respond at the same time to generate a volley of outgoing impulses in the motor nerve. This motor volley activates the corresponding muscle cells to produce the synchronized mechanical response that jerks the lower leg.

It was at one time supposed that reflexes depended simply upon the five components of a so-called 'reflex arc', namely a peripheral detector system, a sensory nerve path, a central nervous 'centre', a motor nerve path, and a peripheral effector organ. If any one of these five components is defective in any way, the expected response fails to follow the presentation of the appropriate specific stimulus. This view of the nature of reflex activity is the basis of the use of reflex testing as an aid to diagnostic neurology.

In the case of the jerk reflex, each of the motor units whose activity manifests itself in the observed jerk response either develops, or does not develop, the whole of the activation cycle of which it is capable. Variations in the briskness of repeated taps with the hammer are accounted for in terms of the number of motor units that contribute to the response. For this reason the physician needs to train himself to standardize the intensity of his blow with the tendon hammer. When this is done, it is found that characteristic changes occur in the sizes of the responses when certain parts of the central nervous system have been damaged by injury or disease, even when these parts are not themselves components of the reflex arc. This finding is interpreted to mean that the 'sensitivity' of the neural 'centres' in the reflex arc is affected by influences from other parts of the central nervous system.

Divergencies from expectation in the response to standard taps thus come to have considerable diagnostic significance.

When a muscle is stretched in some way other than by a sudden tap, the impulses generated in the sensory nerve-fibres by the stretch-receptors in the muscle are not synchronized with one another. There is then no synchronized activation of groups of motoneurons, but the general level of activity in the stretched muscle is in many cases increased by the stretch. This type of response has been called a 'stretch reflex'. It is important to realize the significant differences between these responses to sustained stretch and the response to a sudden stretch. The jerk reflexes play no part in the normal behaviour of balance and locomotion, while the true stretch reflexes are all-important, especially in the way the responses are altered by outside influences. Most of the muscle activity involved in converting the loosely jointed assembly of the bones of the skeleton into a springy framework capable of supporting the weight of the body is derived from stretch-reflex mechanisms. Several stages can be distinguished in the overall coordinating mechanism.

MUSCLES AS ADJUSTABLE SPRINGS

It is the stretch reflex that is responsible for the ability of a muscle to act as a spring. We have already seen, in an earlier chapter, that a muscle can, when activated, behave in one or more of three ways: it will shorten if it can; it will develop force against a resistance; and it will show an increased resistance to extension. In the absence of direct activation by an experimenter, the activity of each muscle cell depends on the arrival of an impulse, or of a succession of impulses, in the motor nerve-fibres serving that muscle. When a limb is being used to support the body, the compression stress on the limb tends to flex the various joints, thus stretching the extensor muscles. This stretch pulls upon the stretch-receptors in the muscles and these in turn send neural messages to the central nervous system which set off stretch-reflex activity in the extensor muscles, thus developing tension to resist collapse of the limb.

The force developed by a muscle in the body depends on the inter-action between that muscle and the load on it. This may be illustrated by a diagram such as Figure 6.12. The curve AB represents the way the force exerted by a flexor muscle (e.g. biceps) varies with the angle at the joint (elbow) when the muscle is stretched by an external agency. For simplicity, most of this curve is drawn as a straight line, rather than as a hysteresis loop such as that in Figure 4.18 since, in the neighbourhood of the working point, even a curved relationship can be specified in terms of two parameters, the slope of the tangent and the

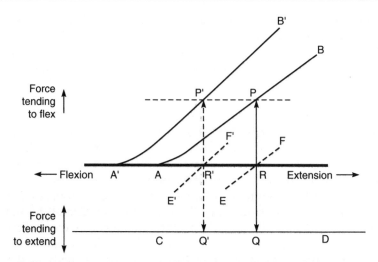

Figure 6.12 Interaction between muscle force and external load, and the way this changes with an increase in stretch-reflex sensitivity.

intercept this makes with one of the axes. The horizontal line CD represents a load which exerts the same extending force at all positions. The muscle will support the load, in equilibrium, at the position R since, if the joint is further extended, the muscle force exceeds the load and produces flexion whereas, if the joint were to flex from the position R, the load would exert more force than the muscle, thus extending the joint. The broken line ERF indicates the stiffness with which changes in the angle at the joint are resisted.

If the sensitivity of the stretch reflex in the muscle we are considering is increased by the influence of activity elsewhere in the nervous system, the relationship between tension and extension for that muscle will be altered. Suppose the new relation to be represented by the curve A'B'. The equilibrium position shifts to R' where the force tending to extend, R'Q', is equal to the muscle force tending to flex, R'P'. The effect of the external influence is to change the angle at the joint even though it has no direct action on the muscles operating at that joint. The stiffness of the resistance to changes in joint angle from the new position is now represented by the broken line E'R'F'. The change in sensitivity produced by external influences can affect either or both of the two parameters expressing the tension–extension relationship at the working point. It is this mechanism that is responsible for most of the postural adjustments involved in balancing activity and in locomotion.

These activities are accomplished by coordinated regulation of many muscles to control the attitude of the limbs and the forces exerted both between the limbs and the supports and between the limbs and the trunk. It is possible to study the overall coordination mechanism in terms of contributory components that can be looked at separately. Some of these components have the status of reflexes, like the stretch reflex just described, insofar as they can be demonstrated in 'reduced preparations', i.e. in animals that have been surgically prepared, under appropriate anaesthetic, in such a way as to eliminate the possibility either of any spontaneous behaviour or of any form of conscious sensation. Reflex behaviour can be regarded as 'automatic'.

The full range of coordinated activity cannot be accounted for in terms of reflexes alone. Some components in the coordinating process call for a degree of detailed 'awareness' of aspects of the conditions in which the animal happens to be placed that cannot reasonably be expected on the basis purely of inherited structure. Component reactions of this type cannot be demonstrated in reduced preparations. They depend on processes of learning that involve conscious sensory experience at some stage even if, once established, the patterns of behaviour are performed without the animal, or the person, being aware of what is going on. This description of apparently 'unconscious' semi-automatic reactions fits the description of the class of actions that are commonly referred to as 'habits'.

As already mentioned, the stretch reflex makes it possible for a muscle to act as a variable spring. The required variations are achieved by altering the sensitivity of the neural 'centres' where the messages from the stretch receptors in specific muscles are converted into the motor commands to those same muscles. The effect is that forced extension of a particular muscle is resisted by the development of more tension. There has to be a limit to such an increase in tension since, if the tension is allowed to become too great, the tissues will be ruptured. This occasionally happens in athletes where a sudden movement may 'pull a muscle'. Excessive stretch is normally avoided by the limited range of movement available at the joint across which the muscle operates.

MODES OF REACTION

Muscles are not called upon to resist extension always in the same way. If someone pushes against us, we may respond in various ways. We may yield, giving way to an imposed movement; or we may resist, standing our ground and refusing to budge. Alternatively, we may actively push back, forcing the other person to yield. Each of these response patterns can be achieved by adjusting the two parameters of slope and intercept characterizing the tension–extension relation of individual muscles. These three modes of motor control are used in combination to produce changes in posture and in the attitudes of the limbs, as well as to oppose external forces.

If a limb is free, it can be moved relative to the trunk. The muscular forces to produce such movement have to take account of changes in the relative positions of the centres of gravity of the limb segments as well as to accelerate the masses at the start of the movement and to bring the masses to rest when the desired new attitude has been arrived at. This means that adjustments have to be made in the activity of the trunk musculature and in that of the muscles linking the limbs to the trunk as well as in the limb muscles themselves. Thus even a small free movement of a finger will involve adjustments in the control of most of the skeletal muscles in the body.

If a limb is restrained, by contact with the environment, or if it encounters resistance to movement, a different pattern of control is required from that which suffices for simply **resetting** the attitude. The limb may be called upon to apply force to an obstruction, overcoming the opposing resistance and **driving** the obstacle to a new position. It may then be called upon to **hold** the new position in spite of external forces tending to dislodge it. Alternatively, it may be called upon to **yield**, absorbing momentum from an external object. These alternatives may be illustrated by an example.

When we extend our hand to another person, this involves **setting** the limb to a new position. If the other person takes the proffered hand and shakes it in greeting, the limb is required to **yield**. However, if the other person offers a cup and we accept it, the attitude of the limb has to be **held** to support the weight of the cup together with that of any fluid poured into it. Alternatively, we may offer a hand to assist another person in moving a load, in which case the change in attitude of our arm has to **drive** against the load. The movements of the limbs in locomotion involve phases in each of the modes of setting, yielding, holding, and driving.

STRETCH REFLEXES IN THE DECEREBRATE PREPARATION

The reflex behaviour of a single muscle can be studied in a reduced preparation. The decerebrated cat is suitable for experiments of this type. The animal is first prepared, under full surgical anaesthesia, by cutting across the brainstem between the colliculi and removing all the brain tissue in front of the plane of section. After the cerebral hemispheres have been removed in this operation, the animal can no longer carry out any of the detailed interpretations of sensory information that are necessary for consciousness, nor can it initiate voluntary movement. Its mental life has been abolished so that, to all intents and purposes, the animal is dead. In spite of this, and provided that suitable precautions have been taken to control haemorrhage, many of the routine functions of the body continue to operate normally: the heart beats and respiratory movements continue; regulation of blood pressure and of ventilation, and the processes of secretion, digestion and excretion all appear to be unaffected. As the reduced preparation is incapable of feeling anything, let alone pain, the anaesthetic can be discontinued after completion of the operation. This leaves the lower parts of the nervous system in a near normal condition with full powers of reflex activity.

INTERACTION BETWEEN STRETCH REFLEXES

The bony anchorage of the muscle to be studied is immobilized by attaching it to a rigid framework and the tendon is dissected free and detached from its insertion. Care is taken during this preliminary work to preserve the innervation and the blood supply of the muscle and to prevent the exposed tissues from drying up. A pulling device can then be connected to the tendon with suitable monitoring of changes in length, tension, or electrical activity. In such a preparation, both jerk reflexes and stretch reflexes can be elicited and studied in detail. When a single tendon is pulled upon, it is only the attached muscle that shows a visible response. However, if the stretch-reflex sensitivity of other muscles is tested at the same time, it can be shown that a stretch applied to one muscle enhances the stretch-sensitivity of synergic muscles. This **load-sharing** effect can be seen not only in other muscles acting at the same joint, but also in muscles that cooperate by acting at adjacent joints. For example, ankle extensors may be affected by stretching knee-joint extensors and *vice versa*.

A related interaction can be shown to operate between flexors and extensors. When an extensor muscle is pulled upon to elicit its stretch reflex, the stretch-reflex sensitivity of the antagonistic flexor muscles is reduced, and if a flexor muscle is reflexly responding to stretch, the stretch-sensitivity of the antagonist extensors is reduced. This phenomenon of **reciprocal inhibition** has an important part to play in voluntary movement since, without it, any attempt to change the angle at a joint would be opposed by the tension reflexly generated in the muscles that are stretched by that movement.

When a limb is called upon to contribute to weight-bearing, a complex set of interactions is involved. Unless it is aimed voluntarily in one direction or another, an unsupported limb will dangle limply. Its joints can be freely manipulated by an experimenter and present no resistance. In Figure 6.13(a), a small dog is supported at head and tail. The limbs all hang limply in moderate extension. The sandbag slung over the dog's back shows that the back muscles are also relaxed.

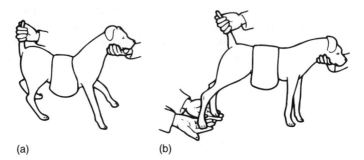

(a)   (b)

Figure 6.13 Effect on muscles of the back of eliciting a supporting reaction in the hindlimbs. The dog is held in the air by its head and tail, with a sandbag laid across its back. (a) Feet hanging free: the back is concave upwards; (b) supporting reaction elicited by pressing on the soles of the hindfeet: the back is straightened and the neck is arched. Because the hindlegs are extended at the hip joint, the forelegs are extended, although still hanging free. (After Rademaker, 1931.)

However, if a supporting surface is brought up against one of the feet, a number of changes occur not only in the muscles of the affected limb but also in the trunk musculature. In Figure 6.13(b) a second experimenter has brought his hands into contact with the dog's hind paws. At once the hindlegs are stiffened and push strongly downwards. The muscles of the back are also tensed so that the back no longer sags under the weight of the sandbag. This **supporting reaction** is initiated by the splaying of the digits that occurs on contact with the potential supporting surface. In the horse, which has only one functional digit in each foot, a comparable effect is initiated by the displacements occurring at the joints between the distal phalanges. If the horse's hoof is held in a fully flexed position, the extensor stiffness of the limb melts away and the foot can readily be lifted in the hand. Similarly, if the dog's paw is curled in flexion by the experimenter's hand, that limb can be folded up without resistance.

If, in addition to bringing his hands into contact with the underside of the dog's paws in the arrangement of Figure 6.13(b), he also gives a brief upward push against the foot, the leg will respond with an extra downward thrust. This **extensor thrust** reaction is produced by the stretch-reflex response to rate-of-change of extension.

The activity of the extensor muscles in the supporting reaction is sufficient to bear the weight of the animal. Indeed it can support considerably more compressive stress than the body weight. This can be demonstrated by putting one hand on the top of the dog's pelvic region while pushing against the foot with the other hand. Considerable resistance will be felt. As the applied force is gradually increased, however, there comes a moment when another reflex mechanism takes over. All resistance suddenly melts away and the limb collapses. The effect is referred to as the **clasp-knife reaction** since the experimenter's sensation resembles that felt when closing the blade of a large pocketknife.

Another reaction that involves all the muscles in a limb is the **withdrawal reflex**. If any part of the skin of a limb suffers a sharp injury, as by pricking or by coming too close to something hot, the whole limb is suddenly and very rapidly folded up to withdraw from the painful contact. The reaction often occurs so quickly that the limb has already moved before any sensation has had time to develop. The withdrawal movement involves strong activation of the flexor muscles together with simultaneous inhibition of the activation of extensors. Thus, although the flexion of the joints of the limb stretches the extensor muscles, no stretch-reflex response is generated to impede the withdrawal. If any activation of extensors is in progress at the time of the painful stimulus, that activation promptly ceases.

A consequence of the abolition of extensor activity during the withdrawal reaction is that the withdrawn limb is, for a time, unavailable to contribute to weight-bearing. In automatic compensation, the extensor activity is increased in the corresponding limb on the opposite side, in the **crossed extensor reflex**. In addition, changes also occur in the other two limbs. Weight-bearing support is enhanced in the other limb of the same side and is diminished in the limb diagonally opposite to the limb being withdrawn. This leaves the main burden of weight-bearing to be carried on a diagonal pair of legs.

WEIGHT-TRANSFER

After the initial sudden reaction, the weight may be redistributed so that all three of the legs unaffected by the painful stimulus contribute to carrying the weight. The redistribution is brought about by altering the aiming of the legs with respect to the trunk. As the feet remain in contact with the ground during this adjustment, the effect is to move the trunk over the ground so that its centre of gravity thereafter falls more securely within the triangle of support.

In the discussion in the previous chapter of the stability of a four-legged table placed on a tilted surface it was explained that, in addition to resisting compressive loading, the legs also need to be able to resist forces tending to alter the angles at which they are attached to the tabletop. Similar considerations apply to the legs of an animal. The angles between the legs and the trunk are stabilized by appropriately sited muscles. It is these muscles that have to be adjusted to achieve the **weight-transfer** referred to above. It should be noted that during weight-transfer the changes in all the limbs that are in contact with the ground have to be accurately coordinated with one another and with changes in the trunk musculature.

When the trunk is moved over the ground by changing the aiming of the legs, the upthrust exerted by each of the legs has to be altered to take account of the shift of the centre of gravity. To preserve equilibrium, and to avoid toppling in one direction or another, the turning moments exerted by the limb thrusts on the two sides of any axis through the centre of gravity have to balance one another. The turning moment of a particular thrust depends on the offset distance from the axis as well as on the magnitude of the thrust. If the vertical line through the centre of gravity moves closer to one of the feet, that leg will have to exert a larger thrust, while a movement of the projection of the centre of gravity away from one of the feet allows the thrust exerted by that leg to be reduced. The coordination of the muscle activity in the limbs and trunk has thus to take care of compressive thrusts as well as of the torques associated with changing the aiming of the legs.

The adjustments in the upthrusts exerted by the legs are achieved by altering the sensitivity of the supporting reactions. The accompanying effects on the trunk musculature are dependent on the orientation of the legs. This influence can be illustrated by the following manoeuvres which, like the demonstration illustrated in Figure 6.13, call for a fairly small dog that is reasonably docile and well used to being handled. Such an animal can, for instance, be supported on the hindlegs alone, with the dog's thighs held in the experimenter's hands as in Figure 6.14, which illustrates the influence on the back musculature of the orientation of the hindlegs. If the experimenter holds the dog's thighs in the attitude shown in Figure 6.14(a), the trunk and neck hang limply downwards. The forelegs are also flaccid in moderate extension. The experimenter now rotates the dog's thighs downwards and forwards round an axis through its hip joints. As the thighs pass through the vertical the back muscles begin to tense, and when the thighs are pointing forwards from the hip the stiffening of the back and neck is sufficient to support the weight of the forequarters and head in an attitude not very different from the 'normal' resting posture (Figure 6.14(b)). The forelegs are fully flexed.

A corresponding influence on the back is exerted by the orientation of the forelegs, as shown in Figure 6.15. The experimenter takes hold of the dog's forepaws and lifts gently. The hindlegs are strongly extended to support the dog's weight, while the forelegs extend passively (Figure 6.15(a)). As the experimenter continues to lift, the proportion of the dog's weight that is carried on the arms gradually increases until the dog's hindfeet come clear of the ground and the whole of the weight is taken on the forelegs (Figure 6.15(b)). The

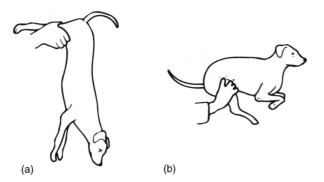

(a)   (b)

Figure 6.14 Effects of changing the angle at the hip joint. The dog is supported entirely by its thighs, held in the experimenter's hands. (a) Hip extended: the body hangs limply downwards, forelegs extended; (b) hip flexed: the back is arched and stiffened, supporting the weight of the forequarters, and the forelegs are flexed. (After Rademaker, 1931.)

stretching of the muscles linking the forelegs with the trunk initiates changes in all the muscles of the limb as though in an attempt to take the weight on the forepaws with the foreleg vertical. The forelegs are strongly flexed at shoulder and elbow, the back is stiffened, the hindlegs are held out horizontally, and the neck is strongly ventriflexed. The changes in the neck, back and hindlegs all contribute to the attempt to bring the projection of the centre of gravity nearer to the support. However, this **hauling up reaction** does not completely succeed without assistance from the hindlegs because of the difficulty in bringing the shoulder forward over the elbow. A further stage in the reaction can be seen if the experimenter grasps the dog by the upper arms to bring the shoulders forward over the elbows (Figure 6.15(c)). The forward extension of the head and neck goes a long way towards the objective of bringing the centre of gravity over the area of support. If the hindfeet are allowed to push against a suitable resistance, as when scrambling over a wall, the full **push up reaction** develops and the objective is achieved.

NECK REFLEXES

It was mentioned earlier that it is possible to recognize a 'normal' attitude of the head which is that commonly taken up when the animal is alert but not doing anything in particular, such as scrutinizing some feature of the environment that is engaging its attention. A consequence of this behaviour is that the relationship between head and neck may vary. For example, in Figures 6.16(a) and 6.16(b) the attitude of the cat's head is the same in relation to the vertical in both cases. In Figure

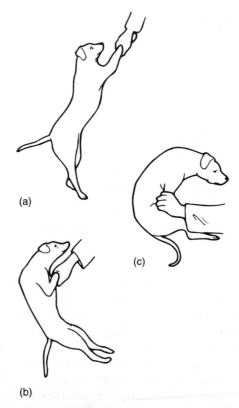

(a)

(b)

(c)

Figure 6.15 Effects of changing the angle at the shoulder joint. (a) The experimenter lifts the dog by the forepaws. Extension at the hip, in conjunction with the supporting reaction in the hindlegs, produces hollowing of the back, flexion of the elbow, and active backward movement of the upper arm on the shoulder to take the weight. (b) When contact at the feet is broken, the back is arched and the pelvis is tucked under. Ventriflexion of the neck is in this case produced by labyrinth reflexes. The forelegs are strongly flexed to haul up the body and the forequarters are hunched forwards. (c) The experimenter's support has been shifted to the lower arms, which are held vertical. The hauling-up seen in (b) is replaced by pushing-up of the hunched forequarters to raise the centre of gravity even further. (After Rademaker, 1931.)

6.16(b), however, the head is ventriflexed on the neck while in Figure 6.16(a) the head is dorsiflexed on the neck. The changes in angle between head and neck produce effects on the limbs in a group of reactions referred to as the **neck reflexes**. Dorsiflexion of the neck produces forelimb extension and hindlimb flexion (Figure 6.16(a)), while ventriflexion of the neck produces forelimb flexion and hindlimb extension. These effects are not dependent on the supporting contact at the feet, as may be seen from Figure 6.17 which shows side views of

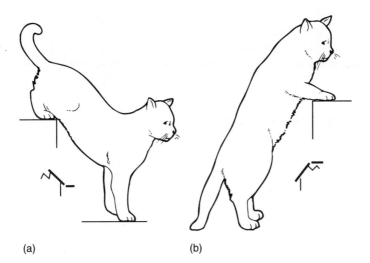

(a)   (b)

Figure 6.16 Lateral views of a cat to show the effects of the neck reflexes on the limbs. The head is in the normal position in each case. (a) Dorsiflexion of the neck produces forelimb extension and hindlimb flexion; (b) ventriflexion of the neck produces forelimb flexion and hindlimb extension.

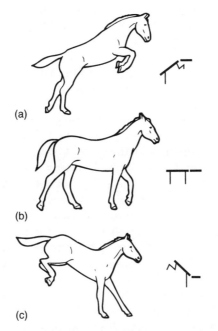

(a)

(b)

(c)

Figure 6.17 Poses to illustrate the neck reflexes acting alone in the horse. The head is in approximately the same position throughout. (a) Neck ventriflexed, the horse is taking off for a jump; (b) normal, during quiet walking; (c) neck dorsiflexed, the horse is landing after a jump.

a horse at a jump. Figure 6.17(b) shows the normal attitude during quiet walking. In Figure 6.17(a) the horse is taking off for a jump, while Figure 6.17(c) shows a stage in the landing after a jump. The attitude of the head is the same in each case. The neck·reflex effects on the limbs are the same as in Figure 6.16, as illustrated by the stick figures.

STABILIZING REFLEXES FROM THE LABYRINTH

The 'normal' attitude of the head results from a set of **stabilizing reflexes** initiated from the balancing organ in the inner ear. This organ is often referred to as the 'labyrinth' on account of its complex shape. The anatomy and physiology of the balancing organ will be discussed in detail in a later chapter where we examine the mechanics of the various transducers involved and the sorts of signals that are generated. For our present purposes, however, we will confine ourselves to the effects observed, while noting that the relevant receptors are located within the skull. If the skull is tilted in any direction out of its 'normal' attitude, effects can be observed both in the muscles linking the skull to the neck and in the way the limbs are deployed in stabilizing the trunk. The effects on the limbs can be revealed by tilting the head without altering the relationship between the skull and the neck. Figure 6.18 shows side views of a dog in three positions where the relation between the skull and the neck is the same in each case. In Figure 6.18(b) the head is in the 'normal' position and the weight is distributed evenly between forelegs and hindlegs. In the accompanying stick figure, the neck is shown as straight, with the head component horizontal to represent the 'normal' posture. Figure 6.18(a) shows the head tilted towards nose-up, with the neck straight. The hindlegs are extended while the forelegs are flexed. In Figure 6.18(c) the head is tilted towards nose-down and the neck is straight. This time it is the forelegs that are extended while the hindlegs flex.

It is instructive to compare the **labyrinth reflex** effects on the limbs shown in Figure 6.18 with the limb responses in the neck reflexes, with the head in the normal position in each case, as shown in Figure 6.17. It will be noticed that a comparable effect on the limbs can be produced either by bending the neck forward with the head in the normal position (Figure 6.17(a)) or by tilting the head back with the neck straight (Figure 6.18(a)). Similarly, foreleg extension with hindleg flexion can be produced either by bending the neck back (Figure 6.17(c)) with the head in the normal position, or by tilting the head forward with the neck straight (Figure 6.18(c)). Another way of looking at the comparison is illustrated by Figure 6.19. Figure 6.19(a) shows a dog with neck 'straight' and head in the 'normal' position. Figure 6.19(b) shows the head tilted back with the neck straight: foreleg flexion and hindleg

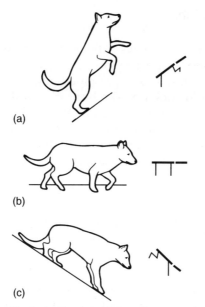

Figure 6.18 Poses to illustrate the labyrinth reflexes acting alone in the dog. The neck is in the same attitude ('straight') in each case. (a) Head up, the dog is about to take off from a ramp to jump up onto a raised platform; (b) normal, during a straight walk; (c) head down, the dog is stationary on an inclined platform.

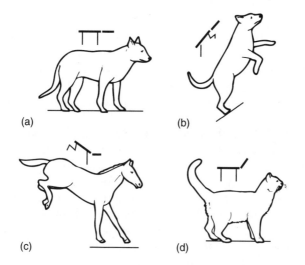

Figure 6.19 Characteristic poses, to illustrate the relationship between neck reflexes and labyrinth reflexes. (a) Head normal, neck straight, weight evenly distributed; (b) head tilted back, neck straight, hindlimbs extended, forelimbs flexed ('prepare to jump'); (c) head normal, neck bent back, hindlimbs flexed, forelimbs extended ('prepare to land after jumping'); (d) head tilted back, neck bent back, weight evenly distributed.

extension. Figure 6.19(c) shows a horse with its head in the normal position and the neck bent back: foreleg extension and hindleg flexion. The two different stimuli are presented together in Figure 6.19(d) which shows a cat looking up. The head is tilted back and the neck is also bent back. The tilt of the head should produce hindleg extension and foreleg flexion (Figure 6.19(b)) while the bending of the neck should produce the opposite effect, namely hindleg flexion with foreleg extension (Figure 6.19(a)). The legs cannot be both extended and flexed at the same time. What happens is that the conflict is resolved centrally so that the animal can move its head freely in any direction without altering the disposition of the limbs.

In addition to providing the animal with freedom to move its head, the combination between the neck reflex effects and the effects from the labyrinth on tilting the head serves to keep the trunk upright when the supporting surface is tilted. Suppose that the support is tilted down at the head end. If the neck were to remain straight, a downward tilt of the head would produce forelimb extension and hindleg flexion, which is just what is required to keep the body upright. If, on the other hand, the head were held in the normal position, a similar uncomplicated forward tilt of the support would involve bending the neck back, thus generating foreleg extension and hindleg flexion as before. The combination thus serves to stabilize the trunk, although the detectors used in assessing the orientation relative to the behavioural vertical lie in the skull, not in the trunk.

The nature of the responses in the neck reflexes can be summarized in the rule that the changes in the limbs are such as would tend to move the trunk to straighten the neck. The corresponding rule for the reflex effects in the positional reflexes from the labyrinth upon the legs is 'downhill limbs extend', with the implication that the uphill limbs flex.

The effects of tilts in the median plane are summarized in Figure 6.20 which shows, in a set of nine stick figures, three positions for the neck – dorsiflexed, normal, and ventriflexed – and three positions for the head – tilted back, normal, and tilted forward. Neck reflex effects alone, with the head in the normal position, are shown in the middle column, while labyrinth reflex effects alone, with the neck straight, are shown in the middle row. Neck reflexes and labyrinth reflexes act in opposite senses in (a) and (i), leaving the leg lengths unaffected, while in (c) and (g) the two reflexes reinforce one another. Such reinforcement is illustrated in Figure 6.21. Figure 6.21(b) shows a dog landing after a drop, with the head tilted down, in contrast with the horse in Figure 6.17(c) where the horse is looking straight ahead. There is a similar contrast between the dog taking off for a jump (Figure 6.18(a)), leading with its head, and the horse in Figure 6.17(a) where

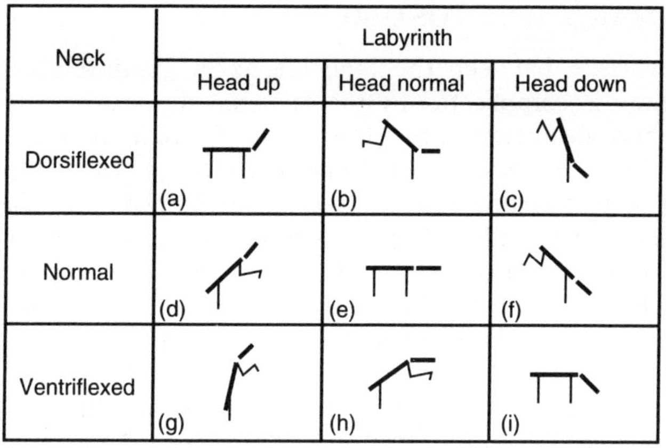

Neck	Labyrinth		
	Head up	Head normal	Head down
Dorsiflexed	(a)	(b)	(c)
Normal	(d)	(e)	(f)
Ventriflexed	(g)	(h)	(i)

Figure 6.20 Scheme of stick figures to illustrate the interaction between positional reflexes from the neck and from the labyrinth (right lateral views).

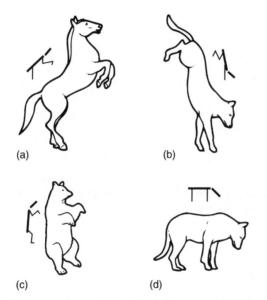

(a)   (b)

(c)   (d)

Figure 6.21 Further examples of characteristic poses. (a) Horse rearing; (b) dog about to land after jumping down from a high platform; (c) bear sitting up; (d) dog looking down.

the head is in the normal position, looking straight ahead. The head-back, neck-straight, attitude occurs in the horse when rearing (Figure 6.21(a)). The pose with head back and neck ventriflexed (Figure 6.20(g)) is characteristic of bears in zoos (Figure 6.21(c)).

THE HUMAN ERECT POSTURE

The comparison between the limb effects in quadrupeds and those seen in man is complicated by the fact that the shape of the human skull has become altered during the course of evolution to accommodate the great enlargement of the cerebral hemispheres. The anterior part of the skull, including the face, is bent forward relative to the occipital part, which remains aligned with the long axis of the vertebral column. Thus, in the erect position (Figure 6.22(a)) the posterior part of the skull is tilted back, with the neck straight, corresponding to Figure 6.20(g). All the weight is taken on the hindlegs, as in the kangaroo (Figure 6.22(b)). To achieve the 'neck straight, head normal' position in man it is necessary to tip the head forward. This produces the all-fours pattern characteristic of the human infant (Figure 6.22(c)). Figure 6.23 shows the array of stick figures from Figure 6.20 completed with the corresponding animal profiles.

LATERAL TILTS

The rules given earlier for predicting the limb effects of neck and labyrinth reflexes in the median plane also apply to lateral tilts of the skull and to axial twistings of the neck. The front views of Figure 6.24 are traced from photographs of an experiment with a decerebrated cat. The head and trunk of the cat are supported separately with the limbs hanging free. The atlanto-occipital and atlanto-axial joints are denervated by cutting the first two cervical nerves on each side, and the axis vertebra is fastened to a third support. With this arrangement, it is possible to produce lateral rotations about suitable axes either of the skull alone or of the axis vertebra, while keeping the trunk stationary. Because the first two intervertebral joints have been denervated, a movement of the skull with the axis vertebra held sta-

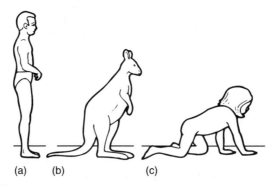

(a) (b)   (c)

Figure 6.22 Effects on posture of the shape of the human skull.

Neck	Labyrinth		
	Head up	Head normal	Head down
Neck dorsiflexed			
Neck normal			
Neck ventriflexed			

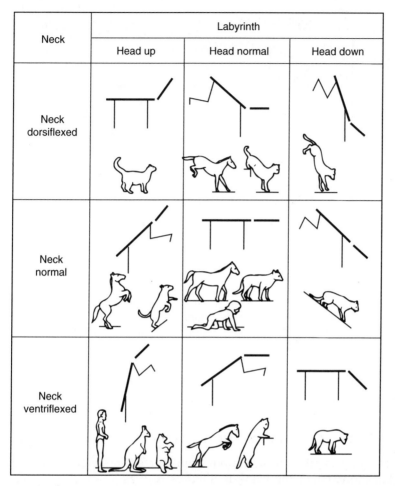

Figure 6.23 Summary diagram of the interactions between neck reflexes and labyrinth reflexes.

tionary produces uncomplicated labyrinth effects, as shown in the upper pair of drawings. Side down tilting of the head alone to either side produces foreleg extension on the 'downhill' side, together with foreleg flexion on the opposite side. In contrast, when the clamp supporting the axis vertebra is rotated, with the skull stationary, the forelimb attitudes alter in the opposite sense. Side down tilting of the axis vertebra produces forelimb flexion on the 'downhill' side with forelimb extension on the opposite side. The cutting of the first two cervical nerves on each side inevitably reduces the intensity of the neck reflexes but there remains no doubt about the direction of the effect. If the trunk were free to move, the nature of the changes in the limbs

Right side down		Left side down
	Head alone	
	Neck alone	

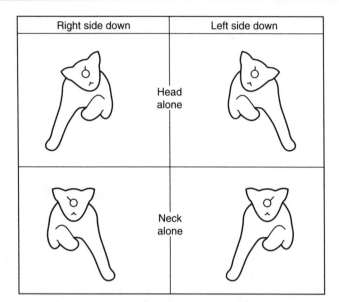

Figure 6.24 Front views of the effects on the forelimbs of separate lateral tilting of the skull (above) and of the axis vertebra (below) in a decerebrate cat in which the joints between the axis vertebra and the skull had been denervated.

during the neck reflex responses to lateral twisting is such as to tend to push the trunk round to straighten the neck.

A MODEL TO CLARIFY THE EFFECTS OF INTERACTIONS

Figure 6.25 is taken from a model constructed to illustrate the various interactions when the trunk is tilted as well as the head or when the supporting surface is tilted. In the model, a common axis supports parts representing the head and the trunk, together with a pointer indicating the direction of the behavioural vertical and a carrier to which the limbs are pivoted. Two sets of mechanical linkages tilt the limb-carrier in opposite directions:

1. by the angle between the skull and the trunk;
2. by the angle between the skull and the behavioural vertical.

Markers on the edges of the moving parts help to draw attention to their relative movements.

Tilting the trunk segment towards right side down while the head remains aligned with the behavioural vertical (Figure 6.25(a)) simulates the neck reflex response: the right leg extends and the left leg shortens. Tilting the head segment also towards right side down, through the

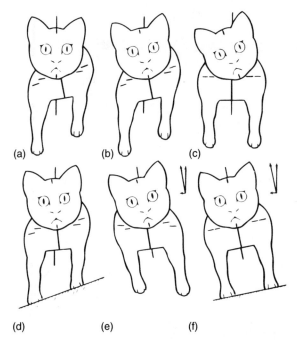

Figure 6.25 Front views of a model constructed to show the effect on the limbs of the interaction between neck reflexes and labyrinth reflexes in relation to the direction of the behavioural vertical and to the inclination of the supporting surface.

same angle as the tilt of the trunk (Figure 6.25(b)), simulates the labyrinth reflex responses with the neck straight: the right leg extends while the left leg shortens. Tilting the head segment alone (Figure 6.25(c)) simulates the normal behaviour of the animal, which can move its head freely without necessarily changing the posture of the limbs. By manipulating the model one can quickly develop a feel for the outcome of the interaction of these two sets of reflexes in a variety of conditions. In the absence of such a model, the reader may find the following argument helpful.

We may refer to the positions of the various parts of the model, according to the scheme of Figure 6.26, in terms of the angles of roll with respect to some arbitrary reference such as the gravitational vertical, these angles being measured as positive in the direction of right side down. As explained earlier, the behavioural vertical does not necessarily correspond with the gravitational vertical. In steady-state conditions, the direction selected by the animal as the behavioural vertical corresponds with the direction of the vector representing the supporting thrust. We call the inclination of this vector V. Similarly,

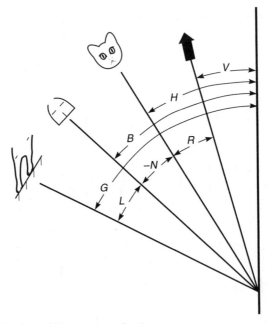

Figure 6.26 Naming of the angles of roll.

the inclinations of the head and body may be called respectively
H and B.

The stimulus for the positional reflexes from the labyrinth is $(H - V)$,
which we may call R (for roll). The responses take the form of asymmetrical changes in the limbs. The degree of asymmetry is represented
in the model by the inclination of that part of the model to which the
legs are fastened by pin-joints. If the feet were on the ground, the tilt
of this leg-carrier would be the same as that of the supporting surface,
which we indicate as G (for ground). The nature of the response is then
given by $(G - B)$, which we may call L.

The stimulus to the neck reflexes is $(H - B)$, which we call N. The
response is an asymmetry which tends to straighten the neck (Figure
6.25(a)). For simplicity, let us represent this response as

$$L_1 = -k_1 N$$

bearing in mind that a tilt of the body towards right side down with
the head stationary has the same effect on the neck as a tilt of the head
towards left side down with the body stationary. In the positional
reflex from the labyrinth it is the downhill limbs that extend. We
represent this response as

$$L_2 = k_2R$$

The combined effect of the two sets of reflexes acting together is given by

$$L = L_1 + L_2 = k_2R - k_1N$$

We are now ready to consider various sets of conditions.

Case A: neck reflex alone.

$$V = 0, H = 0, B = b$$
$$R = 0, N = -b$$
$$L = k_2R - k_1N = k_1b$$

The limbs of the right side extend (Figure 6.25(a)).

Case B: labyrinth reflex alone.

$$V = 0, H = a, B = a$$
$$R = a, N = 0$$
$$L = k_2R - k_1N = k_2a$$

The limbs of the right side extend (Figure 6.25(b)).

Case C: head tilt alone, i.e. head tilted, body upright.

$$V = 0, H = a, B = 0$$
$$R = a, N = a$$
$$L = k_2R - k_1N = (k_2 - k_1)a$$

This means that, if no change occurs in the limbs, as is usually the case (Figure 6.25(c)), k_1 must be equal to k_2. The mechanical linkages in the model have been so designed as to produce this equality, and the head segment may be freely tilted without affecting the legs.

Case D: uneven ground.

$$G = c, V = 0, H = a, B = b$$
$$R = a, N = a - b$$
$$L = k_2R - k_1N = k_2a - k_1(a - b) = kb$$

if

$$k_1 = k_2 = k$$

and

$$G = c = L + B = b(1 + k)$$

or

$$b = c/(1 + k)$$

so that

$$L = kc/(1 + k)$$

which is independent of a, and the head may take up any position free from reflex restraint, while the body is tilted less than the ground. The combination of reflex effects thus serves to stabilize the trunk (Figure 6.25(d)).

Case E: lateral acceleration constant.

$$V = v, H = a, B = b$$
$$R = a - v, N = a - b$$
$$L = k_2R - k_1N = k(a - v) - k(a - b) = k(b - v)$$

Since this is independent of a, the head may take up any position. In Figure 6.25(e), the tilt of the body is shown as less than that of the support vector, while the head is tilted further towards right side down. Here the stimulus to the neck reflexes is greater than that to the labyrinth reflexes, whose effect, if acting alone, would be to extend the legs of the right side, this being the 'downhill' side with respect to the support vector. The greater effect of the neck reflexes results in extension on the left side, that is to say, the legs are adjusted in such a direction as to tend to push the body round to line it up with the support vector.

The legs will be symmetrical if $b = v$, that is if the inclination of the body is the same as that of the support vector. Now

$$G = L + B$$

so that, if the surface supporting the feet is at right angles to the vector representing the direction of the supporting thrust, the legs will be symmetrical (Figure 6.25(f)); the head is still free to move. This situation corresponds to that of the narrow prism balanced on a platform that is swung in a circle, as in Figure 6.1.

The behaviour observed in intact animals corresponds closely with that predicted by the model for the interactions between reflexes of fixed gain. It follows that, although animals move their heads freely, this does not imply that the signals from their labyrinths are disregarded. On the contrary, neck reflexes and labyrinth reflexes complement one another. If one reflex calls for more extension in a particular limb, the other reflex calls for less, and *vice versa*. The combination of reflexes has the effect of transferring the influence of the directional sensor from the skull to the trunk. The limb adjustments are carried out in such a way as to reduce deviations of the orientation of the trunk from its 'normal' position relative to the vertical, even though the relevant sensor, the otolith apparatus, is contained in the skull and not in the trunk. The interaction is effective for tilts in any direction, lateral or fore-and-aft.

In addition to adjustments in the lengths of the legs there are adjustments in the angles at the proximal joints. The limbs are maintained in attitudes approximately lined up with the direction of the support force, even though the trunk may be tilted by different amounts at different times according as the tilt of the supporting surface is varied. This orientation of the limbs is the result of **sway reactions** initiated by the torques developed at the proximal joints.

SWAY REACTIONS

The supporting reaction in a leg is appropriate to the situation in which the resultant force transmitted by the leg to the trunk lies in a line running through both the proximal joint (hip or shoulder) and the foot. The supporting surface in contact with the sole of the foot need not be uniform, or even smooth, so long as there are no sharp places. A dog can stand as well on gravel as on a polished floor, but it will withdraw its foot promptly from a sharp-edged stone. Here the localized cutaneous stimulation initiates a withdrawal reflex with consequent far-reaching adjustments in many parts of the body.

It is not really very precise to speak of a limb which is exhibiting the supporting reaction as being converted into a 'rigid pillar'. The nature of the limb, composed as it is of loosely articulated bones pulled upon by muscles, implies a certain compliance even to longitudinal stresses. Because of the way the stretch reflexes behave, the limbs are much less compliant in compression than they are on release. Each of the legs of a dog is capable independently of supporting about one-and-a-half times the animal's body weight before giving way. When overloaded, the leg collapses suddenly, showing the clasp-knife reaction. If a moderate extra load is added suddenly, the leg at first gives a little, as would be expected for any elastic structure, but then usually extends again, often to carry the load at a slightly greater length than it had before the extra load was applied. If the supporting surface under one foot is gradually lowered, that limb extends with, at first, little reduction in the force. Thus the limb provides the support called for, within limits, in a highly efficient and flexible manner. It is because the legs do not bend progressively under increasing loads that they give the appearance of rigidity.

The amount of load which a particular leg will carry depends on the load which the other legs are carrying at the same time. If one of the hindlegs of a dog is in contact with a support while the opposite leg is hanging free, then the application of a load to the standing leg will impose pressure on the sole of that foot and will elicit the positive supporting reaction in that leg. At the same time the opposite, hanging, leg will be actively flexed. If, now, the sole of the foot of the free leg is pressed upon, to provide that foot in turn with a potential support, the active flexion in that leg gives way to active extension. This leg then develops a supporting reaction of its own and takes some of the load off the other leg. If the positions of the supports are now suitably adjusted, the whole of the load may be transferred to what was previously the free leg. When this happens and the load is taken completely off one of the legs, the supporting reaction in that leg melts away and the leg is lifted up in active flexion. A similar effect can be seen if the hindquarters of a standing dog are gradually but firmly pushed first to one side and then to the other. The weight is transferred to the leg towards which the body is being pushed, and the other leg is lifted in flexion. When the direction of pushing is reversed, the roles of the legs are interchanged. This behaviour is referred to as the **lateral sway reaction**.

The interaction between the legs of the two sides of the body in the sway reaction is reminiscent of the 'crossed extensor' reflex, in which flexion in one limb in response to noxious cutaneous stimulation (withdawal reflex) is accompanied by extension in the contralateral limb. In the sway reaction, we have flexion in the contralateral limb accompanying reflex extension in the limb that is showing the positive supporting reaction. Both in the withdrawal reflex and in the active flexion of the free leg in the sway reaction, the activation of the flexor muscles is accompanied by inhibition of the extensors. We see then that reflex activation of extensor muscles in one leg can lead to inhibition of the extensors in the contralateral leg, in crossed flexion. At least some of the effects appear to be mediated by the cerebellum, but all the pathways involved are not yet precisely known.

BUTTRESSING, STEPPING AND HOPPING

When the supporting surface is tilted, two effects would be produced if the body were an inert system, like the table in Figure 5.7:

1. the vertical projection of the centre of gravity would move relative to the feet, so that the legs carry different proportions of the body weight;
2. the legs would tilt over so that torques would be developed at the

fastenings to the body, thus providing paddle action to prevent collapse.

Accordingly, when the sway reaction is initiated in an animal by a tilt of the supporting surface, this affects the muscles controlling paddle action as well as those for pure propping. These two control systems interact in ways that can be illustrated by the behaviour of a dog when the sideways push to elicit the sway reaction in the hindlegs is continued beyond the point where the nearside leg is lifted from the ground. The dog executes a series of rapid movements to preserve its equilibrium. The free nearside leg is quickly set down just beside the standing leg, the weight is changed over from one leg to the other, the offside foot is lifted, its leg is abducted, and the foot is set down again a little to the side. The supporting reaction then redevelops in the offside leg. Further gradual pushing will now elicit another sway reaction and then another lateral step.

If the free leg is trapped by the experimenter's hand and prevented from taking the weight, no normal stepping sequence is possible. Nevertheless, the lateral movement of the offside leg is still carried out, this time being preceded by a sudden increase in extensor thrust which throws the body upwards momentarily in preparation for a sideways hop. If the lateral push to the body is started from a rest position in which the feet are fairly close together, an outward hop of the offside leg will be executed without the nearside leg being lifted. With the feet now further apart than normal the abducted limb is well placed to act as a buttress to resist lateral forces.

The reactions of **hopping** and **buttressing** are very important for the maintenance of the equilibrium of the body when the centre of gravity is above the feet. They also provide two examples of ways in which the supporting reaction is modified by alterations in the magnitude and direction of the force acting between the limbs and the trunk. As has already been mentioned, the supporting reaction is appropriate to the conditions in which the line of action of the resultant force between the limb and the trunk passes both through the proximal joint (hip or shoulder) and through the area of contact between the foot and the ground (Figure 6.27). In these conditions there is no resultant couple acting between the limb and the trunk, that is to say, any couple arising from vertical forces when the foot is not vertically below the proximal joint is offset by an opposing couple arising from horizontal forces on the trunk together with friction between the foot and the ground. An increased compressive load on the limb in these conditions is strongly resisted by stretch reflexes, sometimes with readjustment of the attitude of the bones of the limb in order to improve the mechanical advantage at which some of the muscles are acting.

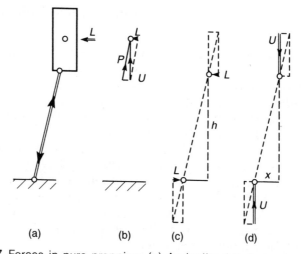

Figure 6.27 Forces in pure propping. (a) An inclined limb exerts a horizontal force against the ground equal to the horizontal force applied to the trunk by some other support. (b) Effects at the centre of gravity. The resultant of the compression force P in the limb with the externally applied lateral force L gives an upthrust U to oppose the pull of gravity. (c) The horizontal forces on the limb are offset by a distance h, producing a couple Lh tending to rotate the limb anticlockwise. (d) Vertical forces on the limb: the upthrust U from the ground together with the downward force exerted by the trunk produce a couple Ux tending to rotate the limb clockwise, where x is the horizontal projection of the limb. From inspection of the figure it may be seen that $L/U = x/h$, or $Ux = Lh$, so that the two couples balance out.

If the relative positions of the ends of the limb are altered, either by shifting the support or by forcibly moving the body, the animal may respond by paddle action of the limbs. Where a limb is used thus in a combination of prop and paddle actions it may be preferable to use the term 'buttressing', reserving the term 'propping' for conditions in which the limb is acting purely in compression.

The choice between buttressing and stepping appears to depend on signals from receptors in the joints. For a particular limb in a given set of conditions there will be a certain inclination of the limb in which equilibrium is achieved by propping action alone even though the limb may be either shortening or lengthening. If the position of the limb deviates from this inclination, some paddle action will be called for. If the leg length is increasing and at the same time this deviation is also increasing, the supporting reaction will melt away and the limb will execute a **reflex step**, bringing the limb nearer to the position for pure propping. Other combinations of changes in leg length and in limb angle result in buttressing (Table 6.1 and Figure 6.28).

The conditions for stepping may be illustrated with a dog standing

Table 6.1 Responses to changes in length and orientation of a leg

Leg length	Deviation of limb position from the inclination appropriate to pure propping		
	Increasing	Steady	Decreasing
Increasing	Step	Prop	Buttress
Steady	Step	Prop	Buttress
Decreasing	Buttress	Prop	Buttress

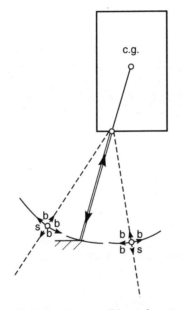

Figure 6.28 Scheme to illustrate the conditions for stepping as opposed to buttressing. The limb is represented as a strut at the inclination appropriate for pure propping. Two other positions of the foot relative to the trunk are shown, together with the possible ways these positions might alter (Table 6.1). Relative movement of the foot into a quadrant marked '*b*' will elicit buttressing. Relative movement into a quadrant marked '*s*' results in reflex stepping, provided another support is available, otherwise a hop will be executed.

on a smooth table. A large card is placed under one of the dog's feet, say a hindfoot. The experimenter slides the card about to alter the angle at the hip while the dog continues to carry its weight more or less evenly distributed between all four legs. In spite of the changes in the angle at the hip most of the movements of the relative position of the foot do not interrupt the propping action of that leg, with one exception. When the experimenter moves the card to carry the foot backwards away from the hip, there comes a point at which the dog lifts that foot and performs a forward step, the foot landing ahead of the normal rest position. Further movement of the card in the same backward direction eventually elicits another step. Using a set of over-lapping cards the experimenter can elicit a series of forward steps by a single leg, the other legs of the dog meanwhile retaining their stationary posture.

If the card is moved forwards, a corresponding set of backward steps will be performed. Similar stepping of a single leg can also be elicited in the forelegs, and also in the sideways direction, though this is less easy to demonstrate.

At the moment of take-off for the step, the supporting reactions in all four legs are adjusted. The trunk first sways a little away from the leg that is to be lifted; the other three legs increase their thrust, to take over the supporting function of the leg that is to be lifted; the activity of the extensor muscles in the stepping leg is switched off to permit that leg to be folded up and swung into a new position; with the new aiming, the leg extends again to resume contact with the support. When contact has been re-established, the supporting reaction develops again in the stepping leg to resume a contribution to weight-bearing; and the trunk sways back to its original position with its centre of gravity roughly over the centre of the area of four-point support.

If no other leg is available to support the weight during the per-formance of a reflex step, the upthrust exerted by the leg that is to be lifted is suddenly increased to throw the weight upwards momentarily, to allow time for the step to be executed during the ensuing period of free fall. This combination of responses constitutes a **reflex hop**. The choice between stepping and hopping depends on the availability of alternative supports for the weight of the body.

Forced hopping on a single leg may be demonstrated in the dog. The experimenter takes the dog in his arms, trapping three of the paws in his hands and leaving one foreleg hanging free. The experimenter now lowers the dog down towards a table. As soon as the dog's paw touches the tabletop the free leg develops a supporting reaction, the force exerted being dependent on how high the dog's body is held up by the experimenter. The dog can take most of its weight on the one leg. Indeed, the leg is actually capable of supporting a load greater than the dog's full body weight, but in this situation some of its weight is necessarily being taken on the experimenter's hands. The experimenter now moves the body of the dog horizontally so that the supporting leg is tilted over. For small tilts, the leg continues to develop the supporting reaction. Larger horizontal movements, to increase the tilt further, lead to hopping. Hops may be induced by sufficiently large movements of the body in any direction.

The sway reaction and the reactions of buttressing, hopping and stepping can all be seen in the responses of the forelegs as well as hindlegs and to applied forces in any direction, forwards, backwards or sideways. Figure 6.29 illustrates the sway reaction in the forelegs. The dog's right foreleg rests on the experimenter's hand with most of the weight of its forequarters taken on its left foreleg. When the experimenter moves the right forefoot towards the left, this displaces the dog's body to the left, and during this displacement the dog's right foreleg flexes and presents no resistance to the experimenter's hand. When the body is similarly displaced to the right, the right foreleg is strongly abducted and extended, and presents considerable resistance to pressure from the experimenter's hand.

Figure 6.30 illustrates a corresponding interaction between forelimbs and hindlimbs. The dog stands with its forefeet on a table and with its hindfeet on one of the experimenter's hands. When the body is moved forwards over the forefeet, the hindlegs flex and do not show much supporting activity. When the body is moved backwards, the hindlegs are strongly extended and push against the experimenter's hand. Here the behaviour of the hindlimbs is altered by changes in the angle at the shoulder joint. Corresponding changes in the behaviour of the forelimbs can be produced by altering the angle at the hip joint. In each case it is probable that it is the out-of-balance couple acting at the joint which is the effective stimulus rather than the joint angle as such. The out-of-balance couple is related to the rate-of-change of joint angle.

Once the response has developed, the unbalanced couple will be neutralized and the joint angle will cease to change. Equilibrium may be reached in a number of positions each of which will show a particular value of joint angle and a particular degree of extension of

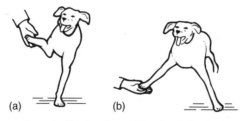

(a)   (b)

Figure 6.29 Sway reactions in the forelegs. The dog's body is supported by the experimenter, leaving most of the weight on the dog's left forefoot. The right forefoot rests on the experimenter's hand. (a) Body displaced to the animal's left: the right foreleg is flexed. (b) Body displaced to the animal's right: the right foreleg is strongly abducted and extended. (After Rademaker, 1931.)

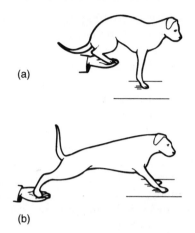

(a)

(b)

Figure 6.30 Effect on the hindlegs of the attitude at the shoulder. The dog stands with its forefeet on a table and with its hindfeet on one of the experimenter's hands. (a) Hindfeet moved forward to displace the body forwards over the forelegs: the hindlegs are flexed. (b) Hindfeet moved back to displace the body backwards over the forelegs: the hindlegs are strongly extended. (After Rademaker, 1931.)

the responding limb. Taking these two together might lead to the idea that the response depends on the magnitude of the joint angle. However, it is the rate-of-change of joint angle that is related to the unbalanced couple and it is this that must therefore be of prime importance in determining the character of the response.

Up to this point, the sway reactions and the interaction between neck reflexes and the positional reflexes from the labyrinth have been described in terms of a quadruped. The same account is applicable to a human in the all-fours position.

LATERAL MOVEMENTS OF THE HEAD

The neck is capable of lateral flexion as well as of twistings and movements in the median plane. Where lateral flexion of the neck occurs about a vertical axis, the resulting horizontal rotation of the skull does not generate positional reflexes from the labyrinth. The effects of the neck reflexes are unopposed. What happens is that the legs are extended on the side towards which the head is turned.

When the head is turned towards the right side about a vertical axis, the mass of the head is carried to the right side of the midline. This affects the position of the centre of gravity of the body as a whole and calls for increased supporting thrust in the legs of the right side. It is just such an increase in thrust that is provided by the neck reflex response to lateral flexion of the neck. The increased propping action in the limbs of the right side is accompanied by paddle action which tends to shift the trunk to the left so that the vertical projection of the centre of gravity is restored to a safer position nearer to the centre of the area of support. This behaviour corresponds to the rule given earlier, that the neck reflex effects on the limbs are in such a direction as to tend to push the trunk round to straighten the neck.

In the erect position, in man, a lateral flexion of the neck will tilt the head out of its normal orientation with respect to the behavioural vertical. This tilt generates positional reflexes from the labyrinth, resulting in extension in the 'downhill' limbs. Thus a tilt of the head, ear to shoulder, towards right side down about a horizontal axis, produces extension of the legs of the right side, with flexion on the left. In this situation, neck reflex effects reinforce reflex effects from the labyrinth to provide the increased supporting thrust on the right side appropriate to the shift in the centre of gravity.

FACTORS OBSCURING THE STABILIZING RESPONSES

In some conditions, in which the general level of excitability of the stretch reflexes is altered, the effects of the neck reflexes may be obscured until supplementary tests are applied. For example, an animal decerebrated by a brain section between the colliculi may hold all four limbs rigidly in extension and no flexion may be apparent when the neck is moved. However, the inhibition of extensors, which is part of the obscured flexor response, shows up as a reduction in the load-carrying capacity of the affected limbs. Again, an animal which is held in the air with its feet off the ground may hold all four legs in flexion with little marked change on moving the neck. The extensor facilitation produced in response to the neck movement will show up, however, as a change in the strength of the supporting reaction when this is elicited in the appropriate limbs by applying pressure to the soles of the feet.

The extension of both limbs of one side, which occurs when the head is turned towards that side, has its counterpart in the response of the vertebral column when the two limbs of one side are simultaneously extended in the buttressing reaction. If lateral pressure is applied to one side of the trunk of a standing dog, the two legs of the opposite side resist the push by developing the buttressing reaction. At the same time, the vertebral column becomes arched sideways, concave towards the legs that are acting as buttresses. This is the same direction of lateral flexion as that which produces extension of these same legs in the neck reflex.

The buttressing reactions in the legs can produce confusing results when one is testing for the neck reflexes to head rotation. The effect of these reactions is to resist displacement of the trunk by adjusting the supporting forces in the appropriate legs. If the head of an intact standing dog is grasped and forcibly rotated to turn the lower jaw towards the animal's right side, the response expected from the neck reflex as set out above would be an extension of the limbs of the right side with flexion on the left. In fact it is the left legs which are strongly extended in this case, and they successfully resist rotation of the body by the force applied to the head. What is happening here is that the buttressing reactions in the limbs of the left side obscure the effects of the neck reflexes. If the same experiment (forced rotation of the head) is attempted in a dog which has recently had its cerebellum removed, and in which the buttressing reactions are for this reason temporarily reduced, the unopposed neck-reflex effects appear, and the body is reflexly rotated to follow the head. (At a later stage after the operation, the buttressing reactions return, usually with somewhat enhanced vigour.)

REFLEX EFFECTS WITHIN THE VERTEBRAL COLUMN

In addition to the effects on the legs, neck rotation also produces reflex rotations in the rest of the vertebral column. The effect is, as it were, to share out the angular displacement among the various intervertebral joints. Thus, the clockwise rotation (looking down the axis of the vertebral column) imposed on the head in the experiment we have just been considering (turning the lower jaw towards the animal's right side) tends to produce clockwise rotation of the forequarters, if the pelvis is held, or anticlockwise rotation of the pelvis, if the shoulders are held. To see these responses clearly, we have to avoid the interfering effects of reactions elicited by contact between the limbs and the supports.

In suitable conditions, it is possible to demonstrate reflex effects passing also in the opposite direction along the vertebral column, rotation of the pelvis leading eventually to rotation of the neck in the same sense. In all these rotational responses of the vertebral column each of the displacements of one vertebral body upon the next is in the same direction, so that the spinous processes, for example, come to be arranged in a smooth helix. It is for this reason that, when the movement is restrained by the shoulders, the head and the pelvis rotate in opposite directions, whereas if one end of the vertebral column is held, the intermediate portion rotates in the same direction as the free end. There is, of course, only a very small relative rotation at each of the individual intervertebral joints, because of the anatomical arrangement of the articular facets.

In the more flexible portion of the vertebral column in the neck, because of the special nature of the atlanto-occipital and atlanto-axial articulations, it is possible for more complex movements to occur than those we have considered so far. Although one naturally thinks of long-necked animals such as the swan in this context, even comparatively short necks are capable of some sinuous movements, although these are only of small amplitude. There is no detailed analysis available at present of the responses to complex movements of this type.

Before leaving the vertebral column, some additional reflexes should be mentioned. The first of these is called the 'vertebra prominens reflex'. It is elicited by pressing downwards on the spinous processes of the lower cervical vertebrae. When this is done the animal at first resists the pressure by propping with the forelegs and arching the back; then, suddenly, all supporting reaction melts away in all four limbs and the animal collapses to the ground. Corresponding downward pressure applied to the spinous processes just in front of the sacrum leads to a reflex tilting of the pelvis (tail up) with enhancement of the supporting reaction in the hindlimbs. This may be enough to prevent the animal from lifting either of its hindfeet. The response may be made use of by veterinarians to discourage a cow from kicking. It is interesting that dorsiflexion of the vertebral column just a little further forward, at the junction between the thoracic and lumbar vertebrae, usually leads to collapse of all four limbs. It is because of these various reflex effects which may arise from time to time from pressure on the spinous processes that it is necessary for saddles to be carefully shaped to avoid pressure on the midline of the back.

FLUCTUATING FORCES

The various factors that interact with the supporting reaction exert their influence against a background of continual small-scale fluctuations in muscle tension. These arise because the repetition-frequency of firing in motoneurons is not usually high enough to produce smooth tetanic fusion of the mechanical responses in the relevant muscle cells. The development and decay of tension in individual muscle cells follow a very rapid time-course (Chapter 4). Furthermore, the composition of the group of motor units that are contributing to the generation of force in a specific tendon at a particular time changes continually, as individual units cease firing and others are recruited to take their place. The tension in the tendons shows less marked fluctuation than that in individual muscle-fibres since, of the many units contributing to the overall tension, some will be developing increasing tension at the same time as the tension developed in parallel units is falling. In spite of this smoothing mechanism, the support thrusts developed by each of the limbs do inevitably show some sporadic fluctuations. Because of these fluctuations, the point of application of the resultant of the thrust against the ground moves about, and this leads to small-scale topplings of the trunk. Some disturbance also arises from the movements of respiration which alter the disposition of the internal forces between body parts. Yet another source of disturbance is the pumping action of the heart with its periodic propulsion of the contained blood and consequent reaction thrust against the rest of the body. If the balance is to be maintained, any tendency to toppling has to be arrested and reversed by active adjustments of the supporting forces just as we need to move our hand when balancing the inverted broom of Figure 5.12. We can make ourselves aware of these active adjustments in thrust if we pay attention to the sensations from our feet. We may feel that, from time to time, more weight is taken on one foot or the other. When standing on one leg we can feel the bones of the foot moving to press down more firmly on one side and then on the other as the semi-automatic balancing adjustments are being made in the torque exerted at the ankle. The consequences of these fluctuations can also be seen in suitable force-plate recordings.

THE MOVING VECTOR DISPLAY

The indications from suitably-placed transducers in the force-plate can be combined in various ways to yield an oscilloscope display of a moving vector representing, at any instant, the magnitude, direction, and point of application of the resultant of the stress forces exerted against the force-plate at that moment. Additional markers can be added to the display to show the relative horizontal movements of the head and of the hips. It is most instructive to watch the movements of this display when a subject stands on the force-plate and performs various manoeuvres. (A vector with an arrowhead pointing upwards indicates the supporting force exerted by the force-plate. If the arrowhead points downwards, as in Figure 6.31, the vector indicates the force with which the subject pushes against the support. The shank of the arrow is the same in each case.)

The force against the ground is not the only thing that has to be adjusted. If the line of action of the force against the ground does not pass through the centre of gravity of the body, a rotation of the trunk will be generated unless torque is developed at the hip. If there is actual tilting, this angular movement will eventually have to be arrested and reversed. The forces controlling such tilts of the trunk about the hip are not revealed by the oscilloscope display.

Another complication is that, if the hips are to be moved over the ground by an inclined thrust through the centre of gravity of the trunk, the flexibility of the body will allow the head to lag behind that movement until active bracing of the muscles of the trunk and neck transfer to the head a suitable proportion of the horizontal component of the force applied at the hip.

SWAYING MOVEMENTS IN QUIET STANDING

In quiet standing, the movements of the displayed vector arise both from the spontaneous fluctuations in muscle tone and from the active changes initiated as part of the strategy of maintaining the posture. The display shows changes occurring both in the inclination of the thrust vector and in its point of application, but it is not possible to distinguish active changes from those arising from fluctuations in muscle force. Since the amplitude of the movements of the thrust point is greater than that of the horizontal displacements of the trunk, which are necessarily very much slower, the vector indicating the line of thrust tends to tilt over in sporadic fashion to one side or the other. An inclined thrust generates lateral acceleration which, if unopposed, would shift the trunk over the feet, with the possible consequence that the vertical projection of the centre of gravity might be brought close to the perimeter of the available area of support. This would present a threat of overbalancing since measures to move the centre of gravity back towards a safer position call for the active development of appropriately inclined thrusts, and the maximum degree of inclination is governed by how far the vertical projection of the centre of gravity is from the edge of the available area of support.

The swaying movements in quiet standing are of several different kinds. At some times the trunk remains stationary while the thrust line moves without tilting over. This involves a transfer of weight, as from one leg to the other, with corresponding adjustment of the torque exerted between legs and trunk. Here it is convenient to refer to a shift of the point of application of the resultant upthrust as a shift in the 'centre of pressure', even though the thrust is contributed to by more than one foot. At other stages in the swaying, inclined thrusts are developed, a shift of the centre of pressure being followed by a movement of the trunk over the feet. During such a movement, the trunk may remain upright, or it may tilt. If the head moves further than the hips in such a tilting movement in the fore-and-aft direction, this may give the impression that the whole body is pivoting about the ankle. A scrutiny of the timing of the movements reveals, however, that the head movement lags behind the movement of the hips, so that this is not a true pivoting movement.

Swaying movements are not usually very large. They may easily escape casual observation. For this reason, it is helpful to expand the horizontal scales in the display by a factor of four, as compared with the vertical scales. When the subject stands on a soft surface, such as a block of foam rubber, larger adjustments of the supporting forces are seen in the moving vector display, even when the displacements of the body are not much more marked than with the subject on a firm base. There is little change in the general character of the adjustments, apart from the increased amplitude.

STANDING ON A MOVABLE SUPPORT

Another technique for enhancing the swaying for the purposes of analysis is to have the subject stand on a force-plate mounted on a light platform that is free to move. This can be achieved by suspending the platform from a high ceiling (e.g. 3.6 m) in a parallel swing. Some care is needed in experiments of this kind since, if the subject happens to raise one foot while the other is not vertically under his centre of gravity, the inclined thrust developed will push the platform aside and the subject will fall. This is just what happens if one steps out of a car onto an inclined road surface that turns out to be covered with black ice. Maintaining one's balance on ice is notoriously difficult. It emphasizes the importance of friction to provide horizontal forces at the feet. The swinging platform has to be firmly tethered while the subject is stepping onto it and again when he is ready to step off. Once the subject is standing securely and has acquired some confidence, the tethers can be released. The inclined thrusts developed during swaying now have the effect of displacing the platform instead of shifting the trunk. The centre of pressure is then maintained vertically below the subject's centre of gravity although the feet are moving with the platform. It is now permissible for the experimenter to impose small tentative movements on the platform in order to observe the subject's responses. It is surprising how large an imposed movement of the support can be tolerated by even a comparatively inexperienced subject once he has overcome his initial, natural, apprehension. The subject's trunk remains in one place while his feet necessarily move with the platform. A comparable behaviour can be observed with a subject standing on a turntable. Rotations of the turntable by several tens of degrees may be tolerated, the subject's trunk meanwhile continuing to face in the same direction throughout.

Figure 6.31 shows a timed sequence of snapshots of the moving vector display in a test in which a fairly brisk but small lateral movement was imposed on the swinging platform. The platform movement is indicated by the displacement of the horizontal bar that also serves

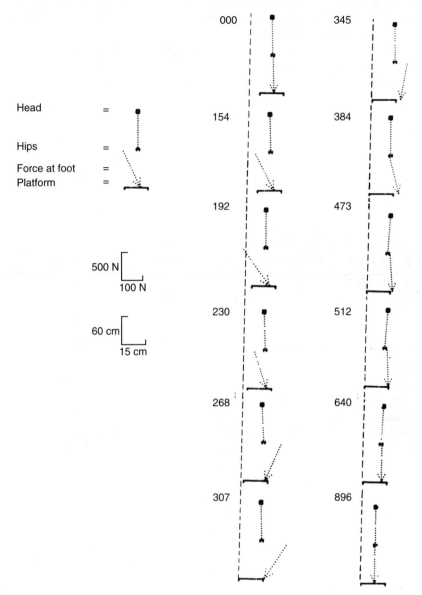

Figure 6.31 Successive appearances of the moving vector display, at the times indicated in milliseconds, during a brisk leftward movement of the platform through 6.5 cm.

as a 15 cm calibration for lateral displacements. In the figure, a broken vertical line has been added as a common reference point for successive frames. The elapsed time from the start of the movement is shown, in milliseconds, at the top left of each frame. The platform is moved, in about 300 ms, through a distance of 6.5 cm, to the left in the figure. This distance does not, in itself, present a serious threat of over-balancing. Because of the inertia of the subject's body, the forced displacement of his feet encounters the resistance of the elastic deformation of his legs and a horizontal force is accordingly developed at the feet. This is indicated by the tilt of the displayed vector, which here shows the force developed by the subject against the platform. During the movement of the platform, the centre of pressure stays, at first, vertically below the midline of the trunk, as indicated by the marker at the hips, while the feet are carried along with the platform. As the line of thrust does not, at this stage, pass through the subject's centre of gravity (which, for practical purposes, may be taken as close to the hip marker), torque must be being developed across the hips. This torque has two effects:

1. it transfers the line of action of the force on the body upwards to the hips, thus accelerating the trunk to the left;
2. it produces a small anticlockwise leftward tilt of the trunk, visible at 268 ms.

After the platform has come to rest, the leftward motion of the trunk has to be arrested by exerting an opposing torque at the hips, so that the vector indicating the force exerted against the platform tilts clockwise (frames at 268 ms and at 307 ms). At 345 ms, the leftward movement of the trunk has ceased, although the distance travelled is less than that moved through by the platform.

At this point the feet, which have been carried to the left by the platform, are not symmetrically disposed about the subject's midline. A 'rescue movement' is initiated, at 384 ms, to correct this asymmetry and to reduce the mild threat of overbalancing posed by the approach of the centre of pressure towards the perimeter of the area of support. The centre of pressure is flung out to the right, to provide a purchase for a leftward acceleration, with the thrust line passing through the centre of gravity. The inclined thrust gradually moves the trunk leftwards until, at 896 ms, the body is once again upright over the feet, but now in the new position of the platform.

During the first brisk movement of the platform, the mass of the subject's head and trunk appears to be largely uncoupled from the horizontal movement imposed on the feet.

The changes shown in Figure 6.31 indicate the subject's response to an external perturbation applied with the platform restrained. A related set of adjustments in thrust may by used by the subject to set the unrestrained suspended platform into motion. He first gently shifts his weight over his feet towards the right, that is to say in the opposite direction to the shift produced in the sequence from 384 ms to 896 ms in the figure. He then relaxes the supporting thrust for a moment, to allow his weight to sink briefly, shifts his weight rapidly onto the other foot while pushing back up to his normal stance height, checks his relative movement over the platform briskly, using a sequence resembling the first 350 ms of Figure 6.31, and resumes normal weight-bearing. The sudden check of the lateral movement of the body transfers some of its momentum to the platform and thus sets the platform into motion. The amplitude of the subsequent swinging excursions can thereafter be considerably increased by further repetitions of the same sequence, with appropriate regard to timing. Corresponding manoeuvres applied at a different phase of the oscillation can be used to bring the swinging platform to rest. A movement of the platform can also be produced by the same manoeuvre when the platform is supported on freely moving wheels.

DECIDING ON THE DIRECTION OF THE BEHAVIOURAL VERTICAL

At the beginning of this chapter it was pointed out that the avoidance of falling was not necessarily related to the direction of the gravitational vertical, but rather to the direction of a vector representing the upthrust supporting an inert body, such as the narrow prism of Figure 6.1. We have now seen how the direction of the vector representing the upthrust on an animal or on a human subject is normally far from steady.

This highlights the problem of determining from moment to moment whether or not any change needs to be made to the current pattern of outgoing neural commands by which the central nervous system is controlling the animal's musculature. The forces actually developed, in terms of thrusts and torques, depend on interactions between neural activations of muscles and the loads against which those muscles work. It is important to be able to decide whether the forces currently being deployed are succeeding in having a stabilizing effect or whether their effect is destabilizing and the commands need to be changed. The decision depends on what is happening to the animal's centre of gravity in relation to the area of support.

There are several sources from which an animal can derive information relevant to determining the direction and point of application of the force currently being developed between the body and its supports. These include cutaneous receptors at the area of contact, proprioceptors throughout the body, and the specialized detectors forming the balancing organ of the labyrinth in the inner ear. Each detector system involves its own inherent frame of reference, which is dependent on the structure of its receptor mechanism. Furthermore, different frames of reference are applicable to the skull, to the trunk, and to the environment, so that the interpretation of the signals from the sense organs has to take account of changes in the relations between all these different frames of reference. As well as the instantaneous values of the required parameters, it is also necessary to know how these parameters are changing. Visual information about movement of the skull can also be taken into account. What is still needed, however, is some reference standard with which to compare the current deployment of force.

For an inert system, it is possible to define a rest position and to determine, as a reference, the direction and line of action of the supporting thrust in this position. For an animal, the situation is less simple because there is no 'rest position'; there is always some sway.

The dependence of successful balancing on the integrity of the sensory apparatus of the labyrinth indicates that this is an important source of information. The structure of the detectors in the labyrinth (to be described in detail in Chapter 8) suggests that they function as accelerometers, so that they might provide clues to the stress gradients arising in the skull as a result of various forces transmitted to the skull by the muscles and skeleton of the neck. Since these forces are likely to fluctuate even more widely than the forces exerted by the limbs against the supports, it becomes even more important to consider how the decision is arrived at as to what direction is to be taken as the behavioural vertical for purposes of aiming the limbs in balancing behaviour. Giles Brindley devised a set of experiments that are most instructive on this point.

Brindley was interested in the familiar observation that a cat will usually land on its feet. To do this the cat needs to know, while it is in the air, which direction will be the best one in which to aim its legs, and it must so twist about in the air as to produce the appropriate aiming of the legs. As a first step in his study, Brindley confirmed that a cat will land on its feet, if allowed sufficient time in free fall during which to rearrange its limbs, no matter what orientation the cat was held in prior to release, and even if it was first thrown upwards feet first into the air. Other animals behave similarly. In these procedures, the supporting force prior to release was always parallel to the gravitational vertical.

Brindley then went on to study how animals orientate themselves in the air when released after being supported by a force that was inclined to the gravitational vertical. To achieve an inclined supporting force, three different experimental procedures were employed. In each the experimental animal was placed in a box whose floor consisted of two doors, sprung to make them open quickly, like a trapdoor, when a catch was released by remote control. At a predetermined interval after the start of the exposure to the inclined support thrust, the trapdoor was opened and the animal was photographed during its fall onto a suitably placed cushion. Rabbits were used in preference to cats for these experiments because they are less likely to move about in the box during the experiment. The rabbit's reaction to unusual conditions is usually to freeze, whereas the cat tends to make exploratory movements.

In one system, the box was suspended by wheels running freely along a track sloping gently from near the ceiling on one floor of the laboratory, through a conveniently-placed open stairwell, down to near the floor on the level below. This arrangement provided an inclined run, up and down, lasting several seconds from a catapult start. Longer exposures to an inclined thrust were obtained by suspending the box in a car driven rapidly in a circle on a disused airfield. To obtain an even steeper inclination of the support force, the box was suspended in a large centrifuge and then moved inwards to the axis of rotation just before the moment of release of the trapdoor.

On the inclined track, the supporting force must be at right angles to the track since the wheels cannot exert any force in a direction along the track. Movement in a circle requires an inwardly directed force as well as a vertical support, giving an inclined resultant like the force exerted by the strings supporting the platform swung in a circle in Figure 6.1.

In separate runs, of each type, the trapdoor was released at different times from the start of the exposure to the inclined thrust, and the attitude thereafter adopted by the falling animal was recorded on ciné film. If the release occurred during the first few seconds, the aiming of the animal's limbs was vertical, just as for the simple drops from a stationary starting position. If the release was further delayed, the aiming of the limbs was more nearly aligned to the support vector prevailing before the release.

The timings measured in the inclined thrust experiments indicate that it takes some 8 s for the animal to 'make up its mind', so to speak, about which direction is the best one in which to aim its legs in preparation for landing. The processes by which this decision is arrived at must be presumed to be quite complicated.

'SHIFTING THE WEIGHT'

The maintenance of balance, in the sense of the successful avoidance of hitting the head on the ground, involves continual management of the direction and magnitude of the thrusts against the supports. In this context the expression 'to shift the weight' turns out to be ambiguous. It does not necessarily imply a movement of mass or even of the centre of gravity. One can shift one's weight from one foot to the other without any apparent motion of the trunk. In this action we adjust the thrusts exerted by the legs against the ground. What we feel is a shift of the centre of pressure. Such a shift normally produces a horizontal acceleration of the trunk but the extent of actual displacement depends on how long the acceleration is persisted in before another adjustment is made in the limb thrusts to arrest the incipient movement. It also depends on whether or not the movement of the trunk is restrained by external forces. One may 'throw one's weight into it', pulling strongly against a rope in a tug-of-war, with very little movement of the mass of the trunk. On the other hand, the shift of weight over the feet illustrated in the later part of Figure 6.31 is achieved gradually without any particularly marked horizontal forces being developed.

Relatively small shifts in the location of the centre of gravity of the body can be produced by altering the disposition of the limbs, but this is not what is usually meant by a 'shift of the weight'. Examples are the forward movement of an athlete's centre of gravity at the top of the pole vault, where the athlete faces the bar with his back arched and his legs, arms and head bent strongly forwards. A shift in the opposite direction occurs in the Fosbury Flop technique for the high jump. The athlete leaps with his back to the bar, hollows his back and bends his legs, arms and head strongly backwards. The effect on the position of the athlete's centre of gravity in these manoeuvres is not very great. However, since the work done during the take-off is expended primarily in lifting the athlete's centre of gravity, and the competitive athlete aims to exert his maximum effort as effectively as possible, these small changes in the relative position of the centre of gravity can be important in affecting the clearance over the bar.

REACTIONS ON OVERBALANCING

It is appropriate now to consider the way balancing behaviour is organized in the face of variations in the direction of the support vector. The animal needs to take account of two possibilities:

1. the changes may arise from the activity of the animal's own muscles;
2. they may be imposed by the environment, as when an animal is supported on a moving platform.

One principle to be observed is that the forces exerted against the supports must always be so arranged that their resultant falls within the available area of support. If the point of application of the support thrust moves towards the edge of the area of support this constitutes a threat of overbalancing which has to be met by semi-automatic **rescue reactions** such as stepping or hopping. It is instructive to examine the circumstances in which such rescue reactions are initiated.

We may do this experimentally using a person standing on one leg with the other leg tethered. A convenient form of tether consists of a long strap, one end of which is fastened round the subject's waist. The subject bends his knee and loops the strap round his raised ankle, holding the free end in his hand (Figure 6.32(a)). Such a tether is readily released by the subject if he should become apprehensive. The subject stands on one leg on a force-plate and various manoeuvres are employed with the aim of overbalancing him (Figure 6.33). At the point of overbalancing, the subject executes a hop. The force-plate indicates that two different kinds of hop can be distinguished (Figures 6.32(b) and (c)).

FORCED HOPPING

In each case the moment of take-off is preceded by a sudden increase in the thrust against the force-plate. This brief upward push serves to project the subject's weight into the air to provide time, during the subsequent free-fall phase, for the supporting leg to be repositioned. When a hop is executed on command, this sudden upthrust is always preceded by a dip in the trace (Figure 6.32(c)). What seems to be happening during this dip is that the subject momentarily relaxes the upthrust in the supporting leg. This permits the body to fall a little, stretching the extensor muscles at the time when they are being re-activated for the take-off. This manoeuvre takes advantage of the muscle

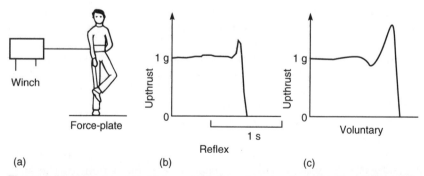

(a)   (b)   (c)

Figure 6.32 Time-courses of representative changes in upthrust during a hop. The subject stands on one leg on a force-plate and is gently unbalanced by a rope attached to a winch (a). In some cases (c) the upthrust decreases momentarily before the hop, in which case the subject is aware of a need to hop. In other cases (b) the upthrust rises without a preparatory dip.

properties reflected in the shape of the force–velocity relation for lengthening (Figure 4.10) and has the effect that more tension is developed by each motor unit.

If the subject is asked to make a voluntary hop, the time-course of the upthrust is always of this second type, with a preparatory dip. It turns out to be extremely difficult to produce by any voluntary manoeuvre a trace in which the dip is absent. If the subject is asked to start with the knee straight and the heel on the ground, voluntary hopping without first bending the knee becomes very difficult. However, provided that the subject is standing on a firm base, some form of hop can always be induced by gently winding in a rope attached to the subject's waist.

It will be convenient to use the expression 'reflex hop' to refer to those hops where the increase in upthrust is not preceded by a dip, the others being called 'voluntary hops'. Where the reflex hop is performed with the knee straight, the trunk is thrown upwards by tilting the pelvis. Other movements of the trunk, shoulders and arms also occur, but these have not been analysed.

THE STIMULUS FOR HOPPING

In a search for the 'adequate stimulus' responsible for initiating the hop, several possibilities have been considered. The crucial changes might be those occurring at the foot, at the hip or at the head. At the moment of toppling the head undergoes horizontal, vertical and angular accelerations, any of which might provide the stimulus to hopping by their action on the receptors in the labyrinth. Take the vertical acceleration first. This arises when the supporting limb, by its inclination, ceases to provide an adequate opposition to the pull of gravity. If this vertical acceleration is the stimulus, we should expect a hop to be elicited when the head is accelerated vertically downwards in other situations as well, for example, in an elevator at the start of a descent. In fact, no hopping behaviour is elicited by downward acceleration in an elevator, or even in a dropping apparatus in which the whole body suddenly goes into free fall at the release of a catch ('hangman's drop') (Figure 6.33(a)).

Horizontal acceleration arises when the trunk topples over a stationary foot. However, there is no observable difference in the hopping behaviour when we compare pulling the body by a rope attached to the subject's shoulders with the responses to movement of the supporting platform while the shoulders are tethered by a stationary rope (Figures 6.33(b) and (c)). The skull moves horizontally when we pull the shoulders, but not when we restrain the shoulders and pull the platform away. Angular accelerations of the skull might arise as a

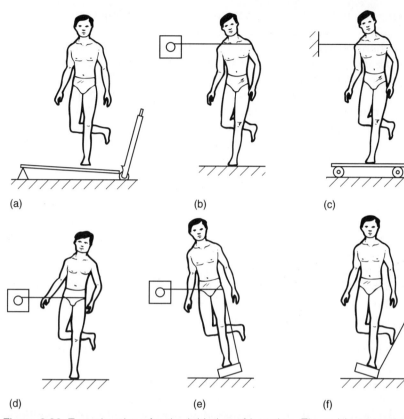

Figure 6.33 Test situations for the initiation of hopping. The subject stands on one leg in each case. (a) Sudden drop, platform released by a catch: (b) lateral pull applied by winching in a rope attached to the shoulder: (c) shoulder tethered to the wall while the platform moves away: (d) lateral pull applied at the hip: (e) foot support tilts with the subject: (f) tilt of foot support alone. Hopping occurs identically in conditions (b), (c) and (d), but not in conditions (a), (e) and (f). In condition (e), two phases can be distinguished. When the body at first begins to tilt over, the thrust line remains within the support area of the foot, so no reaction is elicited. As the body tips further, the lateral force at the foot diminishes, the subject falls, and strong rescue reactions begin to develop, though they may not be successful because of the delay.

consequence of either a horizontal or a vertical acceleration. All three types of acceleration of the skull now seem to be eliminated.

We can also eliminate the hips as the site of the adequate stimulus by comparing the effect of pulling the hips with that of pulling the shoulders. On pulling the hips the change in inclination of leg to trunk makes the body convex in the direction of hopping (Figure 6.33(d)), whereas pulling on the shoulders moves the hips the other way, making the profile concave in the direction of hopping (Figure 6.33(b)). The observed hops are similar in the two cases.

At the foot, we need to consider both the conditions at the ground contact and the movement at the ankle. The appropriate test here is to have the subject stand on a block of wood about the same size as the sole of his shoe (Figure 6.33(e)). The block is fitted with a long handle which can be loosely tethered to the subject's waist. Now, when the rope to the hips is wound in, the block tips over with the body, so that the foot remains at the same angle to the leg throughout. The normal hop does not occur, and it may be advisable to use a safety harness as otherwise the subject may suffer an awkward fall.

The absence of normal hopping when the foot support tilts with the body suggests that the changes occurring at the foot are crucial to the initiation of the hop. However, there is another simple manoeuvre still to be tried. The subject stands on one foot on the block as before, but this time the block alone is tilted by moving its handle (Figure 6.33(f)). This tilting of the block reproduces those conditions, both in ground contact and in ankle angle, that formerly were associated with the initiation of the hop. But now no hop takes place. The subject remains balanced in the upright position in spite of the imposed rotation of the block.

We have now examined all three alternative sites for the initiation of the hopping: head, hips and foot, and each has been eliminated in turn. We are forced to conclude that, for the stimulus to be 'adequate', at least two sites are involved together. The trigger mechanism must involve a quite complex recognition process to distinguish conditions in which a hop is appropriate from others in which it is not.

If we record the horizontal force at the foot as well as the upthrust and combine these into a display of the resultant vector, we find that, in all the cases where a hop is induced, the support vector first tilts over in the direction in which the hop will be executed. The tilt develops quite slowly in the experiments where a winch is used to force the subject to hop. The presence of a horizontal component of force in the direction of the hop implies that the rope must be slack, because it can exert tension but not thrust. There is usually no movement of the head on the trunk at this stage. This means that the recorded support vector at the foot must be identical in direction and related in amplitude to the support force on the skull. It may thus be used as an index of the stimulus to the otolith organs in the labyrinth.

The adequate stimulus for the initiation of a hop may now be identified as the combination of a change in the direction of the vector representing the support force on the skull together with a corresponding change in the tilt of the leg over the foot. The situation in which the subject fails to make a hop, when standing on a block that moves with his foot, is comparable with the situation of the narrow prism balanced on a platform that is being swung in a circle as in Figure 6.1.

We have seen that several factors contribute to the adequate stimulus for the initiation of hopping, yet each of these factors may be eliminated by suitable experimental design without abolishing the hopping response. This leads one to conclude that the crucial recognition process involves the detection of a 'gestalt' where this expression denotes a pattern that is identifiable even when some of its constituents are missing. This is an important idea to which we shall return later in this book.

ANTICIPATORY PRE-EMPTIVE ACTIONS

It may be noticed that in the experiments on forced hopping described above, the conditions giving rise to the hop show a gradual development, building up towards the threshold for the initiation itself. When we compare the thresholds for the reflex hop with the thresholds for voluntary hops, a most interesting fact emerges. The voluntary hops occur at a smaller inclination of the support vector than the threshold value needed for the initiation of a reflex hop. The voluntary hop is thus an example of an **anticipatory pre-emptive action**: anticipatory, in the sense that the gradual change in sensory information is recognized as indicating the imminence of a specific environmental change; pre-emptive, in the sense that, once the action has been generated, the trend in conditions is altered and the threshold is not reached for setting off the reflex mechanism that would have been brought into play if the trend had been allowed to continue further.

Once we have come to recognize the concept of anticipatory pre-emptive actions, other examples come to mind beyond the field of balance and locomotion: for example, the movements of the tongue and cheeks that avoid their being trapped between the teeth during mastication, and the normal movements of quiet respiration that can be suspended for a time to permit speech, swallowing, or breath-holding for underwater swimming, provided that the pre-emptive ventilation remains adequate to keep the accumulating carbon dioxide concentration below the threshold for reflex breathing.

The form of the hop produced as an anticipatory pre-emptive action in response to forced overbalancing closely resembles the form of a voluntary hop produced on command. If the subject is at all apprehensive or if the test follows a number of recent trials, the forced overbalancing may produce only hops of 'voluntary' type. The subject in these circumstances is usually able to report that he was aware of the need to hop. All of this points to the voluntary nature of the act, and emphasizes the distinction from reflex activity.

The promptness and somewhat stereotyped pattern of motor activity in the responses to forced overbalancing suggest that we are dealing with an action that has been learned. We suppose that, in the course of earlier experience, the sensory patterns associated with overbalancing have been followed by reflex movements. The motor patterns generated in these reflexes produced effects that were at any rate in the right direction, even if they did not always develop quickly enough to avoid falling. The reflex responses can thus act as prompts to the animal. If a corresponding motor pattern happens to be emitted early in the development of the sensory signs of the imminence of overbalancing, the animal receives a reward in so far as the punishing effects of overbalancing do not occur. These are the conditions in which learning is known to take place.

Learning is consolidated by repeated rehearsal, and conditions involving a liability to overbalancing recur very frequently, particularly in the course of locomotion. The well-rehearsed responses thus soon come to have the status of habits, in that their successful performance is no longer dependent upon active conscious supervision. An example of a pattern of motor behaviour which, once learned, continues to be performed successfully without conscious supervision is the relaxed riding of a bicycle. Where close attention is called for, as in the avoidance of obstacles, the act of bicycle riding is not strictly habitual, but is more properly classified as a skill. There is no possibility that bicycle riding is reflex in nature.

EFFECT OF LIFE-STYLE ON BALANCING BEHAVIOUR

The balancing behaviour to be expected on a tilted support is not quite the same in the cat as it is in the dog because of differences between the animals' life-styles. In a reaction to disturbance the dog gets to its feet, ready to run. In contrast the cat, when disturbed in a tree, tends to crouch down and grasp the supporting surface with its claws. The grip of the claws allows the cat to pull against the support, exerting tension in a way not available to the dog. Accordingly, if a cat is placed on a support that can be tilted, it responds to a tilt not only by extending the downhill legs as described in the foregoing account, but it also makes grasping movements with the uphill forepaw. The combined action of downhill and uphill legs provides a couple which acts on the trunk to counteract the overbalancing effect of the tilting support.

TILTING THE SEATED SUBJECT

Grasping reactions on the uphill side can also be seen in rescue reactions of the human subject seated on a tilt-table with the legs hanging free. It is necessary, for these tests, to blindfold the subject to exclude the important influence of visual cues. In this situation the blindfolded subject cannot defend against overbalancing by stepping or hopping. Nor can he successfully compensate for the sideways tilt of the support by extending the downhill leg as would a standing subject. What happens (Figure 6.34) is that he tilts his pelvis and bends his spine sideways so that his shoulders are much less tilted than his seat. The flexibility of the neck is then sufficient to allow the head to remain stabilized in the upright position. The neck flexion may over-compensate, as in this illustration, bending sideways in the same direction as the bend in the trunk. With the hands resting on the subject's knees, the arms show downhill extension and uphill flexion in accordance with the pattern seen in the legs when the subject is standing on a tilted support. Meanwhile the lower legs, which are hanging free, are swung towards the uphill side of the tilt.

This sweeping movement of the legs has two effects. If one of the legs encounters an obstacle during the sweep, paddle action can be developed against the obstacle, and this provides torque at the hip with which to resist the overbalancing effect of the tilting. If no obstacle is encountered, the lateral movement of the legs produces a small shift in the position of the centre of gravity of the whole body in a direction that contributes to an increase in the security against overbalancing. None of these reactions occur in blindfolded patients in whom the labyrinths are not functional, by reason of disease or as a consequence of surgery (Figure 6.35).

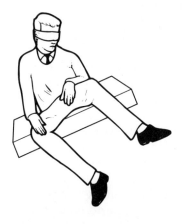

Figure 6.34 Normal subject seated on a tilting apparatus. (After Purdon Martin, 1967.)

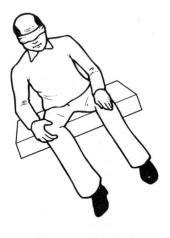

Figure 6.35 Labyrinth-defective subject seated on the tilting apparatus. There is no stabilization or compensation. The subject is about to overbalance and his right arm is beginning to move out to break the fall. (After Purdon Martin, 1967.)

RESCUE REACTIONS

If the angle of tilt of the support is large enough, both normal subjects and labyrinth-defective subjects alike are overbalanced. In each case similar reactions are initiated. From this we may conclude that the initiation of the rescue reactions on overbalancing, like that of the forced hopping described earlier, is not dependent on the labyrinth alone, but involves the recognition of a gestalt contributed to by information from many sensory sources.

   If the legs are available, the simplest defence against overbalancing is straightforward stepping, as described earlier. This involves a smooth transfer of weight to take advantage of the extension of the area of support provided by swinging one or both of the legs to a new position. Stepping calls for a preliminary adjustment of the distribution of the weight between the legs to free a leg so that it can be lifted. If the prevailing posture makes this difficult for any reason, the rescue reaction takes the form of **staggering**. This consists of a series of small hops by the downhill leg to extend the area of support. If a standing subject is unexpectedly pushed sideways strongly, say to the left, staggering will be initiated in the left leg before the sway reaction has reduced the upthrust in the right leg completely to zero in preparation for a step. Staggering may be performed in any direction, backwards, forwards, or sideways. If only one leg is available, the response is a hop, as in the experiments on forced hopping.

The rescue reactions of stepping, staggering and hopping are not available to the seated subject. The next reaction to be recruited is the reaction of **sweeping**. Any limb not already engaged in supporting the body will be used in a rapid sweeping action as an inertia paddle. Here the muscular action to impart momentum to the free limb also applies reaction forces to the trunk, imparting opposite momentum to it and thus helping to arrest the tendency to fall. If the free-moving limb encounters an obstacle, or if its inertia is suitably increased by holding a tightrope walker's balancing pole, the action of these muscular forces serves to oppose the external overbalancing force and the body's equilibrium is regained.

The loss of balance carries with it the threat of impending collision with the ground. If staggering and sweeping both fail, the **fall-breaking reaction** is invoked. This brings in very forceful movements of the limbs. All other activities of the limbs are abandoned, restraints are forcibly overcome, and one or more limbs are flung out in such a direction as to save the head from hitting the ground. The circumstances in which balance was lost provide sensory cues as to the direction from which impact is threatened. The fall-breaking reactions extend the limbs to absorb this impact. If the limbs are trapped, the trunk will be moved so as to take the impact on the shoulders. The movements are organized as though to avoid impact with the skull at almost any cost. The arm may be flung out protectively through fire or broken glass. The risk of peripheral injury is automatically preferred over the liability to injury to the head. Figure 6.36 shows a blindfolded labyrinth-defective patient overbalancing when the seat is tilted. His

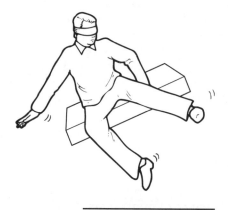

Figure 6.36 Labyrinth-defective subject overbalancing on the tilting apparatus. The transient stabilization and compensation shown by this patient is presumably of cutaneous or proprioceptive origin. (After Purdon Martin, 1967.)

right arm is flung out in fall-breaking; his left hand clutches at the support; both legs execute strong sweeping movements.

VISUAL CUES FOR BALANCING

It was mentioned earlier that, at one stage in the analysis of the reactions on overbalancing, it is necessary to blindfold the subject to exclude visual cues. The reason for this is that we normally rely quite heavily on visual information in ways that are not immediately obvious. With the eyes open we have the impression that we are surrounded by an extensive 'visual field'. In fact, only a surprisingly small portion of this field is actually seen in any detail at any one time. For example, at a normal conversational distance, the part of the face of the person spoken to that is visible in clear detail is not big enough to include both his eyes at the same time. The small size of the area of clear vision corresponds to the small size of the fovea compared to that of the rest of the retina. The extensive non-foveal part of the retina is concerned with detecting movement of contrast details rather than with their identification.

The peripheral retina contains mechanisms for the detection both of the direction and of the speed of movement of contrast details in the retinal image. By comparing signals from different parts of the retina the image-streaming can be classified as lateral, vertical, axial, rotational, or some combination of these. These classes of image-streaming over the peripheral retina correspond to movements of the skull relative to the perceived details of the visual surround.

The subject learns to distinguish those patterns of image-streaming that are associated with his own head movements and with his locomotor progression through the environment. Streaming patterns that differ from this set of self-generated patterns indicate either the relative movement of external objects or some unanticipated relative movement between the subject's skull and the surround. This last category of inferred motion comes to be associated with the various penalties of overbalancing, such as impact with the ground. In consequence, the early signs of involuntary relative movement between the skull and the surround come to be used as a warning of impending loss of balance, and thereafter trigger off appropriately corrective postural adjustments.

THE 'MOVING ROOM' EXPERIMENT

An experiment to demonstrate this effect was devised by Lee and Lishman in the Psychology Department of Edinburgh University. They constructed a 'moving room' consisting of a framework of three large panels decorated with patterned wallpaper and furnished with wall-brackets and pictures to resemble the interior of a suburban living room. The whole assembly was suspended from the high ceiling of a lecture hall with the 'walls' just clear of the floor. The subject stands inside the 'room' facing the end wall so that the whole of his visual field is taken up by the hanging panels, together with a small area of floor, which was deliberately featureless. Very young subjects, just learning to stand, were very readily overbalanced by quite small imposed movements of the 'room'.

To show the effect clearly in more sophisticated adult subjects, it was found necessary to introduce an additional constraint to make the balancing task more difficult than usual. The subjects were asked to stand on a narrow beam about 5 cm wide. This balancing task presents no problem to a normal adult so long as the visual field is stationary. Quite a small movement of the 'room', however, is sufficient to over-balance the subject in these conditions.

In a complementary experiment, by Roberts in Glasgow University, subjects were asked to stand on the lightweight platform suspended from a high ceiling that has already been referred to. The subjects had an unobstructed view of the walls of the laboratory. When the platform was surreptitiously moved by the experimenter (manipulating the controls of the motor drive to the platform), the subject's head and upper body retained their position in space, relative to the room. That is to say, the subject readily allowed his feet to be moved under him while his head and body remained stationary. This effect involves considerable changes in the activity of the limb musculature, since both the distribution of the weight and the aiming of the legs have to be altered when the trunk moves over the feet. The subjects were apparently unaware of these changes in their limbs.

One can conclude that the changes in the legs occurring on the moving platform have the effect of reducing the retinal image-streaming that would occur if the body and head were to be carried along with the swing. In the moving room, a corresponding set of adjustments to the leg musculature, again to minimize retinal image-streaming, is inappropriate to the maintenance of balance, and this is why the subjects fall over.

The effect revealed in the moving room experiment can be demonstrated more simply, as follows. The subject stands on a narrow base, as before, and the experimenter holds up a large open newspaper at a convenient reading distance in front of the subject's face, keeping the newspaper as still as possible to allow the subject to become accustomed to the conditions. The newspaper will almost completely fill the subject's visual field. A small, gentle, sideways movement of the newspaper by the experimenter is usually effective in overbalancing the subject.

The mechanism for maintaining balance by using visual clues from streaming of the retinal images is supplementary to, and integrated with, the other balancing mechanisms that are dependent on labyrinth signals and on proprioception.

SUPPLEMENTARY PROPRIOCEPTIVE CUES

The task of retaining one's balance on a restricted or precarious support is made very much easier if one is allowed to touch some stable object with one's hand. If a substantial force is exerted through the hand, this has the effect of extending the effective area of support, but this is often not necessary. Even a very light contact can be sufficient to produce a very marked improvement in stability. When the body moves, the subject can feel, with his hand, the relative movement of the stable support. The posture of the arm is adjusted to retain contact, and this change in posture affects the proprioceptors in the arm. Signals from the proprioceptors and from receptors in the skin at the area of contact become incorporated into the continually varying gestalt that forms the basis for active balancing behaviour.

TILT OF THE SUPPORT VECTOR

We are now in a position to consider the effect of imposed horizontal forces on the balancing behaviour of animals and to compare this with the effect on an inert system. The comparison is illustrated by Figure 6.37. The upper row of diagrams shows the effects of horizontal forces applied to a body supported by legs standing on a fixed base. The bottom row shows the effect of forces applied to the supporting platform. The effects on an inert system are shown to the left for comparison with the responses of an active system to transient (centre) and to sustained (right) lateral perturbing forces.

A leftward lateral push to the body of an inert system deforms the attachments of the legs so that they develop clockwise torque (Figure 6.37(a)). The horizontal force at the feet, arising from the frictional resistance to movement, is thus transferred upwards to the body to combine with the vertical upthrust, giving an inclined vector buttressing against the disturbing force.

In an animal, any lateral displacement of the body is rapidly detected and opposed by the stabilizing reactions, which develop clockwise torque by paddle action of the legs without significant tilt (Figure 6.37(b)). The effect of this torque is the same as in the inert system: an inclined thrust buttresses against the disturbing force. If the lateral

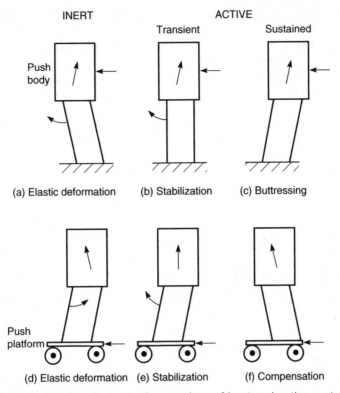

INERT

ACTIVE

Transient   Sustained

Push
body

(a) Elastic deformation   (b) Stabilization   (c) Buttressing

Push
platform

(d) Elastic deformation   (e) Stabilization   (f) Compensation

Figure 6.37 Comparison between the reactions of inert and active systems to a horizontal disturbing force. Top row: on a fixed support, with the force applied to the body. Bottom row: on a moving platform, with the force applied to the platform. An inert system ((a), (d)) is deformed in opposite senses in the two cases. The active system of an animal's body shows the same stabilizing reactions to transient disturbance on the fixed and on the movable supports ((b), (e)). On a fixed support, the body buttresses against a sustained disturbing force (c). On a moving platform subjected to a sustained horizontal force, the buttressing reaction fails to maintain balance because the platform moves away from under the body. Stepping and hopping reactions are elicited to reposition the feet, and thereafter the body adopts a compensatory pose that transmits the disturbing force to the body and aligns it with the new direction of the behavioural vertical.

force is sustained, the attitude of the limbs is altered. They tilt over to provide inclined thrust with little paddle action (Figure 6.37(c)).

If the disturbing force is applied to the supporting platform rather than directly to the body, the attachments of the legs of the inert system are again deformed, but this time they develop anticlockwise torque (Figure 6.37(d)). The resultant inclined vector accelerates the body to the left.

A transient horizontal force to the platform at first affects the animal in the same way as the inert system, but the onset of lateral acceleration of the animal's body is rapidly detected so that stabilizing reactions develop. These are in the same direction as for a force applied directly to the body (Figure 6.37(e)). This time, the clockwise torque of the paddle action of the legs allows the feet to move to the left while the trunk remains almost stationary.

In the face of a sustained horizontal force applied to the platform, the persistence of behaviour like that in Figure 6.37(e) would lead to overbalancing. What happens is that the animal repositions its feet so that the legs are tilted over to develop inclined thrust without paddle action (Figure 6.37(f)). This inclined thrust acccelerates the animal's body to the left so that it can now retain its station on the platform, with a new direction for the behavioural vertical. The animal can thus preserve its balance in spite of large movements of the platform.

THE MAGNET REACTION

The maintenance of balance does not depend solely on adjustments of the aiming of the legs and of the thrust they can develop. It is also necessary that the legs should have a suitable purchase on the supports to provide a firm base against which to develop the necessary thrust. We have seen that, in many situations, pressure on the sole of one of the feet, by splaying the digits and stretching the interosseus muscles, elicits the supporting reaction in the corresponding limb. In an animal with intact cerebral cortex a similar sequence of responses can be elicited by even light touch to the skin of the sole of the foot. The first effect is an extension of the limb, and this may press the foot against whatever it was that touched the skin to elicit the response. As a result, the supporting reaction may follow. However, if the skin contact is provided by the experimenter, and if he withdraws the stimulating object as the limb extends, no splaying of the digits will occur. Nevertheless, the extension of the limb continues and the angle of the limb is adjusted as necessary to retain the skin contact. This means that if the experimenter gently touches the foot of a freely hanging limb with his finger and then moves his finger away, the animal's foot follows the experimenter's finger and keeps up the contact even when this finger is moved about. This aspect of the behaviour leads to its being referred to as the **magnet reaction**.

The magnet reaction can be elicited in any or all of the four limbs when they are hanging free. When a limb is showing the magnet reaction this involves changes in a large number of muscles. Flexion of the limb is resisted; the angle with the trunk is firmly fixed; changes occur in the trunk musculature and in the other limbs just as for the supporting reaction. The magnet reaction is particularly well seen in animals from which the cerebellum has been removed several weeks previously. In such animals many of the inhibitory influences arising from the cerebral cortex appear to be of reduced effectiveness and there are consequently fewer factors to obscure the response in the magnet reaction. If an animal is supporting the whole of its weight on the forequarters, as in the hauling-up and pushing-up reactions (Figures 6.15(b) and 6.15(c)), or if it is supporting all its weight on the hindquarters as in Figure 6.14(b), then a light touch to the sole of one or both of the freely hanging feet produces a dramatic change in the posture. The muscles which are tensely holding up the body are gradually relaxed while the touched limbs extend, as though the animal is letting down its weight in the expectation of finding additional support from the touched limbs. It is easy to see that the magnet reaction must be of great importance to animals walking on rough ground where there may be rocking stones or loose branches which have to be used as footholds.

POSTURAL REACTIONS FROM THE SKIN

Just as the intensity of the supporting reaction in a particular limb is influenced by the attitude of the head and of the other limbs, so it is with the magnet reaction. In addition, there are a number of situations in which stimulation of the skin in other parts of the body produces inhibitory effects which suppress the response in the magnet reaction. In particular, certain types of stimulation of the skin of the back produce generalized inhibition of the extensor activity of all four limbs. Thus, if an intact animal is laid on its back, it usually holds all four limbs in flexion and does not give the magnet reaction, whereas, if it is held upside down in the air, supported at shoulders and pelvis by the experimenter's hands, the magnet reaction can usually be elicited in all four limbs.

The inhibitory effect of stimulation of the skin of the back can also be demonstrated in the intact dog or cat by grasping a fold of loose skin in the hand. If the skin over the shoulders is grasped and squeezed, the forelegs collapse. Squeezing a fold of skin over the pelvis produces collapse of the hindlegs. Squeezing the skin of the middle of the back leads to the collapse of all four limbs. If the animal is held in the air by the skin of the back, all four limbs are held in partial flexion. It may be observed that, while the animal is being gradually lifted up from the lying position which it adopts when the skin is first grasped, the paws retain their contact with the ground as long as possible, even though this involves considerable extension of the limbs. This is an example of the effect of the magnet reaction. Once the contact with the ground has been broken, the limbs move into flexion, and it is difficult thereafter to elicit the magnet reaction. The inhibitory influence of the skin of the back is reduced in animals from which the cerebellum has been removed some weeks previously. In such animals, magnet reactions can be obtained both with the animal on its back and when the animal is held in the air by folds of the dorsal skin.

In some animals the skin of the abdomen also generates inhibitory effects. If a tight bandage is tied round a cat's abdomen, the hindlegs are drawn into flexion and the animal is virtually immobilized. A similar reaction occurs in the cow where it may be made use of in casting the animal. The usual procedure is to attach one end of a rope to the cow's head, either by the horns, or to a halter. The rope is then run in three half-hitches round the animal, once round the neck, once round the thorax, and once round the abdomen. When the rope is pulled upon, the hindquarters begin to sway and then the animal collapses. Because the rope also pulls the head round to one side, the collapse occurs first on the opposite side, as a result of the influences of the neck reflexes to lateral flexion.

RIGHTING WITHOUT LABYRINTHS

The skin of the sides of the body generates a group of responses called the 'righting reflexes from the body'. These reflexes interact with the reflexes from the labyrinth and from the neck described earlier in this chapter. They are therefore best studied in animals whose labyrinths have been destroyed some time previously. The responses involve the musculature of the limbs and of the trunk, and produce movements of the head, forequarters and hindquarters. If a labyrinthectomized animal is laid on its side on a horizontal surface, it brings first the head and then the body into an approximately upright position. The movement of the head generates neck reflexes which would assist in bringing the body into the upright position to straighten the neck. However, if the head is restrained in the side-down position, the body is still brought into an approximately upright position. Here the neck reflexes are acting in the opposite sense and must be over-ridden by the righting reflexes from the body. If the forequarters are restrained in the side-down position, the hindquarters are righted so far as is anatomically possible.

The righting reflexes from the body do not occur unless the stimulation of the skin of the sides of the body is asymmetrical. In a labyrinthectomized animal lying on its side, no righting reflexes arise if a weighted plank is laid on the body to give similar stimulation on the upper side to that on the lower side.

If a labyrinthectomized animal is laid on its side on an inclined surface, the effects of the righting reflexes from the body will tend to bring the animal into a position with the median plane of symmetry at right angles to the supporting surface. In this position the vertical projection of the centre of gravity is displaced from its safe position over the centre of the area of support. There is consequently a tendency for the body to slide downhill. This tendency is resisted by the buttressing action of the downhill limbs and the final position is somewhere midway between the true vertical and the position at right angles to the support.

GRASPING REACTIONS

In arboreal animals, such as cats and monkeys, the response to contact with the underside of the paw may take a different form from that described above. Contact with a flat surface leads to the magnet and supporting reactions already described. Contact with an uneven surface, such as a branch of a tree, or the experimenter's finger, produces, particularly in the forelegs, a grasping movement, with flexion of the digits and, in the cat, protrusion of the claws. The grasping movement is often followed by strong flexion of the limb. This pattern is especially well marked in conditions where the stabilizing reflexes call for flexion of the limb under test. If contact is broken during this response, as it may be, for example, by the claws pulling out from the bark of a tree, the flexion is abruptly halted and the limb is extended in a sweeping movement to re-establish contact, as in the rescue reactions on overbalancing. If need be, a number of sweeping movements will be made in rapid succession. The grasping reflex can be elicited in cats from which the cerebral hemispheres and cerebellum have been removed. It does not occur in the decerebrate preparation.

PLACING REACTIONS

It has been convenient to suppose, up to this point, that when the feet of an animal are on the ground, the attitude of the digits and the nature of the ground surface have been such as to result in a fairly even stimulation over the sole of the foot. When the feet are set down after a reflex stepping or hopping movement, the attitude of the digits is governed primarily by the fact that the muscles used to lift the limb produce, as an indirect consequence of the anatomical arrangement of the tendons in relation to the joints, a particular pattern of extension of the digits. Thus it comes about that, where the ground is not too uneven, a reflex stepping movement will place the foot in an appropriate attitude on the ground for it to play its part in the next supporting reaction.

In the normal life of an animal, however, it will often happen that, owing to unevennesses in the ground or for other reasons, one foot or another will fail to land squarely on a suitable supporting surface. If no correcting movement were made, the foot might then slip off the edge of its supporting stone or branch, and the animal would stumble. As a result of experiences in early life, each animal learns a set of appropriate correcting movements. These are called **placing reactions**. They occur with such stereotyped regularity that one might be tempted to call them reflexes. It can be shown, however, that they are learned responses and not true reflexes.

The essential part of the response in the placing reactions is that the foot is neatly placed upon the supporting surface with the digits disposed in such a fashion that the foot is ready to support the animal's weight. If the area of the supporting surface is only just big enough to accommodate the foot, then the position of the limb is adjusted until the foot is placed sqarely upon the support without overhanging in any direction. If the animal is standing on a smooth table and the experimenter, by sliding the animal about, pushes one of its feet off the edge of the table, the animal promptly picks up the displaced foot and replaces it upon the table. If one foot is pulled out from under the animal by the experimenter, the animal struggles to free its limb and, on succeeding, promptly and neatly replaces the foot on the support.

If an animal is held in the air by the forequarters and then gently lowered until its hindlegs touch the ground, then, as soon as contact is made, the animal makes backward running movements with the hindlegs to bring the hindfeet under the centre of gravity, ready to take the weight. If any of the hanging legs is touched, particularly on the back of the paw, that leg is lifted up and the paw is accurately set down on the object which touched the leg. This **contact placing** leads into the magnet reaction when the area of contact is brought, at successive trials, round onto the sole of the foot. If the touched leg is restrained by the experimenter, the contralateral foot will be lifted and placed on the touching object, unless that leg is already engaged in supporting the animal. If the attitude of the foot on the ground is altered by the experimenter, for example by his flexing the digits so that the animal stands on the backs of the toes or fingers, then as soon as the paw is released, the animal corrects the posture of the foot.

These placing reactions depend on cutaneous stimulation. However, if the skin has been denervated, similar responses can still be performed if the animal is allowed to see the tested foot. The tests are accordingly best carried out with the animal blindfolded.

Another group of placing reactions arises from contact with the head. Here again similar responses can arise from visual cues and it is more difficult to exclude vision by blindfolding while retaining access to the skin of the head for the tests. For example, if an animal is held upright in the air with its legs hanging free and is allowed to see objects within its reach, it will adjust its posture and stretch out the nearest paw to touch the objects and to test them as possible supports. This **visual placing** response is particularly well seen in the forelegs if the hindquarters are at a higher level than the shoulders.

The reactions from cutaneous stimulation of the head have been demonstrated in blinded animals. If the chin is touched, the blinded animal lifts both forepaws and places them beside the chin on the touching object. This response is followed by extension of both forelegs to lift the head clear. If the animal is not blinded but the forelimbs are restrained to avoid visual placing, then, as soon as the chin is touched, the animal makes very strong movements to free the forelegs, places the forepaws beside the chin and lifts its head. In blinded animals it can be shown that placing of the forepaws followed by extension of the forelegs can also be elicited by touching the vibrissae.

Placing reactions of the forepaws similar to those elicited by contact with the chin can also be obtained from touching the skin of the breast, and corresponding hindlimb responses can be obtained from touching the skin of the belly. Note that in these hindleg responses, as in the responses to contact with any part of the anterior aspect of the hindlimb, the foot is moved forwards to make contact with the support, whereas in the responses to contact with the tail, back of thigh or hindfoot, when the animal is being held by the forequarters and is being lowered into contact with the ground, the foot is moved in the backward direction.

In each of these situations where the limbs of both sides are involved, when one limb finds a support it develops the magnet reaction and stiffens against the support. If the other limb of the pair does not at once find a support, it may make one or two sweeping movements as though seeking contact, and then it will be drawn up into flexion, showing the crossed influence of the magnet reaction now present on the opposite side.

POSTURAL REACTIONS IN THE NEWBORN HUMAN BABY

The placing reactions are absent in the newborn human baby. The grasping reflex is present, but if the baby is held by the hands and is lowered gently to bring the feet into contact with a table, the feet are lifted away from the contact, instead of moving into a position where they can support the weight. These responses may be associated with the human baby's dependence on its mother and with the primitive need for the baby to cling on to its mother to avoid separation. The changeover to the adult pattern of response occurs when the baby is about six months old, at about the same time as the reversal in sign of the response in Babinski's test (scraping the sole of the foot near its outer edge produces dorsiflexion of the toes in the newborn infant and plantar flexion in the adult).

If the weight of the baby is taken round the chest, instead of on the arms, a different pattern of responses appears when the body is gently lowered to bring the feet into contact with the table. The legs now show supporting reactions although the force developed is not sufficient to carry the weight of the body. If the experimenter now gently carries the baby forwards with the feet still touching the table, the legs will execute reflex stepping movements, in alternation, as though the baby were walking.

The placing reactions extend the usefulness of the magnet reaction in ensuring that the feet are each securely placed on a firm foothold. The supporting reactions, with their interactions between the four limbs and between limbs and trunk, ensure that the forces necessary to support the weight are suitably distributed between the limbs.

In this chapter we have seen something of the complexity of the task of coordinating the activities of the large number of individual muscles whose tensions stiffen the loosely-jointed skeleton. Various types of threat to the animal's balance are met by appropriate automatic or semi-automatic 'reactions' which help to keep the animal upright. We now turn to the way these reactions are modified to enable the animal to move from one place to another in various modes of locomotor progression.

There is a school of thought that holds that locomotion is driven by some sort of central rhythm generator. In my own view, the evidence I present in detail in the next chapter leads to the conclusion that a dependence on a central generator is unlikely.

Locomotion

7

The components of motor organization that are employed in the maintenance of balance in the upright posture also form the basis for active locomotion. In the previous chapter we saw that, even in quiet standing, there is always some movement. In consequence there are continual changes in the position of the vertical projection of the centre of gravity of the body in relation to the perimeter of the available area of support. In this context, the expression 'vertical' has to be taken to mean the direction judged by the animal to be currently the best one in which to aim the limb thrusts against the ground in order to avoid falling over and hitting the head on the ground. The strategy for remaining upright includes adjustment of the limb forces in both propping and paddle action to arrest and reverse unwanted movement of the weight over the feet.

Locomotion is achieved by active revision of the direction of the behavioural vertical to produce a desired shift of the animal's weight. There are, in fact, several ways in which locomotor activity can be organized, the distinguishably different 'ways of going' being referred to as 'gaits'. Before embarking on a detailed consideration of the techniques of gait analysis it may prove helpful to look at something that is familiar to all of us, namely the bipedal locomotion of man.

Although the activity itself is familiar, we are not usually aware of the way in which the progression is achieved. In forward progression, advantage is taken of the fact that, if not adequately supported, any object will tend to fall towards the centre of the earth under the action of gravity. If an object is partially supported by an inclined strut, the action of gravity produces horizontal acceleration as well as falling, as explained in Chapter 5 in relation to the task of balancing an inverted broom. The horizontal acceleration leads to forward progression if the falling component of the action of gravity can be dealt with by a succession of controlled bounces.

CONTROLLED BOUNCING

An instructive example of controlled bouncing may be seen in acrobatic performances in which the acrobat lies on his back and bounces a barrel upwards with his feet (Figure 7.1). Here the object to be bounced may be adequately treated as a rigid body. (The rotations have to be taken into account as well as the simple up-and-down motion.) The free-fall movement of the centre of gravity of the barrel has a parabolic time-course. What happens when the barrel lands on the acrobat's feet depends on the behaviour of the acrobat and on the positions of the points of contact in relation to the centre of gravity of the barrel.

In one mode, the acrobat adjusts the musculature of his legs to absorb all the momentum of the falling barrel, both vertical and angular, bringing the barrel to rest in a single catching movement, which ends in maintaining a constant upthrust to balance the weight of the barrel. In another mode, the acrobat develops extra thrust in his legs, throwing the barrel up into the air and at the same time imparting rotation about either a vertical or an inclined axis. In a third mode, a brief catching action is closely followed by a strong throwing action, so that the barrel is bounced repeatedly, often rotating in a different way during successive free-fall phases.

The bouncing movement involved in locomotion resembles this third mode of acrobatic barrel-bouncing, with the modification that, in the erect posture, it is the mass of the animal's body that is bounced instead of the barrel. Three different stages occur in each cycle, distinguished by the direction of acceleration and by the nature of the

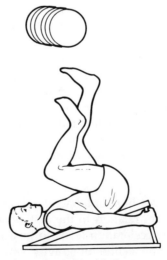

Figure 7.1 Acrobat bouncing a barrel on his feet.

accelerating forces. A free-fall stage, accelerating downwards under gravity, is followed first by the deceleration of catching and, later, by an active upward throwing effort. In these two stages of upward acceleration, different relations apply between force and displacement.

The behaviour of the musculature of the legs is adjusted voluntarily to produce the desired overall motion of the trunk. The momentum of movements in undesired directions is absorbed and other movements are imparted either to propel the body over the ground in a selected direction and at a selected speed or, alternatively, to regain the upright posture and to maintain it in a succession of quiet swaying movements.

RIDING THE POGO-STICK

Some of the essential features of locomotor activity can be illustrated by describing the process of riding a pogo-stick. This device consists of a long hollow handle, normally held upright, which is fitted at its lower end with a crossbar on which the rider stands. Inside the handle there is a spring-loaded plunger which extends downwards for some distance below the crossbar. When the rider puts his weight on the crossbar, with the tip of the plunger on the ground, the spring is compressed. By bending at the knee and hip, the rider can surge his weight up and down to vary the thrust against the crossbar. It is not possible to stay upright while standing still on the pogo-stick because the device is inherently unstable. Skill is, accordingly, essential for the initial mounting, as the rider has to embark immediately on an active bouncing strategy. By surging the weight downwards against the crossbar it is possible to compress the spring until it exerts a thrust considerably greater than body weight. The legs are at this point stiffened to resist compression so that the action of this thrust during the recoil of the spring then throws the body of the rider into the air. His strategy now must be to reposition the tip of the pogo-stick in such a way that, when he lands, the new thrust will counteract any tendency for the body to topple over as a result of the angular momentum acquired at the previous thrust. If a series of repositionings is appropriately chosen for successive bounces, it is possible to continue to ride the pogo-stick for a period whose length depends on the skill and persistence of the rider. As skill develops, the rider can learn to organize his successive bounces into a coordinated locomotor progression, by permitting translation in one desired direction and correcting for deviations from this direction.

During the bouncing progression, the centre of gravity of the body repeatedly rises and falls, remaining at roughly the same mean height above the ground so long as the rider is successful in his performance. The magnitude of the upthrust exerted against the ground varies with time, being zero during the periods of free flight, when the tip of the plunger is off the ground. Since the average thrust over any extended period must balance the body weight, the peak thrust at each bounce must correspondingly exceed body weight. It is this excess that is responsible for throwing the body upwards at each bounce. The individual 'bounces' in the bounding progression are not quite like the bounces of a rubber ball. The heights of successive bounces do not progressively diminish, as do those of an inert ball. It is the activity of the rider that makes this difference.

CATCHING AND THROWING

During the upward part of the free flight phase, the upward momentum of the body diminishes to zero under the action of gravity, and thereafter the body gradually acquires increasing downward momentum as it falls. When the moment for landing approaches, the rider extends his legs in preparation to receive the impact. He then allows his legs to give under the increasing load of the thrust against the crossbar during the compression of the spring. A little later, when the downward momentum has been almost completely absorbed, he extends his legs again strongly, and develops a very strong thrust against the crossbar, compressing the spring further. The increased thrust completes the arrest of the downward movement and propels the body upwards. The legs are stiffened and continue to extend so that the feet remain in contact with the crossbar in spite of the upward movement of the trunk, until all the energy stored in the spring has been converted into kinetic energy of upward motion of the body. The 'bounce' thus contains a 'catching' phase followed by an actively thrusting upward 'throwing' phase. Energy is fed into the system by the rider's muscular activity at each bounce. This makes up for the inevitable losses of energy to friction, and accounts for the maintained heights of successive bounces.

When the area of support is larger than just the tip of the plunger of the pogo-stick, the body can be prevented from falling over without recourse to repeated bounds into the air. It is, however, still necessary to provide a well-co-ordinated series of thrusts against the ground, with suitable adjustments not only of the magnitude of the thrust, but also of its direction and point of application.

INITIATION OF THE SLOW WALK

It is possible to become aware of the nature of the sequence of changes necessary for the initiation of a walk by paying special attention to the sensations from one's legs when changing from quiet standing into a slow forward walk. The routine for initiating a progression at the walk includes several stages. The trunk is first deliberately swayed to one side so that the whole of the weight can be taken on one foot. The other foot can then be lifted. A small excess backward movement of the thrust point now sets the trunk moving forwards (Figure 7.2(a)). The correction that would normally follow such a movement must now be switched off. As the trunk continues to accelerate forwards, the free leg is 'furled' by bending at the knee, and swung forward. The activity of the muscles spanning the hip joint of the supporting leg is also continually readjusted at this time so that, as the leg tips forward, the trunk retains its original attitude without tilting.

The need for some preparatory lateral sway may be illustrated by the following simple experiment. Stand close beside a heavy piece of furniture such as a massive table, adopting a comfortable upright stance with the feet slightly apart and with one hip, say the left, in close contact with the table. You will then find it very much easier to lift your left foot than your right. The reason is that the sway to the left that normally precedes the lifting of the right foot is, in this case, prevented by the presence of the table. To achieve the necessary shift of the centre of gravity you have to lean sideways over the table with the upper body, a manoeuvre that is noticeably unusual.

During the forward tilt of the support leg there is a tendency for the trunk to fall downwards as well as moving forwards. At this point the swinging leg is straightened and aimed at the ground ready to receive the impact of the falling trunk. After the foot has touched down (Figure 7.2(b)), the receiving leg bends to absorb the vertical momentum of the moving trunk but the horizontal momentum continues to carry the trunk forwards. There follows a phase in which the weight is supported on the two legs, one in front of the other, while the body is moving steadily forwards, transferring the weight gradually from one foot to the other until the whole of the weight comes to be carried by

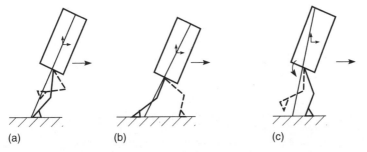

(a)   (b)   (c)

Figure 7.2 Stages in bipedal walking. (a) Forward swing of the free leg; (b) aiming and touch-down; (c) transfer of weight to the new leading leg.

the forward foot. As the weight comes off the previously supporting leg, that leg is furled and swung forward in turn in a stepping action (Figure 7.2(c)). Meanwhile the new supporting leg straightens to restore the trunk to its original height above the ground.

As one leg is swung forward past the other, a new cycle of actions is initiated. The cycle then repeats so long as the walk continues, and one can distinguish four phases in each cycle – two periods of support on two legs alternating with two periods of one-legged support, first on one leg, then on the other.

GAIT DIAGRAMS

One can represent the sequence of events in a linear diagram such as Figure 7.3(a). In this diagram, the horizontal line represents the progress of time, from left to right. Symbols immediately above the line indicate the moments when a foot leaves the ground; symbols below the line indicate moments of touch-down; open circles for the left foot, and filled circles for the right. The row of insets (Figure 7.3(b)) indicate which feet are on the ground in each of the successive phases.

Since the progression is regular, we can adopt a cyclic representation. In Figure 7.4, the line of time progression has been bent round in a circle, the moments of touch-down now being inside the circle and the moments of lifting outside. The succession of support patterns is arranged around the circle, a little further out. In reading a cyclic diagram of this kind, we imagine an arrow moving round the circle like the hand of a clock (Figure 7.5), pointing in succession to the individual

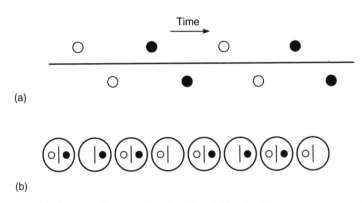

Figure 7.3 (a) Timing diagram for the bipedal walk. Time progresses steadily from left to right. A symbol above the line indicates a moment of lifting, a symbol below the line indicates a moment of foot placement: ○ = left leg; ● = right leg. (b) Sequence of support patterns indicating which feet are on the ground during each epoch of the progression.

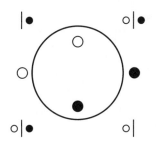

Figure 7.4 Cyclic gait diagram for the bipedal walk. Stages in the locomotory cycle are set out clockwise round a circle like the hour-markings on a clockface. A symbol just inside the circle indicates that it is at this stage in the cycle that the indicated foot is placed on the ground. A symbol just outside the circle indicates a moment of lifting. The plan diagrams arranged further out indicate which feet are on the ground at the corresponding epochs in the cycle. ○ = left foot; ● = right foot.

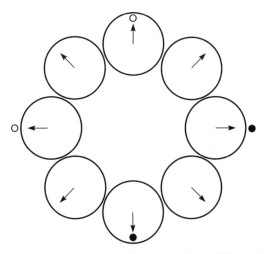

Figure 7.5 Successive appearances of the clockface of Figure 7.4 as the arrow indicating the current moment moves progressively round and points in turn to the symbols marking the events in the cycle.

events as they occur. The arrow makes one revolution for each complete cycle of locomotor progression.

Figures 7.6(a) and 7.6(b), indicate the relative durations of the support by each of the legs. In these two diagrams the durations of the swing phases have been taken as equal to the durations of the phases of two-legged support, though it is usual for the two-legged support phase to be relatively rather shorter than that shown here.

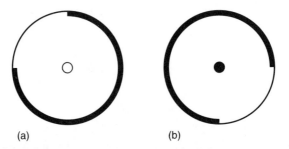

(a)   (b)

Figure 7.6 Relative durations of the support phase (thick line) and swing phase (thin line) during bipedal walking.

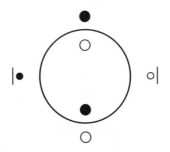

Figure 7.7 Cyclic gait diagram for the race-walk, in which two feet are on the ground together for only a very short time.

As the speed of walking increases, there is an increase in the forcefulness of the straightening of the legs during the phases of one-legged support. This propels the trunk upwards so that its subsequent fall is delayed. Time is thus gained in which the swinging leg can be aimed to reach further forward. Another effect of the increased thrust is that the absorption of the downward momentum and the development of appropriate upward momentum can be achieved in a shorter time. The relative durations of the two-legged support phases can then be reduced. Figures 7.7 and 7.8 represent the sequence in the racing walk, which is the fastest mode of progression available while retaining at least one foot on the ground at all times. Note that, in these cyclic diagrams, it is the **relative** durations of the phases that are indicated, not their absolute duration.

Since the leg thrusts are applied to the trunk through the pelvis and since the hips are set out to the side of the midline, these leg thrusts produce a complex series of accelerations of the trunk at each step. There are pitching, rolling and yawing accelerations as well as accelerations in the vertical and in both horizontal directions, lateral and fore-and-aft.

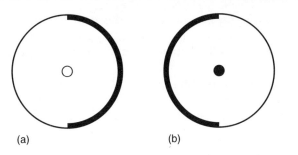

Figure 7.8 Relative durations of the support phase (thick line) and swing phase (thin line) during the race-walk.

TRUNK MOVEMENTS DURING WALKING

The trunk is not a rigid structure, so different parts of the trunk do not execute identical motions. There is considerable apparent twisting of the trunk since the yawing movements of the shoulders are quite different from those of the pelvis. However, most of this relative movement between hips and shoulders is due to sliding of the shoulder-blades over the ribcage rather than to actual torsion of the vertebral column. In rapid walking, strong rolling movements of the pelvis are used to increase the effective length of the thrusting leg in its stance phase. These pelvic movements are in the opposite direction to those expected from the elastic reaction to the thrust force. Thus, where one might expect the sacral part of the pelvis to sink relative to the hip when the weight comes onto that leg, in fact what happens is that the hip is actively pushed downwards, so that the sacrum and vertebral column are lifted relative to the hip as well as being lifted by the upward movement of the hip itself due to the straightening of the leg.

The swinging movements of the arms that are associated with the forward and backward movements of the shoulders serve to generate fluctuating angular momentum of the trunk in yaw to counteract the fluctuating torques about the vertical axis that are exerted by the alternating limb thrusts. Each leg produces an opposite torque at heel-strike from that exerted during the last stage of thrust before take-off.

BIPEDAL RUNNING

To increase the speed over the ground further, it is necessary to increase the stride length, that is to say, the distance between the successive placements of an individual foot. This can be achieved by a further increase in the forcefulness of the thrust by the legs. In running, each leg in turn thrusts the trunk upwards with sufficient momentum to propel the body forwards and upwards in free flight with both feet off the ground before the next touch-down. The corresponding cyclic diagrams and relative support durations are given in Figure 7.9 for a middle-distance runner and in Figure 7.10 for a sprinter.

In the absence of supporting forces, the action of gravity on the mass of a body causes it to accelerate towards the centre of the earth. If the body is supported at a fixed height above the ground, the supporting force must be equal to the product of the mass multiplied by an acceleration of a magnitude equal to that of the acceleration due to gravity in free fall but this time directed upwards. If the support force differs from this value, the body will accelerate, upwards or downwards as the case may be, according to the magnitude of the force.

In the case of the fluctuating support forces involved in locomotion, where the average height of the centre of gravity of the body above the ground remains the same, as it does for periods which are an exact multiple of the duration of the locomotor cycle, the average magnitude of the supporting thrust must also remain the same over the duration of each cycle. In gaits such as running which involve periods in which there are no feet on the ground and where there is consequently no upthrust force available for a time, the average has to be preserved by exerting extra force during those other times when ground contact is available.

The action of the excess upthrust is to accelerate the body upwards and this takes the centre of gravity further and further away from the ground. If the thrust is to be maintained, the thrusting leg must increase in length, but there is a limit to the anatomically possible extension of the limbs. For this reason the period of extra thrust prior to take-off is preceded by a short period during which the body is allowed to sink by flexing the supporting leg. The full thrust can then be exerted for a longer time.

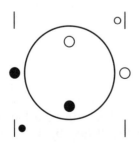

Figure 7.9 Cyclic gait diagram for a middle-distance runner.

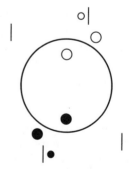

Figure 7.10 Cyclic gait diagram for a sprinter.

When the subject breaks into a run, he must start with a deliberate preparatory flexing of the legs. Once the run is in progress, however, the necessary flexion for each stride is provided in the course of the catching process by which the receiving leg absorbs the downward momentum of the trunk after each period of free flight.

To some extent, the action of the limbs in running resembles the action of a pogo-stick, where in bounding progression the energy developed during the falling phase of each bound is stored in the spring of the pogo-stick and used later to assist in the upward launch into the next bound. Simple bouncing, like that of a rubber ball, is not sufficient for continued progression because of the energy losses due to friction. To maintain the progression some energy in the form of work has to be fed into the system during each successive take-off phase. This energy comes from muscular activity in using a pogo-stick just as it does during running.

The relation between running and the action of a pogo-stick has prompted the invention of a device for assisted running. The operator wears a light framework supporting an arrangement of levers and springs which transmit the thrusts exerted on the pedals indirectly to artificial feet. The effect is to increase the effective length of the legs and, at the same time, to extend the range of lengths over which force can be exerted against the ground. By thus lengthening the time during which thrust can be exerted during the stance phase, the body can be thrown up further at each stride, and this extends the potential stride length and consequently increases the speed over the ground. The springs in the device store energy on compression during the catching phase after each foot has touched down, and release this energy again to assist with the subsequent push-off, just as in the pogo-stick. The device is effective in increasing the speed over the ground but has proved rather cumbersome for mounting and dismounting. Skill is required for steering it.

THE SPRINT START

In sprinting races, the athlete needs to make a very rapid transition from a stationary posture to as great a forward speed as possible, the transition being completed in the shortest possible time. The required acceleration of the mass of the body calls for the exertion of considerable muscular effort but there is no advantage if too much of this effort is expended in lifting the body upwards. The solution is to adopt an all-fours starting position with a good deal of the weight taken on the fingers. The legs are extended backwards, one behind the other, with the feet resting against specially shaped blocks pegged to the track. The function of the blocks is to provide a purchase for a horizontal force against the ground, since to rely on friction alone would involve too great a risk of slipping. When the starting gun is fired, the athlete pushes very strongly against the blocks. The resulting thrust lifts the body so that the hands leave the ground (Figure 7.11(a)). As well as greatly increasing the compressive thrust of the legs in propping, the athlete also exerts considerable torque at the hip, in paddle action (Figure 7.11(b)). At this stage, the athlete's centre of gravity is well forward of his hip joints so that, without this paddle action, the trunk would tend to topple forward over the hips.

The actions of the various forces on the two ends of the leg are shown in Figure 7.11(c). At the foot, the vertical upthrust from the ground is shown as a little greater than body weight. The horizontal force transmitted from the ground, through the blocks, is made up of two components. One of these resists the tendency for the inclined leg to tilt over under the action of the clockwise couple made up of the vertical forces at the two ends of the leg (Figure 6.27). The other resists the clockwise torque applied across the hip. The resultant thrust against the foot is shown as an arrow with two fleches. At the top end of the leg we have a corresponding set of vertical and horizontal forces, together with a torque. The effect of this clockwise torque is to shift the line of action of the thrust against the trunk to the position indicated by the arrow with three fleches. This arrow passes through the centre of gravity of the body. This means that the leg thrust does not impart any rotation to the trunk.

Figure 7.11(d) shows the effect on the body. The leg thrust projects the body upwards and forwards, while the action of gravity accelerates it downwards. Resolution of these two effects indicates, by the arrow with two fleches, that the body accelerates forwards and upwards into a shallow parabolic trajectory, since the upward component of acceleration is comparatively small. It needs to be sufficient only for the subsequent free-fall phase to last long enough for the leading leg to be appropriately positioned ready for the next touch-down. The first few strides at the sprint are similar in principle to the initial take-off stride but, once the athlete has started to move, only a very much smaller horizontal force is available to him from the friction between his shoes and the ground, even with the aid of spikes. The attitude of the sprinter's trunk becomes more upright for the later parts of the race.

In bounding progression, as in running, the avoidance of falling is achieved by adjustment of the aiming of the leg that is to receive the impact of the trunk in its descent after each phase of free flight. This aiming governs the direction along which the next upthrust will be developed between the trunk and the ground. Thus any deviation from the desired course that happens to have resulted from earlier thrusts can be corrected by an appropriate choice of direction for the next thrust. Continued progression calls for an adjustment of aiming

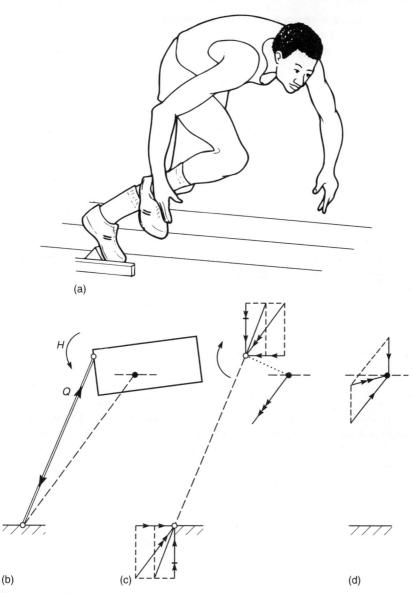

Figure 7.11 The sprint start. (a) The attitude of the athlete: one leg has already left the blocks while the other is thrusting strongly against a point well behind the centre of gravity of the body (after a photo of Tommy Smith by E.D. Lacey). (b) Diagram of the forces in a sprint start: the limb develops a compressive thrust Q by the action of the single-joint extensors such as quadriceps (propping), together with a torque H at the hip developed by two-joint muscles such as the hamstrings (paddle action). (c) Resolution of the forces acting at the two ends of the limb. Note the magnitude of the horizontal force at the ground. The starting blocks provide the purchase for this force. (d) Forces acting at the centre of gravity.

for each successive footfall, and the avoidance of falling depends on continuation of this succession of adjustments. The progression can be brought to a halt by choosing sufficiently strong backwardly directed thrusts.

BIPEDAL LEAPING PROGRESSION

A different style of high-speed bipedal locomotion is adopted by certain arboreal monkeys when crossing an open space on the ground. They proceed in a series of sideways leaps, the two feet landing in rapid succession. This is followed by a strong upward push with both legs, which then leave the ground one after the other. The cyclic gait diagram for this mode of progression is shown in Figure 7.12. During the bounding progression of the monkey, the animal holds both its arms, and its long tail, well up and away from its trunk. The downward momentum of each of these appendages has to be arrested at each landing, and new upward momentum has to be generated in them for take-off. Alteration in the thrusts to produce these individual momentum changes is used in fine adjustment of the attitude of the trunk to take account of unexpected irregularities in the surface of the terrain.

This form of leaping progression is appropriate where the body weight is small compared with the muscular forces available from the legs. It is interesting to observe that when astronauts first walked on the moon, although they were encumbered by spacesuits and the backpacks containing their life-support systems, they spontaneously adopted a diagonal leaping gait for all but the shortest distances. They found that their leg musculature could readily throw the whole mass of their loaded bodies clear of the ground for a leap. Because the gravitational attraction of the moon is so much less than that of the earth, a larger proportion of the muscular effort available to them could

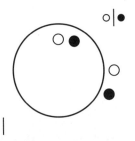

Figure 7.12 Cyclic gait diagram for bipedal leaping progression, as used by certain arboreal monkeys when crossing open spaces on the ground. This gait was also used by astronauts on the moon.

be deployed in generating upward acceleration. Once clear of the ground, the ensuing free-fall phase lasts longer in the reduced gravitational field of the moon than it would on the surface of the earth. This combination leads to a great increase in potential stride length and consequently also in speed over the ground.

The bipedal leaping gait of the monkey differs from that of the kangaroo, in which the two hindlegs operate in very close synchrony.

THE CRUTCH WALK

The heavier primates tend not to use the bipedal leaping gait. They mostly have the habit that, when not actively moving from place to place, they squat on the hindquarters, leaving both hands free of the ground and available for various manipulative tasks. For forward progression, they often lean forward, place both hands on the ground, taking the weight on the knuckles, and then, after surging the weight forward over straight arms, they swing both legs forward together between their hands. The motion resembles that of a man on crutches. The ground can be covered fairly rapidly provided that there are no obstacles. Since contact with the ground is maintained throughout this mode of progression, it is referred to as the 'crutch walk'. If the terrain is very irregular, with much undergrowth and fallen branches, a quadrupedal gait is preferred.

In the slower modes of progression, where there is always at least one foot on the ground, the progression can be brought to a halt during any one of the sway phases, with the centre of gravity positioned somewhere over the area of support provided by the contact with the ground. In man, even a single foot can provide an adequate area of support so that the subject can remain standing on one foot for some time. While he is doing so, a continuing series of swaying actions takes place and the centre of thrust is moved about, remaining, however, all the time within the area of ground contact. The adjustments in the position of the centre of thrust are brought about by changes in the muscle forces that exert torque about the ankle joint.

QUADRUPEDAL LOCOMOTION

The legs and feet of digitigrade quadrupeds offer only very small individual areas of ground contact, and these animals are unable to balance on a single leg. When standing in one place or moving in slow progression the body is supported on a base provided by at least three legs. We need to look now at the tasks involved when a quadruped wishes to initiate a locomotor progression to move from one place to another.

The nature of the problem may perhaps be appreciated by considering the comparable task of moving a grand piano without sliding the feet and without benefit of wheels or rollers. The main mass of the body of the piano is supported, well above the ground, like the trunk of a horse. The legs must perform two functions in supporting the weight. The most obvious is that they must be stiff enough to resist compression along their length. Less obvious, but no less important, is the function of bracing against change in the angle between the legs and the trunk. In the absence of such bracing, the structure is unstable and is readily pushed over, even if the legs are upright. If any one of the legs deviates ever so slightly from being precisely vertical, the weight of the body will tend to tip that leg over to increase the deviation, and the structure collapses like a house of cards.

In a piece of furniture, like a piano or a table, the legs are firmly braced to the 'trunk' by stiff brackets. In an animal, the stiffness of the corresponding bracing can be varied, as can also the the stiffness with which the legs resist compression along their length. It is by such adjustments of stiffness that an animal performs its acts of locomotion.

Movement in opposite directions at any particular joint is resisted by separate sets of muscles so that an adjustment in the bracing stiffnesses on opposite sides of a proximal joint produces an alteration in the aiming of the limb. If the feet are on the ground, a change in the aiming of the legs relative to the trunk implies a movement of the trunk over the ground. You can see an example of this when a horse is grazing. The movement of the trunk over the feet is achieved by adjusting the bracing between the legs and the trunk to alter the aiming of the legs. At the same time, adjustments have to be made in the thrusts developed by each of the legs to take account of the changes in the proportion of the weight that is to be carried on each leg.

The example of the grand piano shows us that three legs are quite sufficient to support the weight. Thus, if four legs are available, then so long as the centre of gravity of the trunk lies over the triangle of support provided by the other three legs, the fourth leg is free to be lifted. It can then be repositioned without the animal falling over.

The trick is to move the centre of gravity over the feet while all four feet are on the ground, transferring the weight from one triangle of support to another. The free leg is then advanced to establish potential support in a new position and the trunk is moved forward, again with all four feet on the ground, until its centre of gravity is safely over the new triangle of support. The cycle can then be repeated, swinging forward another foot in its turn. When you watch a horse performing this manoeuvre while it is grazing, you will find that, with a little practice, you can always predict which leg will be the next one to be moved. It turns out that there is only one sequence in which the legs can be moved without the animal falling over if, when each leg is to be moved forward, full advantage is taken of all possible forward movement of the trunk over the supporting legs so that the moving foot is advanced to the full extent of its reach.

THE 'CANONICAL' SEQUENCE OF LIMB MOVEMENTS AT THE CRAWL WALK

There are various ways in which one can convince oneself as to the uniqueness of the sequence. One way is to consider logical possibilities. In a smooth forward progression, at the 'crawl walk', in which one leg is to be moved at a time, we look at the situation of the limbs at each of the four moments at which a foot has just been placed on the ground. There are four possible relative positions for each foot at such moments.

1. **Full ahead:** The foot is the one that has just touched down, in which case it will be well forward relative to the trunk.
2. **Half ahead:** The foot was the previous one to touch down and the trunk has started to move forwards over it.
3. **Half trailing:** The foot is past the middle of its stance phase but there is, as yet, no urgency about moving it.
4. **Fully trailing:** The trunk has passed almost as far over the foot as it can. This foot must therefore be the next one to be lifted.

If each leg can be in any one of these four relative positions, there are 24 possible support patterns to consider. Other patterns in which more than one foot occupies a particular relative position can be disregarded since this arrangement implies that at some stage in the progression two legs would have to be lifted at the same time. If this were to happen at a slow progression, the animal would fall over.

Figure 7.13 sets out the full set of available patterns, with the potential positions for the feet indicated by small circles and the actual positions shown by triangles for forefeet and circles for hindfeet. Open symbols indicate the left side and filled symbols the right. The head is to the top of the page in each case. The small crosses mark the projections of the centre of gravity of the trunk. In this array, each foot occupies each of the four possible positions in six instances, which differ among themselves in the arrangement of the other three feet.

The group of 24 support patterns can be subdivided into two sets of 12. In one group the next foot to be lifted is a hindfoot, in the other it is a forefoot. The triangle of support by the other three feet when a forefoot is to be lifted always encloses the projection of the centre of gravity. So these 12 patterns are all 'safe'.

When the next foot to be lifted is a hindfoot, the forward apex of the

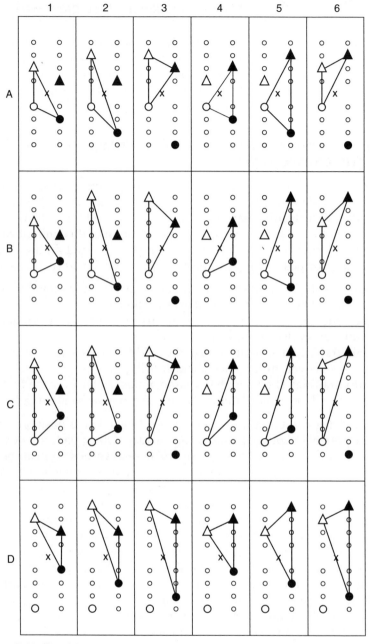

Figure 7.13 The 24 possible support patterns for a quadruped if only one leg is to be lifted at a time and, at each step, the lifted leg is to be swung forward to the full available extent. Each foot can be in one of four positions (indicated by the smaller circles) at the moment at which one of the feet is about to be lifted: full ahead; half ahead; half trailing; fully trailing and about to be lifted. △ = left forefoot; ▲ = right forefoot; ○ = left hindfoot; ● = right hindfoot; × = centre of gravity. (See also Figure 7.14.)

triangle of support provided by the other three legs is the position of the foot that was most recently moved. In the four cases where this was an opposite forefoot, the rearmost side of the triangle of support passes through, or very close to, the projection of the centre of gravity. These four support patterns can accordingly also be regarded as 'safe'. In the other eight cases, the rearmost side of the support triangle passes in front of the projection of the centre of gravity, so these support patterns are unstable. In the figure, the unstable patterns are, by row and column, A3, A6, B6, C6, D1, D2, D3, and D4.

Each of the 24 support patterns under consideration can be linked to another which is produced from the first by a single phase of forward progression. Thus the total of 24 can be subdivided into six sets of four where each set of four consists of patterns passed through in succession during steady forward progression. All but one of these six sets include a 'prohibited' (i.e. unstable) pattern of support at some stage. This leaves a single, unique, sequence of limb movements consistent with the maintenance of stability. The 'acceptable' sequence of support patterns is A5, B3, C1, D5, A5, and so on. The corresponding footfall sequence is: left hind, left fore, right hind, right fore, and so on.

The uniqueness of this sequence can also be demonstrated with a model of a horse, made with jointed legs, the friction at each joint being adjusted so that the attitudes of the limbs can be easily changed by the operator, while the legs are stiff enough to bear the weight of the model. Each foot of the model is pegged down to a track. The demonstrator can then move the model forward over the track, whereupon each joint necessarily adjusts itself to the new posture. As each leg in turn reaches the limit of available extension, its foot is unpegged from the track, the leg is moved forward as far as it will go, and the foot is pegged down again before proceeding with the forward progression of the trunk. No matter what starting position is chosen, one finds that very soon a single sequence of leg movements becomes forced.

One can also experiment for oneself with various sequences of limb movements when crawling on all fours. The unique sequence soon emerges. One can readily understand how it comes about that any young animal, including the human infant, during the initial struggles to maintain balance during forward progression, soon learns to adopt this particular sequence of limb movements as 'preferred'.

It is possible to adopt a different sequence of limb movements if the trunk is not moved forwards at each stage as far as it will go. This can happen in climbing, where the weight is taken on the hindlegs in compression with the forelegs in tension, hanging either from claws or from a hand-hold. The trunk is not advanced over the supporting feet during the forward reach of a foreleg, but only after a secure new grip has been established. The body is then hauled up to relieve the load on the trailing hindleg, allowing it to be repositioned to provide a stable base from which the next foreleg can be advanced. The sequence then may be: left fore, left hind, right fore, right hind and so on. The 'stride length' is necessarily less in this mode of progression than it can be for continuous movement over open ground.

In Figure 7.14(a)–(e), five successive stages in the progression at the crawl walk are illustrated in schematic plan views. At each of these five stages, one of the feet is in the fully trailing position and is about to be lifted. The other three feet that are to provide the support during the next swing phase are linked to show the triangle of support. The forward progression of the trunk is indicated by the sloping line that connects the successive positions of the projection of the centre of gravity. In the lower part of the figure, the horizontal line indicates the progress of time, from left to right, with symbols for the feet shown above the line for a moment of lifting and below the line for a moment of touch-down.

When the left hindfoot is lifted, between stage (a) and stage (b), the body is supported on the triangle ABD. During the forward movements of the left forefoot and the right hindfoot, the projection of the centre of gravity passes across the line CB. The body is stable at all times,

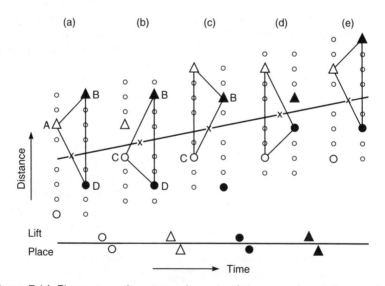

Figure 7.14 Five successive stages in a steady progression at the crawl walk (grazing walk). Symbols as in Figure 7.13.

there being always at least three feet on the ground. The progression can be interrupted at any stage.

CONTINUOUS PROGRESSION AT THE WALK

The horse uses the crawl walk only for the rather intermittent progression associated with the feeding behaviour of grazing. Between steps, the animal remains more or less in one place for a time while cropping the vegetation in the immediate neighbourhood of its head. For continuous progression at the walk the movements of the individual limbs follow one another in an unbroken sequence. The trunk maintains its forward momentum so that, at a transition such as that from the triangle DBC to the triangle ABC in Figure 7.14 (b) and (c), the right hindfoot can be lifted before the left forefoot has touched down, the trunk meanwhile being supported only on two legs. A timing diagram for this progression is given in Figure 7.15.

At the top of the figure the two horizontal lines with associated symbols above and below them indicate separately the moments of lifting and placing of the forelegs (upper line) and hindlegs (lower line). This part of the figure can be compared with Figure 7.3 for the bipedal walk. The movements of the forelegs and also those of the hindlegs resemble those of a walking man, so that the movements of the walking horse resemble those of two men striding along one behind the other, out of step by a quarter of a cycle.

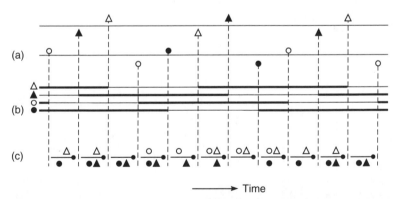

Figure 7.15 Timing diagram for the routine walk. (a) Moments of lifting (above the line) and of placing (below the line) for forelegs and hindlegs; (b) durations of the support phases (thick lines) and of the swing phases (thin); (c) patterns of support, with the head to the right in each case.

In the middle part of the figure the four horizontal lines indicate the durations of the support phases (thick lines) and swing phases (thin lines) for each of the four legs. The time scale is the same as for the upper part of the figure. The cycle is arbitrarily divided into eight epochs at the moments of lifting and placing of the feet.

At the bottom are shown the support patterns in each of the eight epochs. Each pattern shown applies to the whole of the corresponding epoch. It will be noted that epochs of three-point support are separated by epochs in which there are only two feet on the ground, these being alternately diagonal or lateral pairs.

This mode of progression achieves increased speed over the ground at the expense of being able to stop instantly and without notice if circumstances should make this advisable. It is sometimes convenient to refer to this continuous gait as the 'routine walk', to distinguish it from the crawl walk which lacks the unstable phases with only two feet on the ground. The routine walk is the gait adopted by very many animals for unhurried progression from one place to another. It can be executed at a considerable range of speeds over the ground.

Figure 7.16 shows, at the top, the clockface markings for the cyclic

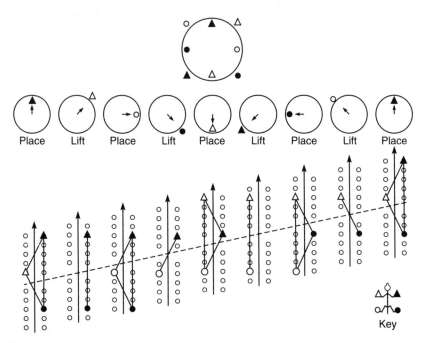

Figure 7.16 Succession of support patterns at the routine walk. Above: moments of lifting and placing arranged like the hour-markings on a clockface to show the repetitive nature of the cycle. Below: support patterns at successive stages.

gait diagram for the routine walk, together with the sequence of appearances of the clockface as the arrow points in turn to the moments of lifting and placing of the individual feet. The succession of support patterns is shown below, for comparison with Figure 7.14. This emphasizes the unstable phases where there are only two feet on the ground and the animal is relying on the forward momentum acquired during the preceding phase of three-point support. Any undesired motion that might develop during a phase of two-point support can be corrected at the ensuing three-point phase.

The full cyclic gait diagram for the routine walk of the horse is shown in Figure 7.17, with the support patterns in place around the central clockface and with corresponding side views of a walking horse opposite the appropriate phases.

Cyclic gait diagrams of this kind facilitate the comparison of one gait with another. They make clear the ways in which the gaits differ from, or resemble, one another. The diagrams also draw attention to the changes that an animal must make in the rhythm of its limb movements to effect the transition from one gait to another. The horseman

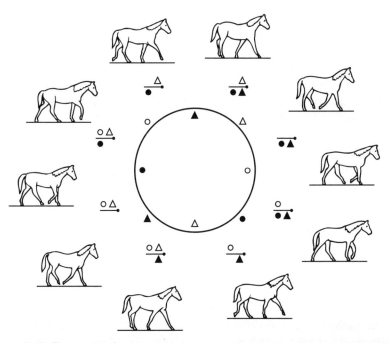

Figure 7.17 The cycle of movements at the routine walk of the quadruped. The support patterns shown in Figures 7.15 and 7.16, together with the corresponding side views, are here set out in appropriate positions around the clockface of Figure 7.16. (Outlines after Muybridge, 1893.)

can learn something here by inferring how he should adjust the selection and timing of the 'aids' by which he indicates to his mount that a specific change of pace is to be carried out.

The fact that the sequence of movements in the quadrupedal walk is similar in a great many animals has prompted some to suppose that the rhythm of the limb movements is controlled by some sort of 'central rhythm generator'. Support for this idea comes from experiments in which rhythmic movements of the four legs in a superficially normal-looking sequence can be elicited in reduced preparations on a treadmill. In these experiments it is usually necessary to support the animal's head in order to steer the progression along the belt of the treadmill. Rhythmic limb movements can also, in certain circumstances, be elicited by electrical or chemical stimulation of a strictly localized region of the midbrain. The underlying mechanism here lies in the combination of some of the reflexes described in the previous chapter.

We have seen that a movement of the trunk over the ground will elicit a reflex step in any limb that has reached a particular critical angle of tilt. We have also seen that flexion and extension in one limb affect the stretch reflex sensitivities, and thus the supporting reactions, in each of the other limbs, in a diagonal pattern of organization, the legs of a diagonal pair tending to be affected in the same sense. If a step is elicited in the right hindleg, the weight will be taken on the diagonal pair consisting of the left hindleg and the right foreleg. When the right hindleg touches down and, by developing its supporting reaction, resumes its contribution to weight-bearing, the thrusts in the right foreleg and left hindleg are reduced. It then becomes easier to elicit a step in whichever of these legs is approaching its critical angle of tilt. On the treadmill, the leg liftings are mechanically constrained to follow the canonical sequence after a few strides, no matter what the starting positions. It can therefore be argued that the apparent 'normality' of the locomotion on the treadmill in the reduced preparation is an artifact of the experimental conditions. The difference between reflex stepping and the stepping of active locomotion lies in the forcefulness of the forward thrusts exerted by the legs. In active locomotion the trunk has to be actively thrown forward at each stride.

A pattern of alternating limb movements may be elicited by stimulation of the midbrain in a reduced preparation with the trunk supported and the legs hanging free. Here there are no thrusts developed by the limbs because no resistance is offered at the feet. The motion is a succession of swing phases. The diagonal pattern of these swings can be attributed to the diagonal organization of the interactions between the flexor and extensor muscles of the four limbs that has already been referred to.

The subdivision of the limb movements in locomotion into 'swing' and 'stance' phases, while adequate for some purposes, is in fact an oversimplification. In normal locomotion each limb is involved, in sequence, in the following discrete processes:

- **Furl:** i.e. discontinue supporting thrust and fold up the limb to lift the foot clear of the ground.
- **Swing:** either passively, as a pendulum under the action of gravity, or at an accelerated speed by paddle action.
- **Aim:** i.e. extend the free limb to direct the foot towards a chosen landing site, and stiffen the limb in preparation for landing.
- **Catch:** i.e. the limb yields but resists compression, to absorb the momentum of the falling trunk, with some loss of gravitational potential.
- **Stance:** i.e. support the body weight after its unwanted downward momentum has been absorbed, and restore its gravitational potential.
- **Sway:** i.e. shift the centre of gravity over the feet to bring it to an appropriate relative position to provide purchase for the next limb thrust.
- **Thrust:** i.e. develop excess force to throw the body upwards and forwards into the next step.

In rapid locomotion, the aiming stage may include paddle action just before touch-down to ensure that the foot itself has no forward momentum that will need to be arrested at ground contact, since such arrest would have a braking effect on the forward movement of the body as a whole. The landing site has to be selected for each touch-down so that appropriate correction is provided for any unwanted component in the current motion of the trunk. It also has to give the appearance of providing a secure foothold. It is by adjustments of the aiming of the swinging legs that the animal achieves changes in course and speed.

THE RUNNING WALK

When considering bipedal locomotion, it was explained that the transition from walking to running is achieved by increasing the forcefulness of the thrusts at take-off in each leg. The increased thrust leads to a shorter stance phase, the liftings of the feet being relatively earlier in the cycle at the run than at the walk. At the same time the swing phase is extended and the placings are relatively delayed. A similar set of changes in timing can be seen in a comparison between the crawl walk and the routine walk in the quadruped, as shown by the linear timing diagrams of Figures 7.14 and 7.15. In both these gaits each foot is brought to the ground before the corresponding foot of the other side is lifted. For example, the placing of the right forefoot precedes the lifting of the left forefoot, and similarly for the other feet.

A further increase in speed, by additional forcefulness of the take-off thrusts, leads to the gait illustrated, in the horse, by the diagram of Figure 7.18. Here each transverse pair of legs, i.e. the two forelegs as a pair and the two hindlegs as a pair, behave like the legs of a man running, as illustrated in Figure 7.9, the foot of one side being lifted before its partner of the opposite side has touched down. However, while the gait of the running man involves unsupported phases with no ground contact, in the gait illustrated in Figure 7.18 there is always at least one foot on the ground. This is because each unsupported phase for one transverse pair coincides with a stance phase for the other transverse pair. It is accordingly appropriate to refer to this gait in the quadruped as a 'running walk'. Because there is always at least one foot on the ground at this gait, the progression does not involve large vertical bouncing. This feature contributes greatly to the comfort of the rider, while at the same time making it possible to cover con-

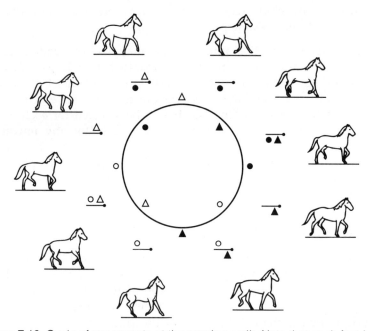

Figure 7.18 Cycle of movements at the running walk. Note that each foot is here in contact with the ground for only three-eighths of the cycle, compared with five-eighths of the cycle at the routine walk (Figure 7.17) and seven-eighths of the cycle in the grazing walk (Figure 7.14). In consequence there are periods where there is only one foot on the ground. There are, however, no unsupported phases. (Outlines after Muybridge, 1893.)

siderable distances quite rapidly and with a minimum of fatigue. Gaits such as this one, which provide comfort for the rider by avoiding undue bouncing, are referred to as 'easy gaits'.

TROTTING

The smooth progression at the running walk depends on a fairly evenly spaced four-beat rhythm of the footfalls. If the footfalls are not evenly spaced, they fall into groups of relatively closely spaced footfalls separated from other groups by larger intervals. There may be two groups in the cycle, as in the trots and in some gallops, or there may be only one group, as in the canters.

In the familiar trot of the horse, as illustrated in Figure 7.19, the two legs of each diagonal pair move more or less in synchrony with one another, so that these two feet come to the ground in rapid succession to provide a stance phase supported on a diagonal pair of legs. The body is then thrown up for an unsupported phase with all four feet clear of the ground before the feet of the other diagonal pair touch down. The gait may be likened to the progression of two men running

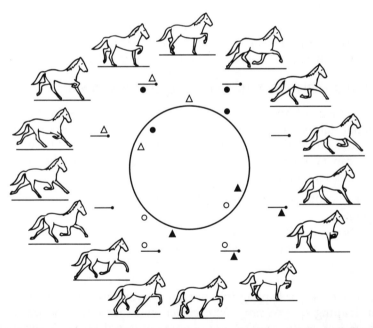

Figure 7.19 Cycle of leg movements and support patterns at the trot. The body is tossed from one diagonal pair of legs to the other. (Outlines after Muybridge, 1893.)

one behind the other almost completely out of step. When the left forefoot is on the ground, so is the right hindfoot also. This type of progression involves a brisk up-and-down bouncing of the trunk. It is this brisk bouncing that justifies the naming of the gait as a 'trot', rather than simply as a 'run'. Because the horse's body has substantial mass, the short period of this vertical oscillation implies that the legs act as very stiff springs and must develop substantial forces. Since the thrusts of foreleg and hindleg are applied to the trunk on opposite sides of the midline, the trunk is subjected to considerable torsional stresses occurring in opposite directions as the alternate diagonals come to the ground.

It is sometimes convenient to refer to this familiar trotting gait as a **diagonal trot** since the leg movements are coupled in diagonal pairs, in contrast with an otherwise similar gait involving coupling in lateral pairs. Here it is the two legs of the same side that swing forward at the same time. This gait is used in trotting races where the horse draws a light carriage called a 'sulky'. A long horizontal strap is fitted to the horse, running round behind the hindlegs just above the hocks and terminating at the front in loops round the forelegs just below the elbows. The effect of this strap is to constrain the movement of the foreleg so that it can be moved forwards only when the hindleg of the same side is also moving forwards. This **lateral trot** is sometimes referred to as the 'pace'. The maximum speed over the ground at the lateral trot is found to be very slightly greater than that at the diagonal trot, while the ride is considerably less comfortable.

PREPARATION OF THE CYCLIC GAIT DIAGRAM

The four legs of an animal may be associated in pairs in three ways: diagonal, lateral and transverse. The changeover of support from one leg to the other of a transverse pair can be effected in different ways. These can be characterized by the names given to the bipedal gaits. The transitions may be:

1. at the **walk**, in which case there is always at least one foot on the ground;
2. at the **race-walk**, where the lifting of each foot occurs just as its fellow of the opposite side is touching down, so that the duration of the phase of two-point support is reduced almost to zero;
3. at the **run**, where each foot is lifted before the other foot has touched down, leaving two unsupported phases in each cycle;
4. in **leaping** progression, where each cycle includes one phase with both feet on the ground and one unsupported phase. Phases with a single foot on the ground may precede take-off for the leap and may also occur during the landing after the unsupported phase.

We now have a number of criteria which can be used in combination to distinguish different gaits from one another and for deciding which gait is being performed by a particular animal at a specific time. The first step is to prepare a cyclic gait diagram. We can then inspect the diagram and apply the criteria in a series of tests. The results of these tests will tell us what gait it is that we are dealing with. The most satisfactory way to construct the gait diagram is to work from slow-motion cine film, or from a videotaped record with superposed time-coding. The record is examined, frame by frame, to determine which frames show each of the eight events that will be used as the basis of the analysis. These events are the moments of lifting and of placing of each of the four feet. A relative frame-number is noted for each event, continuing for as many cycles as are available in the record.

The next stage is to determine how many frames it takes to get from one end of a cycle to the other. If the record covers five full cycles, this gives us 32 values for the cycle duration, in numbers of frames, taking one cycle as the interval between successive occurrences of a particular event, such as a moment of lifting, or of placing, of a specific foot. A statistical test can be used to eliminate runs which are unacceptably ragged, or which are contaminated by gross changes in speed. We can now use a mean value for the cycle duration and, after deciding upon a reference point, such as the moment of placing of the left hindfoot, we can express the relative positions in the cycle of the other seven events of interest on a scale of 60 for the full cycle. The events can then readily be plotted on a clockface, making use of the familiarity of the minute-markings, and setting the reference event, conventionally, at 12 o'clock. To complete the cyclic gait diagram, schematic plan views are added around the circle to indicate which feet are on the ground in each of the phases between the individual events.

The criteria for distinguishing the gaits can now be applied to the gait diagram, seeking the answers to the following questions:

1. Are the footfalls evenly spaced, or are they grouped?
2. If grouped, are there two groups, or only one?
3. If there are two groups of footfalls in the cycle, is it a grouping by lateral coupling, by diagonal coupling, or by transverse coupling?
4. If the footfalls form a single group, is there a phase with three feet on the ground?
5. Considering the forelegs and hindlegs separately, are they walking, running, or leaping?

One advantage of the cyclic gait diagram as an aid to classification is that precise timings are not essential, so long as the sequence of the relevant events is clear. It is not always necessary to have a cine record since the answers to the questions set out above can sometimes be obtained by direct observation. One can then build up the cyclic gait diagram from these answers. For example, the description given earlier of the crutch walk leads to a gait diagram of the form of Figure 7.20. This shows the transverse coupling of the footfalls and indicates leaping transitions. Since there is always at least one foot on the ground, the gait can be characterized as a 'leaping walk'.

THE CANTER

An example of a leaping progression with a single group of footfalls is the canter of Figure 7.21. In this case, the sequence of footfalls is the same as in Figure 7.17 for the routine walk, but the footfalls are all grouped together into one half of the cycle. The liftings are all delayed, in comparison with the walk, but the sequence of support patterns in the lower right-hand part of the figure is the same as in the corresponding part of Figure 7.17.

There is a single unsupported phase, after which the horse lands, first on a hindleg, then on the foreleg of the same side, which is soon joined by the other hindleg to provide a phase of three-point support. During this phase, the weight is rocked forwards over a diagonal pair of legs while the first hindfoot is lifted and its contribution to weight-bearing is taken over by the second forefoot. The two phases of three-point support, together with the intervening phase of support on a diagonal pair of legs, provide a strong combined thrust to throw the body upwards and forwards into the unsupported phase. The legs of the second triangle then lift off in turn. The last to lift in this case is the left forefoot, which is diagonally opposite to the foot that lands first after the unsupported phase. Although the left forefoot is the last to

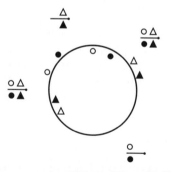

Figure 7.20 Cycle of movements at the crutch walk. The forelegs are lifted and extended together while the weight is taken on the hindlegs. After the forefeet touch down, the hindlegs are swung forwards briskly together between the widely-spaced forelegs.

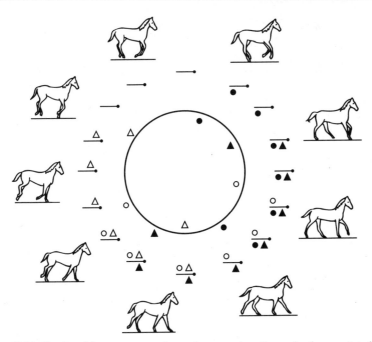

Figure 7.21 Cycle of leg movements and support patterns in the canter. Note that the footfalls occur in the same order as in the walk (Figure 7.17), but that they are here grouped together in time, to leave a single unsupported phase. (Outlines after Muybridge, 1893.)

land as well as being the last to lift off, this leg is referred to as the 'leading leg', because it is held prominently out in front during a large part of the cycle. Canters can be performed with either foreleg as the leading leg.

As already mentioned, increased speed over the ground is obtained by an increased forcefulness of the leg thrusts. This leads to increased stride length. A further increase in speed can be obtained by applying the thrusts in more rapid succession, with consequently shorter ground-contact time. Many animals switch to the canter when wishing to increase speed. The advantage of this change of gait can be seen in the comparison of relative ground-contact times illustrated in Figure 7.22. Here, below the cyclic gait diagrams for walk, trot, and fast canter, are shown the relative ground-contact times (shaded) for each of the four feet. The figure shows that, because the trot involves two unsupported phases, as compared with the single unsupported phase of the canter, relatively less time is spent by each foot on the ground at the trot than at the canter. To obtain the same impulse from a shorter thrust duration implies the exertion of a greater force. The increased speed of the

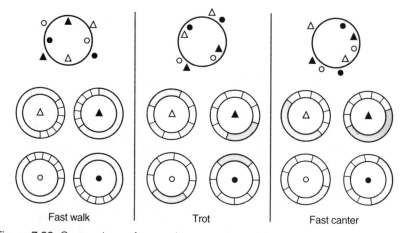

Figure 7.22 Comparison of ground-contact times for walk, trot and canter.

canter is thus obtained without demanding too great an increase in force.

THE GALLOP

As the speed increases at the canter, the footfalls of the diagonal pair that form the pivot for the main thrust tend to come closer together. At this point it is a simple matter for the placings of these two feet to become interchanged. The result of such an interchange is that the coupling changes from diagonal to transverse (Figure 7.23). It is then possible to obtain an additional increase in stride length by bringing into play the flexion and extension of the back that characterizes the gallop. The change from canter to gallop is smooth and gradual and the resolution of slow-motion cinematography is required for elucidating the intermediate stages.

Once the transverse coupling has been established, the gallop can be performed in various different ways. The canter and the various forms of gallop are all 'leaping gaits'. The horse, at the gallop, takes off from a foreleg, as in the canter, so that during the unsupported phase all four legs are carried close together under the body. He then lands on the hindlegs. The cat, on the other hand, takes off from the hindlegs, as for a jump (Figure 7.24), and lands on the forelegs, the body being at full stretch during the unsupported phase, with the legs extended to front and near. Many antelopes gallop in the same way as the cat. The greyhound and the cheetah, both sprint specialists, use a gallop with two, or even three, unsupported phases (Figure 7.25), one with the four feet held close together under the body, as in the horse gallop,

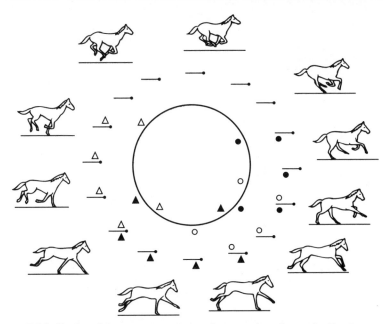

Figure 7.23 Cycle of leg movements and support patterns in the transverse gallop of the horse. In the rotatory gallop the order of landing of the forefeet is the opposite of that of the hindfeet, i.e. RH, LH, LF, RF (or LH, RH, RF, LF) as the case may be, instead of RH, LH, RF, LF (or LH, RH, LF, RF). (Outlines after Muybridge, 1893.)

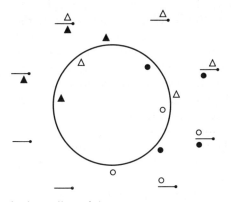

Figure 7.24 Stages in the gallop of the cat.

one at full stretch, as in the cat gallop, and sometimes a third un-supported phase between phases of support on a single forefoot. In these animals the contribution of the flexible back is very obvious to the observer.

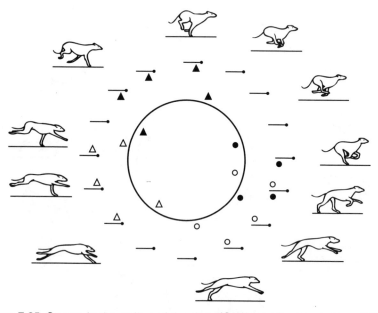

Figure 7.25 Stages in the gallop of the dog. (Outlines after Muybridge, 1893.)

When changing course, either at the canter or at the gallop, animals usually prefer to lead with the inside leg on the turn. For a change of lead at the canter, the hindlegs change over at the same time as the forelegs, as this avoids the risk of a hindfoot striking a forefoot, as might happen if the two transverse pairs were moving out of phase with one another. This risk is rather less at the gallop and, once the transverse coupling has become well established, it is possible to interchange the placings of the forelegs without altering the sequence for the hindlegs. Where the left–right sequence for the forelegs is the same as for the hindlegs, as it is in Figure 7.23, the gait is referred to as a 'transverse gallop'. If foreleg and hindleg placings are in opposite sequence, as in Figure 7.25, this is a 'rotatory gallop'.

In another form of gallop, favoured by certain antelopes, all four feet come to the ground more or less simultaneously, and all push off together to produce marked vertical bounds. It appears that the height of the leaps in this bounding progression, which is known as the 'pronk', serves as a discouraging signal to a potential predator. It shows that the bounding animal is in a high state of athletic fitness so that pursuit might involve more effort than is likely to prove worthwhile.

GAIT VARIANTS

There are many variations in the pattern of limb movements that are adopted by different animals when they wish to travel at a greater speed over the ground than is available at the walk. The four principal gaits already referred to, namely the walk, trot, canter and gallop, by no means exhaust the repertoire of gaits available to the horse alone. Mention has already been made of the lateral trot and of the even-spaced four-beat running walk. In earlier times we find frequent reference to the 'amble', as another very familiar mode of progression. For example, Rosalind in *As You Like It* says: 'Time travels in divers paces with divers persons. I'll tell you who Time ambles withal, who Time trots withal, who Time gallops withal, and who he stands still withal'. However, by the beginning of the eighteenth century, the amble seems to have gone out of favour, and we find that 'riding masters allow only the walk, trot and gallop'.

The range of variation is reflected in the large number of gait names that are in use, about 40 at a recent count. There are, however, considerable problems involved in associating particular names with specific gait patterns.

Although there are obvious disadvantages in using words in senses that can be taken to be ambiguous, it is not really surprising to find that before the advent of photography, there was a good deal of confusion as to what is to be understood by each of the names for the different gaits. One problem has been that the naming of gaits has depended on the judgement of an 'experienced observer'. Thus the analyst takes a specific example, with its label provided by whatever 'authority' happened to be on the spot at the time, and prepares a gait formula to describe it. Thereafter, this formula is intended to define that named gait. It is not usually possible to compare the judgements of different 'experts' in relation to a specific example of a gait performed at a particular time by a particular animal, and we run into the pitfalls of unconfirmable generalization. This leads to a situation in which similar formulations are provided for gaits to which different names have been assigned by different authorities, and different formulations have been derived from instances where different authorities happen to have used the same name at different times. Thus, in relation to one of the gaits of the horse, what A calls a 'rack' on one occasion may not be the same as what B calls a 'rack' on another occasion. Dictionaries, which report earlier usages, are not much help, since they tend to reflect the prevailing confusion, rather than resolving it.

The literature contains a number of gait descriptions of a somewhat theoretical nature, from the Duke of Newcastle (1743) to the present day. Muybridge, in the early 1880s, was the first to attempt detailed characterization of individual gaits from photographs. His monumental and pioneering photographic study, *Animal Locomotion* (1887) and related books, and his public demonstrations with his Zoopraxiscope, are based on more than 100 000 original photographs of a variety of animals, including man. He attempted to distinguish the various gaits on the basis of which feet were on the ground at successive phases in the progression. A number of gait names have been associated, by various authors, with specific sequences of support patterns. Many of these associations are clearly traditional. Others, in contrast, appear to be somewhat speculative in origin.

There are various criteria for distinguishing the gaits: footfall sequence, hoofprint pattern, support sequence, timing, and so on. For horses, the 'definitions of paces and movements', as printed in the British Horse Society's Dressage Rules, distinguish four walks, six trots (if we include piaffes and passages), and five canters, but no gallops, as well as the halt and reinback. Note that all these gaits are referred to in these rules as 'paces'.

The principal criterion used in the Dressage Rules appears to be the rhythm of the sound of the footfalls. Thus we find the walk defined as a 'marching pace in four time', the trot as a pace of 'two time' and the canter as a pace of 'three time'. Further distinctions are based on the personal assessment of a judge from their list of accredited judges. There are, naturally, no references to the 'easy gaits' since these are not used in dressage competitions.

It is not easy to decide, with the naked eye, just what it is that an individual horse is doing when progressing at each of the various gaits. The sequence of footfalls is not of much use to us in distinguishing different gaits since the same sequence is used for practically all the gaits found in the terrestrial vertebrates, with a few exceptions. As has been explained earlier, this sequence is the only one available for a slow walk without overbalancing if one leg is to be moved at a time and only once in each cycle, the trunk being moved forwards at each stage as far as the limb supports will allow, to make use of the full reach of each advancing leg. Exceptions to this sequence arise where two legs are brought to the ground almost simultaneously during more rapid locomotion, allowing minor interchanges in their placing sequence, as in the gallops and bounds, and in the 'crutch walk' of certain primates referred to earlier.

The system of cyclic gait diagrams, paying attention to the moments of lifting of specific feet in relation to the moments of placing of other feet, can be used to establish the classification of all the different gaits. It avoids the complications arising from small variations in the regularity of the cadence or in the durations of the individual support phases. Within each gait category, wide variations in individual patterns can be produced by adjusting the timings. Some of these variations will be obvious from the sound of the footfalls, but they should not affect the classifications, so long as the sequence of support patterns is not changed.

Cyclic gait diagrams prepared from over 200 photosequences of horses in motion reveal 60 discrete gait patterns, using the criteria for classification already set out. Of these, 37 are walks of various kinds (including running walks), 14 are trots, and nine are leaping gaits (canters and gallops).

A glance at the cyclic gait diagram is sufficient to reveal whether we are dealing with an evenly-spaced ('square') gait or whether there is a grouping of limb movements, such as into lateral, diagonal, or transverse couplings. The support patterns distributed round the circle indicate the occurrence of unsupported phases, as in the trots and leaping gaits, and help in the distinction between walking and running gaits.

Detailed scrutiny of the individual samples of locomotion leads to the clear impression that the traditional notion of regularly-repeated limb movements is an illusion. Even in the so called 'symmetrical' gaits, rarely is the pattern of one 'half' of a cycle a precise mirror image of the other 'half'. Furthermore, the relative timing of the movements of a particular limb varies from cycle to cycle. Far from being a locomotor automaton, with a set of gears, driven by some form of internal pattern generator, the horse appears to construct each limb movement individually, being influenced by the nature of the terrain as well as by the moment-to-moment adjustments of momentum essential to the maintenance of balance while regulating course and speed.

In some of the symmetrical patterns, the interval between the footfalls of one pair of feet is less than the interval before the next footfall. Couplings of this kind range from one extreme to the other. In one form of the walk, the footfalls of a diagonal pair of feet are almost simultaneous, as they are in the trot, but in this case all the changeovers are at the walk and there are no phases with all four feet off the ground at the same time, such as are characteristic of the trot. This gait can be referred to as a 'synchronized diagonal walk'. The range extends through gaits with variously-separated footfalls still retaining some degree of diagonal coupling and through gaits with some degree of lateral coupling, right through to gaits in which the footfalls of the two feet on the same side are almost simultaneous, to form a 'synchronized lateral walk'.

In some cases the degree of coupling may be closer in one half of the cycle than in the other, or closer for the placings than it is for the liftings, or there may be a mixture of degrees of coupling. Transverse coupling at the walk, such as occurs in the 'crutch walk' of certain primates, has not been observed in the horse.

An increase in speed over the ground is associated with a change from walking to running, achieved at the cost of reducing the time available for each leg to contribute supporting thrust.

Many of the variants encountered at the walk have their counterparts at faster gaits, in which the transverse pairs of legs make either race-walk changeovers or running changeovers. The variant couplings range from the traditional trot, with synchronized diagonal coupling, through four-beat diagonal trots, running walks, and lateral walks with spaced footfalls, to the synchronized lateral trot.

It is quite common for the actions of the diagonal pair that form the central support in the canter to be separated in time to some extent. This produces a four-beat canter. Even further such separation produces a 'pacing canter' with an extended phase of two-point lateral support.

The vigour of the leg thrusts at the canter varies according to the required speed over the ground. At one extreme, there is no unsupported phase, as the lifting of the leading foreleg is delayed until after the first hindfoot has come to the ground. This gait is a 'walking canter'.

Less energetic forms of the gallop are also encountered. In some cases the leading foreleg does not leave the ground until after the opposite hindfoot has touched down. One might speak of this as a 'walking gallop'. However, since both transverse pairs perform leaping changeovers, and there is no phase in which all four feet are off the ground at the same time, this gait might properly be called a 'leaping walk'.

No conclusions can be drawn as to the relative frequency of occurrence of the individual gait variants found in this study since the set of photosequences examined cannot be said to represent a comprehensive survey.

'GAITED HORSES'

There are a great many gait names in use for the so-called 'easy gaits' of the horse, most of which appear to be varieties of the running walk. It is not clear whether these gait names all indicate different gaits, or whether the same gait is given different names by different people. It appears to be true that different people use the same name for gaits that are significantly different.

Particular difficulties arise with the following terms: amble, pace, rack, running walk, singlefoot, stepping pace, fox trot, jog, flatfoot walk, and slow gait.

The term 'singlefoot' is sometimes said to indicate that 'the feet come to the ground one at a time'. This statement seems rather unhelpful, since it would apply to the great majority of gaits. A more acceptable alternative is to reserve the term for those running walks in which there are phases in which there is only one foot on the ground.

Other gait names to be considered are those associated particularly with three breeds of American 'gaited horses': the American Saddlebred, the Tennessee Walking Horse, and the Missouri Fox Trotting Horse. These breeds to some extent share a common ancestry, but the breed societies insist on sustaining a separation, and emphasize different features of the various gaits called for in their competitive displays. The American Saddlebred is shown at five gaits: walk, trot, canter, slow gait, and rack. The gaits of the Tennessee Walking Horse are named as: flatfoot walk, running walk, and canter. The Missouri Fox Trotting Horse Breed Association requires its competitors to display flatfoot walk, fox trot, and canter, with special emphasis on the fox trot. The descriptions given for each of these gaits in the publications of the breed societies do not make it very easy for the uninitiated to appreciate the distinctions.

The Rule Book of the Missouri Fox Trotting Horse Breed Association describes the fox trot as 'basically a diagonal trot', with 'periods of single leg support as well as periods of lateral support with no period in which all four feet are off the ground. . . . The Fox Trotting Horse is not a high-stepping horse.' The smoothness of the ride is emphasized and this is explained in terms of 'the sliding action of the rear feet'. The contradictions in this description are not resolved by the accompanying diagram of the support sequence, which suggests that the gait involves walking changeovers of the hindlegs with running changeovers of the forelegs.

In another publication of the same association, the fox trot is described in the following terms: 'The horse walks with the front feet and trots with the hindfeet. This extremely sure-footed gait gives the rider little jar since the hindfeet slide into place.' Such a gait, walking in front and trotting behind, is more appropriately referred to as a 'jog'. This gait is typical of an untrained horse under restraint. The horse carries relatively more weight on the forelegs and bounces up-and-down on the hindlegs. This is in marked contrast with the 'collected' condition preferred in dressage, where more of the weight is taken on the hindquarters.

Yet another description of the fox trot suggests that it is a diagonal running walk. Such gaits are performed by horses of all three breeds: Saddlebreds, Tennessee Walkers, and Missouri Fox Trotting Horses, as well as by the Peruvian Paso.

The fully-developed running walk of the Tennessee Walking Horse is equivalent to the 'rack' of the Saddlebred. The emphasis here is on speed over the ground, as well as on the smoothness of the ride. For the Tennessee Walking Horse there is additional emphasis on an exaggerated high-stepping action of the forelegs, often encouraged by fitting the forefeet with weighted shoes.

The 'flatfoot walk' of the Tennessee Walker is described in the breed literature as involving a 'diagonally-opposed movement' of the feet. For the Fox Trotting Horse, it is said to be 'a four-beat gait performed in a square and straight manner'. However, the gait samples offered with the label 'flatfoot walk', of either breed, all turn out to be fox trots, i.e. trotting in front and walking behind.

'Slow gait' is equated, by some, to 'stepping pace', which suggests a lateral walk. However, the small number of samples with the label 'slow gait' all turn out to be either fox trots or running walks.

Several variants of the running walk have been found, if we include all those with one or more of the changeovers of the transverse pairs at the race-walk or run. In the photosequences of this type examined, all degrees of coupling are represented, diagonal and lateral, in addition to examples with equally-spaced footfalls, and those showing various degrees of asymmetry. No obvious correlation has been found between the types of gait pattern and the breeds of the horses concerned. Such distinctions as exist between the gaits of Tennessee Walking Horses and those of the Missouri Fox Trotting Horses appear to depend primarily on the emphasis placed on the degree of elevation of the forefeet, and on the character of the display offered in the show ring.

GAITS OF ANIMALS OTHER THAN HORSES

There is no comparable detailed analysis of gait variants in animals other than horses but there is no reason to suppose that variation in gait pattern is confined to the horse. One needs to remember that, in addition to varying the gait pattern, an animal has to adjust the aiming of each individual limb placement in order to avoid insecure footholds and also to compensate for irregularities in the motion of the trunk occasioned by earlier foot placements. It is hard to see how detailed variation of this kind can be compatible with central control by a pattern generator.

The terminology developed here for distinguishing gait variants is intended to be descriptive rather than prescriptive, since many usages are firmly entrenched in common speech.

An interesting version of the synchronized diagonal walk is used by certain lizards that live in a hot desert environment. These lizards have relatively large feet in which the digits are long, arched, and widely splayed. Ground contact is restricted to small pads on the heels and on the tips of the digits. The animal moves in a series of short sprints at the diagonal race-walk, with little up and down movement. Between sprints it pauses with the body supported only on a diagonal pair of legs. Stability is ensured by the wide spacing of the digits, each foot having the same sort of widely-spaced ground contacts as those of a music stand. The feet of the diagonal pair of legs that are not being used for support are held up well clear of the ground, presumably to take advantage of the cooling effect of air movements. From time to time the lizard changes support diagonals, without moving forwards. This behaviour appears to be an adaptation to the high surface temperature of the sand of the desert. It helps to avoid dangerous overheating of the tissues of the feet.

Hildebrand has collected photosequences of the gaits of a large number of animals and has prepared linear gait diagrams from them. (He was kind enough to provide, from this collection, copies of those linear gait diagrams for the horse that have formed the bulk of the material on which my own analysis is based.) The timings of the liftings and placings of the feet during a single cycle can be expressed numerically in terms of nine parameters derived from the linear gait diagram, namely: the duration of the cycle, and the relative position within the cycle of the moments of lifting and of placing of each of the four feet. By making various simplifying assumptions, Hildebrand reduces to two the number of parameters needed to describe certain symmetrical gaits:

1. the contact time for one foot, as a proportion of the total cycle duration;
2. the proportion of the cycle duration that elapses between the footfall of a hindfoot and that of the forefoot of the same side.

These two variables were plotted on a two-dimensional array for over a thousand samples of symmetrical gaits, ranging over 156 genera, to provide a means of comparing the gaits of different animals. A modified scheme accommodates the asymmetrical gaits, and a further 330 samples of asymmetrical gaits from 79 genera were plotted on appropriate graphs. In the resulting arrays it was found that the points derived from animals in related taxonomic groups formed clusters in restricted regions of the parameter-space. The positioning of these clusters reflects the evolutionary relationships between the various species of animals.

Hildebrand noted that different regions of his parameter-space could be distinguished according to the corresponding sequences of support patterns and proposed a scheme for naming the gaits to correspond with these distinctions. Hildebrand's naming scheme differs from the namings in common use. Some of the gait names used by Muybridge also do not correspond with present-day usages which, as has already been explained, appear to involve a number of ambiguities.

JUMPING

If a quadruped is called upon to make a standing jump, it first moves its weight backwards onto the hindquarters, lowers its shoulders momentarily and then throws up the forepart of its body by thrusting with the forelegs and stiffening the back. The extra load placed on the hindlegs at this stage compresses the hindlimb, stretching the extensor muscles and preparing them for the development of the extra force needed for lift-off. As soon as the forequarters have started to rise, the forelegs are drawn up under the body in flexion and the main thrust for lift-off follows, using a simultaneous drive by both hindlegs. The momentum of the head plays an important part in this manoeuvre. The head is thrown strongly upwards just before the forelegs take off. Some of the upward momentum of the head can then be transferred to the forequarters to help in aligning the trunk with the hindlegs during the main thrust phase. As well as accelerating the body upwards and forwards like a javelin, the thrust of the hindlimbs tips the body forwards, so that it executes a pitching movement in the air and lands on the extended forelimbs.

If there is an obstacle in the path of an animal which is proceeding at a canter, there is a quick changeover from the sequence of limb movements characteristic of the canter, in which the principal effort of weight-bearing is concentrated on a single diagonal pair of legs, to the alternation of forelegs with hindlegs for the jump. The animal thus passes, with only a slight hesitation, from the canter into the movements of a jump.

The hindlegs make an extra half stride just before the jump so that, although the normal take-off at the canter is from the forelegs, at the jump the animal takes off from the hindlegs. The change in rhythm is more noticeable if the jump is approached at the trot, as many novice riders will have discovered with dismay.

When horse and rider are landing after a fence in the show-jumping arena, or in a steeplechase, the impact forces are very considerable indeed. One has the impression that the horse's forelegs are straight, so that the shock must be taken by the bones in longitudinal compression. In fact there are two important shock-absorbing mechanisms. The first resides in the muscular coupling between the scapula and the ribcage that has been referred to earlier. In addition, the hoof is offset forward slightly, from the line of the long bones of the foreleg, by the inclined posture of the pastern bone, so that it is only the hoof itself that is stopped suddenly. The long bones themselves are decelerated more slowly, and the peak stress on them is correspondingly lessened. If a horse lands awkwardly, with all the bones in line, the impact is enough to shatter the pastern. A fresh specimen of a pastern bone from a racehorse withstood a loading of nearly seven tons before giving way in a compression testing machine. This may give some insight into the importance of the attitudes taken up by the various parts of the skeleton when a large animal is moving fast. In the horse, a special ligament crosses the fetlock joint from the suspensory ligaments behind the cannon bone forwards to the front of the distal phalanx so that, when the limb is extended just before landing, the hoof is lifted forward ready to touch down on the sole. If the action of this mechanism is interfered with by an unexpected obstruction, so that the hoof lands toe first, no supporting reaction occurs and the leg collapses, causing the horse to stumble.

During the oscillatory motions of the trunk which occur as a result of the variations in the forces in the limbs in locomotion, the head has to be supported by correspondingly varying forces in the neck. To some extent the inertia of the head at the end of the neck can be used in checking the angular oscillations of the trunk. There are, however, considerable advantages to be gained from keeping the head on an even course, and some of the reflexes described in the previous chapter appear to be directed to this end.

EFFECT OF RESTRICTING THE AREA OF SUPPORT

When one examines the footprints of an animal that has been travelling at speed it will be seen that a line joining the individual footprints always follows a sinuous course. The track of a bicycle shows similar lateral undulations. The reason for this oscillation is that any tendency to fall to one side or the other is promptly opposed by developing an appropriately inclined thrust whose horizontal component arrests the momentum in unwanted directions. The process is analogous to the movement of the support vector to correct the swaying of quiet standing, as revealed by the force-plate studies referred to earlier. The quadruped achieves the required inclined thrusts by setting the feet to one side or the other of the projection of the centre of gravity. The sinuous course steered by the bicycle rider serves the same function. The context of this mechanism prompts the question how it can be possible to walk a tightrope.

When a human subject stands upright without moving his feet, the alternating shifts in the line of the supporting thrust are achieved by altering the torque exerted about the ankle joint. There is a limit to how far the thrust line can be shifted since it must always pass through the area of contact between the feet and the ground. This area can be artificially reduced by having the subject stand on a small plank laid over the upturned edges of two parallel pieces of angle iron laid on the floor. He can stand successfuly if the edges are about 3.5 cm apart (Figure 7.27). He is then instructed to move his weight gradually forwards until the plank lifts off one of the supporting edges. His task is then to balance on the remaining edge.

The usual reaction, in the face of imminent overbalancing, is to alter the torque exerted across the ankle joint, thus shifting the point of application of the supporting thrust, as in Figure 7.26(c), where ankle torque shifts the thrust line from A to U to correct for a movement of the centre of gravity, O, forward of the vertical through the ankle, AP. This adjustment makes it possible to develop an inclined thrust, from U to O, which has an effective stabilizing action.

Changes in the torque exerted at the ankle have no useful effect in the situation we are now considering, since the plank just pivots over the supporting edge without affecting the line of the thrust transmitted to the body. Furthermore, so long as the line of action of the support-

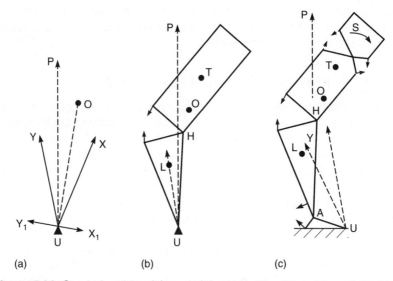

(a)   (b)   (c)

Figure 7.26 Overbalancing. (a) and (b) show the disposition of forces in balancing the trunk on a fixed narrow base. O = centre of gravity of the body; UP = direction of thrust appropriate to equilibrium; UX_1, UY_1 = resolved components, at right angles to UO. These produce rotations about O without displacement. (b) Recovery from the brink: H = hip joint; T = centre of gravity of trunk; L = centre of gravity of legs (toppling to left). (c) Effect of torque at the ankle, A, and of sweeping movements of the arms: S = segment consisting of the shoulders, arms, and anything held in the hand. It pivots on the trunk about the sternoclavicular joint.

ing force passes through the centre of gravity of the body, there is no reason for the nervous system to institute corrective movements, since the neural criteria for stability are then met. However, any casual misalignment of this force relative to the position of the centre of gravity will cause the body to start to fall.

A common rescue strategy involves sweeping movements of the arms. In Figure 7.26(c), the segment marked S represents those parts of the upper body, including the arms and the head, that can be moved relative to the trunk. The sweeping movements of the arms seen in these rescue reactions provide a means of partitioning the angular momentum of the body. When clockwise angular momentum is being developed in the movable segment, S, the anticlockwise reaction torque on the trunk would produce anticlockwise angular momentum in the trunk, if the trunk were free to move. However, angular rotation of the trunk is here obstructed by the presence of the legs, which develop thrust between the hips and the fixed support. The restraint of the leg segment produces a reaction couple exerting a forward force against the ground and a backward force against the trunk. Without this restraint, the three linked segments, S, T and L, would operate like a train of gears, each element rotating in the opposite sense from its immediate neighbours. The backward force against the trunk is just what is required for stabilization. One often sees gymnasts making use of this strategy during exercises on the beam.

The sweeping manoeuvre is not necessarily successful by itself. The moment of inertia of the arms about the shoulder joint is very much less than that of the whole body about an axis through the support at the feet. Consequently a transfer of angular momentum from the arms to the trunk leads to only a small angular movement about the feet. Habitual arm-sweeping does, however, usually accompany attempts to return from the brink. A disadvantage of such sweeping movements when attempting to balance on a fixed narrow base is that the forward pitching of the trunk reappears at the end of each arm movement when the time comes for the angular momentum of the movable segment to be absorbed. This means that each successive stage in the necessary alternation of corrections, first on one side of the support and then on the other, is interfered with by the consequences of earlier arm movements, adding further difficulty to the task, and the subject falls off after only a very few seconds.

THE RETURN FROM THE BRINK

Physical considerations might at first suggest that there is no possibility of recovery once the body has started to topple. Suppose that the direction of support thrust for successful balance lies in the direction

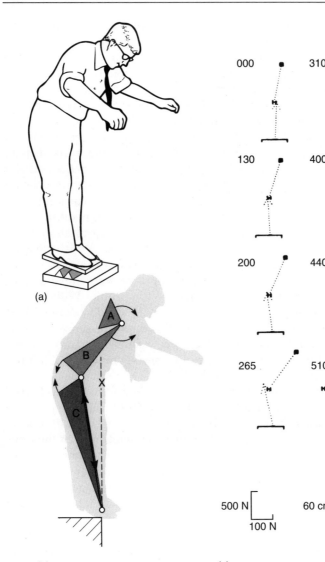

000   310

130   400

200   440

265   510

500 N
        100 N

60 cm
        20 cm

(a)

(b)   (c)

Figure 7.27 Balancing on a narrow base. (a) A subject stands on a board laid over two parallel edges mounted 3.5 cm apart on a force-plate; he gradually moves forward to the point of overbalancing and then rescues himself. (b) Scheme of the body segments contributing to the balancing manoeuvre. (c) Successive appearances of a computer-generated display at the times indicated in milliseconds. The arrow indicates the magnitude, direction, and point of application, of the support force at the foot. Horizontal, but not vertical, displacements of the head and hips are also indicated. Horizontal scales, both for force and for displacement, are exaggerated (×4) with respect to vertical scales.

UP in Figure 7.26(a), while the centre of gravity of the body is at O, i.e. the subject has begun to topple forwards over the edge U. Any thrust applied at U, such as in the direction of X or of Y, will have effects which can be analysed by resolving the applied force into one component along UO and another at right angles to this. The first component can accelerate the centre of gravity of the body only along the line UO. A force in the direction of the second component produces only a rotation of the body about its centre of gravity, with no movement of the centre of gravity itself. Thus there appears to be no way in which O can be brought nearer to UP by a thrust constrained to act through U. It is for this reason that it is necessary to move the hand when balancing the inverted broom, as in Figure 5.12.

The situation of Figure 7.26(a) applies to a rigid body. A different situation arises if the body can change its shape by the action of internal forces, as in the case of the rescue movements of sweeping with the free limbs referred to above. An everyday illustration of another related principle is provided by the way a playground swing is set into motion. When the swing is at rest and the subject is not pulling with his arms, the thrust against the seat is applied vertically below the subject's centre of gravity which, in turn, is vertically below the point of support at the rings fastening the swing chains to the supporting frame. To set the swing in motion, the subject allows his upper trunk to fall backwards, and then arrests this fall by pulling with his arms. At the same time he extends his lower legs by straightening the knees. The resultant of the supporting forces on the subject's body now passes somewhere between his shoulders and his hips at a point depending on the proportion of his weight that is taken on the arms. Since the support point at the tops of the chains is not changed, the effect is that the resultant support force is no longer vertical. Its action can be resolved into two components, one vertical and the other horizontal. This horizontal component of force serves to accelerate the subject's body horizontally in the direction of his feet and thus sets the swing in motion.

When the support point is below the centre of gravity of the body the possibilities illustrated in Figure 7.26(b) become available (see also Figure 7.27). We suppose the trunk, with centre of gravity at T, to be supported at the hip, H, by the combined action of thrust at the hip joint together with torque applied by muscles such as the hamstrings and gluteals. The centre of gravity of the legs is at L, and the legs are supported at the single edge at U. The centre of gravity of the whole body is at O, which in our case lies to the right of UP, indicating that the subject has started to overbalance in the forward direction.

A possible strategy for 'recovery from the brink' in these conditions is as follows. The hip is relaxed. This allows T to fall freely forwards.

The centre of gravity of the legs alone lies to the left of UP, so that in the absence of hip torque the legs will fall to the left like a felled tree, the hips moving to the left and carrying the trunk with them. One can illustrate this effect with a model hinged at the hip with the force at the hip simulated by a thread. The model is propped up in the attitude of Figure 7.27 and, when the thread is cut, the model falls to the left. Thrust against the ground, acting along UL, can move L further to the left so that O also moves to the left, which is the required direction for correcting the overbalancing. Once the desired movement of O has been initiated, the hip torque is turned on again strongly to arrest the fall of the trunk.

Figure 7.27(c) shows a timed succession of snapshots of the moving vector display obtained from a force-plate during this 'recovery from the brink' manoeuvre. The markers for the hip and head show horizontal displacements but not vertical ones. The hip is starting to move backwards (to the left in the figure, which represents a side view) at around 130 ms, while the trunk segment tips progressively forwards. The hip torque is switched off between the frames for 310 and 400 ms and is beginning to be resumed at 420 ms. By 510 ms the main part of the rescue reaction has been completed, leaving only the correction of the excessive forward tilt of the trunk.

The manoeuvre appears well suited to situations where excessive sway has taken the projection of the centre of gravity too close to, or even a little beyond, the edge of the available area of support, with an imminent danger of falling over. It seems unlikely, however, that balance can be maintained by a succession of manoeuvres of this type when supported on a single fixed edge because the body tends to be thrown some way back towards the 'safe' area and, in the case of the single fixed edge, no such safe area exists.

WALKING THE TIGHTROPE

This conclusion suggests that it should not be possible to walk along a fixed line, which is what the tightrope walker appears to do. When the support is reduced to a pair of points or to a number of points in the same straight line, equilibrium with the centre of gravity directly above the support is unstable, because any casual deflection produces a couple tending to displace the body further. However, if the relative position of the support can be altered in some way, it is possible to maintain a dynamic equilibrium, and to avoid falling. The procedure is to initiate a sequence of manoeuvres that repeatedly shift the support from one side to the other of the vertical through the centre of gravity. In this way a couple tending to tip the body to one side of the support is replaced, after a short interval, by an opposite couple which arrests the movement initiated by the previous couple, and which starts to tip the body to the other side. The cycle then repeats in the opposite direction. This is the technique adopted by acrobats on the slack wire. It is occasionally used by birds perching on telegraph wires, and it forms the basis of the equilibrium of a bicycle or of a skater.

When riding a bicycle, the alternation in the relative positions of the points of support is achieved by steering an appropriately sinuous course. It is the acquisition of the necessary habits of steering, with their delicate adjustment of timing, that constitutes the principal task involved in learning to ride a bicycle. A similar strategy is used in skating. In contrast, the necessary movement of the support on the slack wire depends on complex muscular adjustments of posture achieved through a sequence of paddle actions.

The effects of an inertia paddle have already been set out in the context of the sweeping movements illustrated in Figure 7.26(c). The magnitude of the torque that can be developed between the movable segment, S, and the trunk is affected by the moment of inertia of S. This can be increased by extending the arms and, even more so, by holding in the hands an acrobat's balancing pole with weighted ends. As already explained, the torque to generate clockwise angular momentum in S leads to a force against the support, directed towards the right in the figure. If the support is free to move, the effect is to shift the line of the supporting thrust to the right, which is in the correct direction for stabilization.

If a subject, standing on a slack wire, is about to overbalance, say clockwise looked at along the wire, his recovery strategy is to apply torque at the shoulder so as to impart clockwise momentum to his inertia paddle. Torque is at the same time applied at the hip to rotate the leg segment in the opposite (anticlockwise) direction. This moves the supporting wire to the right, from our viewpoint, so that the upthrust now comes to pass to the right of the vertical through the centre of gravity of the body. The risk of overbalancing is thus temporarily averted. The manoeuvre has to be repeated at intervals, in one direction or the other, so long as the subject remains on the slack wire. On a tightrope the strategy is similar, although the lateral displacement of the rope is much less extensive than that of the slack wire.

When an air-resistance paddle is used, such as the tightrope walker's fan or umbrella, or the wings and tail of a perching bird, the effect is to provide an additional point of support, albeit on a temporary basis. Upthrust is obtained from the paddle by imparting downward momentum to the mass of air displaced by the movement of the paddle.

MOVEMENT IN THE AIR

As already mentioned, the principles of conservation of linear and of angular momentum tell us that, even with the expenditure of energy, no system of purely internal forces can change either the total linear momentum of a structure or its total angular momentum about its centre of gravity. The rotations and other motions of birds in flight, of aircraft and of space vehicles, all depend on imparting momentum either to neighbouring air masses or to some other mass that is discarded from the moving body, such as the gas jets from a rocket engine.

Although manoeuvres involving movable segments, and using purely internal forces, can have no effect either on the linear momentum of the centre of gravity or on the total angular momentum about that point, they can be of use to adjust the attitude of the body during free fall, as on the trampoline or in an orbiting spacecraft. While, in the absence of external forces, the total momentum must be conserved, it is possible to arrange, on a temporary basis, the partitioning of this momentum between the various parts of a structure and in this way to achieve a change in the orientation of the body as a whole. It is by manoeuvres of this type that a springboard diver or a trampoline artist can turn in the air, or a cat land on its feet after a fall. The principle on which this manoeuvre depends is that the moment of inertia of an elongated object is less for rotations about its long axis than it is for rotations about any other axis. A torque applied between two bodies will produce equal and opposite changes in the angular momentum of each, and the angular velocities attained after a given time will therefore be inversely proportional to the moments of inertia.

The cat, dropped from a supine position, arches its back so that the longitudinal axis of the head and forequarters (A) is not in line with that of the hinder parts of the body (B). It can then rotate the forequarters about its long axis, by applying torque between the two segments first in one direction and then in the other. Because the moment of inertia of A about its long axis is less than that of B about the axis of A, the temporary partitioning of the angular momentum produces a greater angular displacement of A about its long axis than that of B about the same axis. There is no change in the total angular momentum during this manoeuvre.

The next stage is to rotate B about its long axis. This time it is the moment of inertia of B that is the less, so that B can now be brought round to face in the same direction as the new direction of A. The sequence of manoeuvres produces a change in the orientation, but not in the total angular momentum.

The human body is not capable of so extensive a twisting movement as the cat's and a somewhat different strategy is required, as may be seen in Figure 7.28 (from McDonald's slow-motion film of the Olympic diver Brian Phelps). To describe the motion, we regard the body as made up of three segments: A, the arms and the head; B, the trunk; and C, the legs. The procedure is to rotate both A and C simultaneously so that their axes each describe a cone about the axis of B. These rotatory movements are carried out by a succession of fore-and-aft and lateral bendings, without twisting. The moment of inertia of B about its own axis is less than that of A and C in their conical paths round this same axis. Thus while A and C rotate to the left, the trunk rotates to the right.

Meanwhile, the corresponding rightward twist of the segments A and C is produced by the mechanism described above for the cat. C is

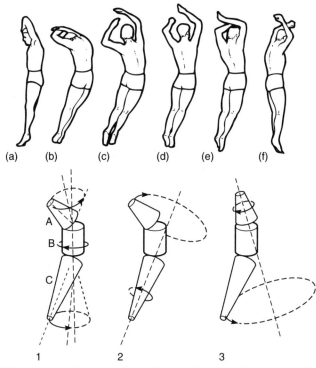

Figure 7.28 Manoeuvre for lateral rotation in the air. Above, (a)–(f): outlines from a cine film of an Olympic diver, Brian Phelps. Below: schematic representation of the component movements. 1: Rotation of the trunk, B, produced by conical counter-rotation of A and C. 2: Twisting of the legs, C, using A and B as an inertia paddle. 3: Rotation of the arms and shoulders, A, using B and C as an inertia paddle. (The outlines (a)–(f) after McDonald, 1961, by courtesy of *New Scientist*.)

first twisted about its own long axis, which is inclined to the long axis of the combination of A and B (stages (b), (c) and (d) in the figure). Thereafter A is twisted about its long axis, which is inclined to the axis of the combination of B and C (stages (c), (d) and (e) in the figure). Using a succession of such manoeuvres, Mr Phelps was able to carry out a 360° turn in a little over half a second, the required direction being shouted to him after he had left the springboard.

To produce the change in attitude from head-up at take-off to head-down for entry to the water, the diver usually relies on angular momentum acquired at the moment of take-off by a suitably directed push against the springboard. For the final adjustment of attitude required for clean entry he may use a procedure that involves the partitioning of angular momentum about a series of horizontal axes.

Again we consider the body of the diver as made up of three segments: arms (A), trunk (B) and legs (C). We start with all three segments in line (Figure 7.29). The moment of inertia of A about the shoulders is less than the combined moment of inertia of B and C about the same axis. A sequence of torques, to produce acceleration in flexion followed by deceleration, will rotate the arms towards the front through a larger angle than the accompanying backward rotation of the rest of the body. In the next phase an upward extension of the arms is accompanied by flexion at the hip. This rotates the trunk forwards about a central transverse axis, producing less backward rotation of the arms and legs about the same axis because the combined moment of inertia of A and C about the central transverse axis is greater than that of B about this axis. Finally, the legs can be rotated by straightening at the hip, because the moment of inertia of the legs about the hip is less than the combined moment of inertia of A and B about this axis.

Another procedure for fine adjustment of pitch attitude involves extending the arms sideways and rotating them so that each describes a cone about the shoulder. The torque needed to set up this rotation imparts to the trunk a pitching rotation in the opposite sense. This technique is used by trampoline artists to adjust the attitude of the feet for the descent, and it forms the basis for some of the sweeping arm movements seen in the reaction to overbalancing.

Somersaults performed during a dive depend on angular momentum acquired from the springboard at take-off. When the arms and legs are fully extended, the moment of inertia of the whole body about a central transverse axis is comparatively large. If the arms and legs are flexed and tucked in close to the trunk, the moment of inertia of the whole body is much reduced. As the total angular momentum cannot be altered in the absence of external forces, this decrease in moment of inertia entails an increase in angular velocity. The slow rotation imparted at take-off is thus converted, in flight, into the more rapid

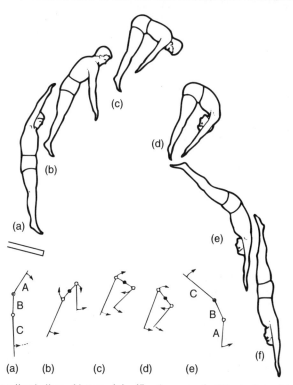

Figure 7.29 The piked dive. Above, (a)–(f): change of attitude from head-up to head-down during a dive. (a): Arms extended above the head after leaving the springboard; ((a)–(b)) rotation of the arms, A, clockwise about the shoulders, produces much smaller anticlockwise rotation of B and C; ((b), (c), (d)) clockwise rotation of B at the expense of some anticlockwise rotation of A and C about the central transverse axis; ((d), (e), (f)) clockwise rotation of C about the hip is offset by a smaller anticlockwise rotation of A and B about this axis. Below: ○ = hinge point; ● = axis of rotation.

rotation of the somersault. Just before entry the diver straightens up again and slows up the rotation.

Comparable manoeuvres, involving the movement of body segments in paddle action, are used by astronauts in the free-fall conditions of an orbiting spacecraft, both for moving about within the vehicle and for extra-vehicular activity, to orient themselves appropriately to the various instruments that are attached in different places to the walls of the spacecraft.

Proprioceptive transducers

8

The accounts of balancing behaviour both at rest and during locomotion, as set out in the preceding chapters, have concentrated on describing what actually happens without going into details of the neurophysiology of the central mechanisms involved. Before examining this question we need to consider what information is available to the central nervous system as a basis for the appropriate organization of motor commands in the form of nerve-impulses sent to muscles.

TRANSDUCERS

There are various possible sources for this information. Sensory receptors are found in the capsules of the joints of the skeleton, in tendons and in association with modified muscle-fibres in the 'muscle-spindles' that are embedded in the skeletal muscles. This group of receptors, together with their sensory nerves and the specialized receptor systems in the balancing organ of the inner ear, are collectively referred to as the 'proprioceptive system'. Contributions to balance are also made by cutaneous receptors reporting skin contact and local pressure, and by that part of the visual system concerned with retinal streaming.

The expression 'transducer' is used to denote a structure which is affected by changes in special features of its local environment in such a way as to generate signals whose intensity is related to the magnitude of the local change that has been detected. All the transducers involved in the proprioceptive system are affected by the mechanical stresses and strains occurring in their local environment. They can therefore be classified as 'deformation-receptors'.

A SIMPLE DEFORMATION-RECEPTOR

The simplest of these deformation-receptors are the 'spray endings' of Ruffini found in the capsules of joints and elsewhere. A drawing of the typical histological appearance of one such receptor (when stained with gold chloride) is shown (inset) in Figure 8.1. The various branches of the spray are distributed in three dimensions. Here the appearances at various planes of focus have been drawn in on a photograph which, by itself, could show only those structures that lie in one particular plane. The structure consists of the fine terminal branches of a nerve cell with their bead-like extensions, all devoid of a myelin sheath. A small part of the parent fibre is shown at the bottom of the inset figure. The thicker appearance here shows the start of the myelin sheath which

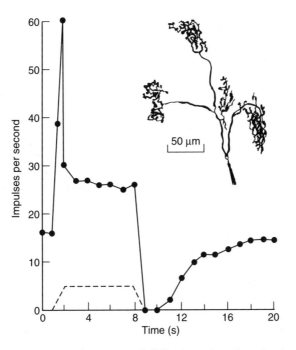

Figure 8.1 Plot of impulse-frequency (full line) against time for the discharge from a receptor in the knee joint of a cat during a change of joint angle (broken line) from one position to another and back again. Note that there is a definite impulse-frequency corresponding to each position and that an exaggerated change in impulse-frequency accompanies the change in position. After the movement, the impulse-frequency gradually settles towards the value appropriate to the new position. (Graph from Boyd and Roberts, 1953, by courtesy of *J. Physiol.*) Inset: typical appearance of a Ruffini spray ending from the joint capsule of the knee joint of a cat. (From a preparation by I.A. Boyd, stained with gold chloride.)

covers the length of the axon, apart from the nodes of Ranvier, all the way from this point right up to the destination of the fibre in the spinal cord. The whole of the spray is embedded in the fibrous tissue of the joint capsule, but the precise relationship, between the nerve fibrils and beads, on the one hand, and the connective-tissue fibres on the other, has not so far been elucidated.

Various functions have been proposed for the similar spray endings that can be found in the skin, but none of these functions is known with certainty. In the case of the spray endings in the joint capsules, electrical recording of nerve-impulses in the sensory nerve reveals that the sense organ is affected by mechanical deformation. Exploration of the capsule with a probe can elicit bursts of action-potentials in the sensory nerve when the probe disturbs that part of the capsule where the receptor lies. This sort of reaction can, however, be obtained from many types of receptor and does not necessarily imply that this type of stimulus has any particular physiological significance. One has to remember that mild deformation of the eyeball can elicit a response in the sensory nerves from the eye. One can confirm this for oneself. With the eyes closed, direct the gaze of the right eye towards the nose and tap gently with the tip of a finger on the outer angle of the right eyelid. A 'flash of light' will be seen though, of course, the tap does not produce any light. What happens is that the sense cells in the retina respond to mechanical deformation as well as to light and consequently they generate impulses in the optic nerve in response to the tap. The actual sensation that arises when these impulses reach the brain depends on the function that is normally served by the nerve-fibres that have been actuated. We interpret the activity in terms of a stimulus by light.

A more 'realistic' form of stimulus to the sense organs in the joint capsules is to change the angle between the bones forming the joint, since it is clearly relevant to the task of organizing balancing behaviour to have information about the disposition of the limb segments. A change in the angle at a joint is inevitably accompanied by some deformation of the joint capsule. It is found that, when recording from a sensory nerve-fibre which can be made active by probing the capsule of a particular joint, a stream of impulses appears when the joint is held at a particular angle. So long as the discharge is perfectly regular, the intervals between successive impulses being equal, we may speak of the 'frequency of impulses in the discharge' in terms of a count over unit time. We then find that different angles at the joint are associated with different impulse-frequencies in the afferent nerve. When we change from one joint angle to another, the intervals between successive impulses cease to be equal to one another. We therefore need a new definition of 'impulse-frequency'.

DEFINITION OF 'IMPULSE-FREQUENCY'

A count of the number of impulses in unit time is not appropriate where the discharge is irregular, or when the level of stimulation is changing. An alternative definition runs as follows: 'the impulse-frequency at a particular time is the reciprocal of the duration of the interval between the last two impulses, or the reciprocal of the time elapsed since the most recently recorded impulse, whichever is the less'. The numerical value of this measure is automatically updated by the arrival of each impulse, and decays to zero when further impulses fail to arrive. Using this definition, we can plot the time-course of the impulse-frequency during and after various test procedures.

THE RESPONSE TO A CHANGE IN JOINT ANGLE

With this technique we find that a particular unit shows a steady frequency of discharge after the joint has been at rest in a particular position for a few seconds. The frequency of this resting discharge depends on the angle of the joint and also on the direction from which this position was reached. When the angle of the joint is altered, the impulse-frequency changes in the direction appropriate to the change of position, but to an exaggerated degree. For example, in the graph of Figure 8.1, when the joint angle was altered from a position in which the resting discharge was at 16 impulses per second to another position where the new resting discharge was at 25 per second, the impulse-frequency rose during the movement to reach 60 per second. After the end of the movement there was a decline in impulse-frequency, the new resting level being reached after a few seconds. A return move-ment, in the opposite direction, produced a reduction in impulse-frequency, the exaggerated response during the movement this time leading to a complete cessation of discharge. This was followed, after the end of the movement, by a gradual recovery to the frequency appropriate to the new position.

The degree of exaggeration in the response during a change in joint angle depends on the speed of the movement, quicker movements producing greater degrees of exaggeration. The decline in impulse-frequency during the few seconds immediately following the cessation of movement is an example of the phenomenon known as 'adaptation'. The two phenomena – exaggerated response during movement and adaptation of the discharge at the end of the movement – can be combined into the idea that, in addition to the 'static' response of the receptor (which contributes towards the observed impulse-frequency a component which depends on the position reached), there is also a 'dynamic' response whose contribution to the observed impulse-frequency is related to the history of previous movements. A plot of the static component against joint angle has to take account of the direction from which the final position was reached, since there is often some hysteresis (though not in the case illustrated in Figure 8.1).

The action-potentials, as recorded from electrodes in close proximity to a nerve-fibre, are the electrical manifestations of transient cycles of activity in the nerve-fibre. The cell membrane of a nerve cell separates the intracellular fluid from the surrounding extracellular fluid. Both these fluids contain electrolytes, but in different concentrations, and they are therefore able to conduct electric currents, while the cell membrane itself is an insulator. The structure of the cell membrane restricts the exchange of particles between the fluids and, as a consequence of the different permeability to molecules of various kinds, together with active pumping to maintain concentration differences in the face of slow leakages, a voltage-difference is normally maintained between the inside and the outside of the cell. The individual permeabilities are voltage-dependent in different ways, so that an imposed flow of electric current leads to a succession of interacting changes in permeability and in membrane potential, resulting in the cycle of electrical activity which is revealed as the recorded action-potential. Since nerve-fibres are long in comparison with their diameters, it is possible for one region to be active when other regions are 'resting'. Because active and resting membranes have different voltage differences across them, electric currents flow, in local circuits, between active and inactive regions of the same cell, both in the intracellular and in the extracellular fluids. Such local circuit currents can activate regions that were previously inactive, and it is in this way that nerve-impulses propagate from one place to another along a nerve-fibre.

Mechanical deformation of the cell membrane affects its permeability and this is how impulses are generated by disturbance with a probe. It is not known in detail what effect the local deformations of the components of a spray ending that occur during the movement at a joint will have on the individual components themselves, but the combined effect can serve to generate sufficient local circuit current to excite the nerve-cell membrane at the nearest node of Ranvier. This node then activates its neighbour, and so on in turn to other nodes, to set up a propagated impulse.

The cycle of activity associated with the action-potential has a natural termination. It is all over very quickly, whereas the local effect of the deformation commonly has a much slower time-course. In consequence, a succession of impulses is generated, at a repetition-frequency which reflects the intensity of the mechanical stimulation. It can be seen from the plot in Figure 8.1 that the correspondence between change in joint angle and change in firing-frequency is not very close, because of the presence of the dynamic component in the response. Comparison between the responses of individual receptors in the same joint reveal considerable differences both in sensitivity and in the range of joint angles over which the units respond. These differences are likely to be associated with the differences in orientation and location of the receptors in relation to the strains produced in the capsule by changes in joint angle.

TENDON ORGANS

Spray endings of somewhat similar general shape, but commonly three to five times larger than those in joint capsules, are found in the dense connective tissue forming the tendinous insertions of the skeletal muscle-fibres. These are the Golgi tendon organs. As the physiological stresses in the tendons are always in the line of the tendon, the deformation of the receptor is normally the result of the application of tension to the tendon. The Golgi tendon organs thus signal to the central nervous system something about the tensions in the various tendons in the body.

The receptors are situated quite close to the junction between tendon and muscle-fibres (Figure 8.2). The tendon consists of bundles of collagen fibres intertwined like an irregularly braided rope. In the region of the receptor, a number of collagen fibres are bound together by a connective-tissue capsule. At one end of this capsule the collagen fibres are grouped into fascicles which serve as the attachments for a small number of muscle-fibres, average between 10 and 11, range 5 to 25.

The main sensory nerve-fibre is a large myelinated axon (Group Ib). A smaller nerve-fibre of unknown function can also be identified. The fine terminal branches of the sensory nerve-fibre are interwoven with the collagen fibres within the capsule in such a way that they become laterally compressed when the tensile stress in the collagen straightens out the waves and spirals of the braiding (Figure 8.3). In this way, applied tension leads to deformation of the cell membrane of the terminal parts of the sensory axon with consequent depolarization, local circuit currents, and the generation of impulses in the afferent nerve-fibre.

Because of the intimate relationship between each particular tendon organ and a specific group of muscle-fibres, the receptors are especially sensitive to changes in the tension in restricted portions of the muscle, rather than to changes in the total force carried by the whole tendon. From the wide distribution of the muscle-fibres making up a single motor unit, it may be taken that most, if not all, of the muscle-fibres attached to a particular tendon organ are members of different motor

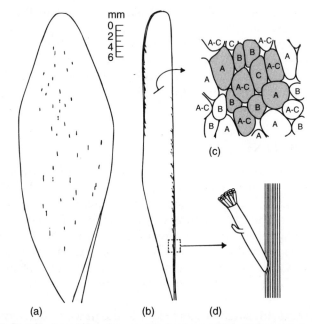

Figure 8.2 Distribution of tendon organs in the medial gastrocnemius muscle of the cat. (a) Surface view. (b) Projection onto a plane at right angles to (a), to show that the tendon organs are located close to the aponeuroses. (c) Typical cross-section of a part of the muscle: individual muscle-fibres are lettered according to histochemical type (A = white, fast twitch; B = red, slow twitch; C = red, fast twitch; A–C = intermediate between A and C); the shading indicates a group of muscle-fibres such as might be connected to a single tendon organ. (d) Manner of attachment of tendon organ capsule between muscle-fibres and aponeurosis. (From Reinking *et al.*, 1975, by courtesy of *J. Physiol.*)

units. Thus if we study the discharge from a single tendon organ by recording from a dorsal root filament while stimulating separate filaments of the ventral root, we see that, although all the motor units in a muscle contribute tension to its tendon, some activate the tendon organ we are recording from, while others do not. Accordingly the relationship between the total force carried by the whole tendon and the discharge pattern generated by a specific tendon organ may vary considerably from time to time according to which motor units in the muscle happen to be contributing to the generation of tension.

While it is clear that the adequate stimulus for excitation of the tendon organ receptor is some function of tension, it must also be remembered that, just as in the case of the receptors in the joint capsules, a change from one level of applied tension to another is

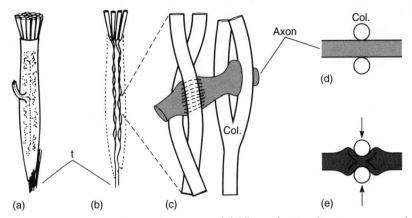

Figure 8.3 Structure of a tendon organ. (a) View of a tendon organ capsule: the Ib afferent subdivides within the capsule into a number of unmyelinated branches. (b) Muscle-fibres enter one end of the capsule and give rise to braided collagen fibres which traverse the capsule and join the tendon (marked t). (c) View under high magnification of a nerve twig lying between spiral strands of collagen (col.); collagen bundles frequently divide and recombine. (d) Unstressed condition. (e) Action of collagen strands to squeeze the nerve twig when the spirals are elongated by longitudinal tension. (From Swett and Schoultz, 1975, by courtesy of *Arch. Ital. Biol.*)

associated with an exaggerated change in the impulse-frequency in the afferent nerve-fibre, followed by a period of adaptation.

THE FROG MUSCLE-SPINDLE

The next type of receptor to be considered is the muscle-spindle. This name is used for a group of receptors found embedded in the skeletal muscles. The sense organs show different degrees of complexity in different muscles and in different species. In each case the nerve ending is associated with a particular group of muscle-fibres, which are bound together by connective tissue to form a discrete bundle within the main body of the muscle. This elongated bundle usually has a small swelling about half way along its length, where the connective-tissue covering separates slightly from the underlying muscle-fibres, leaving a small fluid-filled space (usually referred to as the 'lymph space'). The sensory nerve endings are to be found near this region, and they are very closely associated with the muscle-fibres of the spindle.

In the frog the sensory axon branches near its termination, to form a number of thin, braided strands which run parallel to the muscle-fibres. The bundle forming the spindle may contain about ten muscle-fibres (called 'intrafusal muscle-fibres', to distinguish them from the muscle-fibres forming the body of the muscle), and each of these intrafusal muscle-fibres may have about ten nerve strands associated with it. Each of these nerve strands will be made up of about 100 beads, each 2–3 μm in diameter, linked together by slender cylinders about 4 μm long and 0.15 μm in diameter. Some of the beads lie in depressions in the sides of the muscle-fibres and, at these points, the cell membranes of nerve and muscle come very close together to leave a gap of only 150 Å. (Compare this with the gap of about 300 Å at the synaptic patches under an end-knob at a neuromuscular junction.) With the electron microscope, small bridges can be seen crossing the gap between the two membranes.

Just as in the case of the Golgi tendon organ, the physiological stresses in the sensory region of the spindle are parallel to the direction of the intrafusal muscle-fibres, so that the receptor in the muscle-spindle signals length-changes occurring in the lymph-space region of the spindle. There are various schools of thought about the relationship between these local length-changes and the tension in the spindle as a whole. There can be no doubt that it is the local length-change which is the immediate cause of the deformation of the receptor. The controversy arises over the question whether the spindle as a whole behaves as a length-detector or as a tension-detector.

The spindle as a whole can be thought of as made up of three portions: a short central region bearing the receptor apparatus and two elongated polar regions without receptors. The intrafusal muscle-fibres are continuous and run through all three regions. The extreme ends of the polar parts of the spindle are attached to the connective tissue forming the sarcolemma of neighbouring muscle-fibres. The spindle thus lies anatomically to some extent in parallel with the main tension-generating muscle-fibres of the muscle. Accordingly, if the muscle as a whole contracts, the forces stretching the spindle are relieved and the afferent discharge falls. The spindle cannot therefore signal the overall tension in the muscle because, in these conditions, a rise in muscle tension is accompanied by a decrease in spindle discharge. If, on the other hand, the muscle is passively stretched, there is an increase in the discharge from the spindle. These two observations taken together have given rise to the idea that the spindle signals the overall length of the muscle and it has been called a 'stretch-receptor'.

We may represent the mechanical properties of the different parts of the spindle as in the diagram of Figure 8.4. The receptor region in the middle is represented as a spring-balance, i.e. as a compliant system with a deformation detector on it. The two polar regions are represented as simple springs, to indicate the compliance of those parts of the intrafusal muscle-fibres. The whole is supposed to lie in parallel with

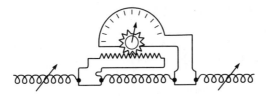

Figure 8.4 Mechanical properties of parts of a muscle-spindle.

the rest of the muscle. If we pull on the ends of this model, all the springs will be stretched, each to an extent dependent on its compliance, and the indicator of the spring-balance can be interpreted equally well in terms of length-change or of tension-change because, for ideal springs, there is a unique relationship between tension and length.

The same considerations apply even if the various compliances are nonlinear. However, if the compliances can be altered, or if there is any hysteresis in the relationship between tension and length, the equivalence of the interpretations in terms of length and of tension is no longer valid. Now, we know that the polar regions of the spindle are made up of muscle-fibres, and although there are certain differences between intrafusal muscle-fibres and other skeletal muscle-fibres, there are many common properties, and there does exist a motor innervation to the intrafusal muscle-fibres. We must, therefore, expect that impulses in the motor nerves to the intrafusal muscle-fibres will affect the activity, and thus the compliance, of these muscle-fibres. When this happens, any relationship between spindle length and afferent discharge which may previously have obtained must now, of necessity, become modified.

In many cases the intrafusal muscle-fibres show modifications in internal structure in the central portions of the fibre that bear the receptor apparatus. In particular, there is usually a marked reduction in the number of the filaments of myosin and of actin which, in other regions, give rise to the cross-striated appearance typical of skeletal muscle. Since it is these filaments that are responsible for the changes in the mechanical properties of the muscle that occur on activation, one may conclude that the compliance of the receptor region of the spindle does not change so much as does that of the polar regions. This leads to the view that the adequate stimulus for the spindle discharge is the tension in the spindle, rather than its overall length.

If electrical recordings are made, in isolated preparations, from a region of nerve very close to the sensory ending, it is possible to demonstrate an electrical effect intervening between the mechanical deformation and the generation of impulses in the afferent nerve. The time-course of this 'generator potential' is related to that of the applied stretch, with a decline at the end of the stretching corresponding to the adaptation curve. The frequency of impulses in the nerve is proportional to the amplitude of the generator potential, giving rise to plots of firing frequency similar in general shape to that shown for a joint receptor in Figure 8.1. If the nerve is treated with cocaine so as to block the formation of action potentials, the generator potential appears by itself. If localized electric currents are applied to the region of the muscle close to the receptor, it is found that the applied current can interact with the current generated in the receptor to produce a combined effect on the frequency of impulses in the nerve. The discharge in response to an applied current does not show adaptation.

From this group of experiments it can be concluded that the form of the stimulus–response relationship is governed by the mechanical properties and anatomical arrangement of the structures forming the receptor apparatus rather than by their electrical properties. Katz has calculated, from the dimensions measured in his electronmicroscope studies, that the most likely site where the mechanical deformations might be effectively converted into generator currents is at the small bridges which join the membranes of nerve cell and muscle cell, i.e. the points of attachment of the beads on the nerve strands to the underlying, modified part of the intrafusal muscle-fibre.

It is necessary to suppose that the effects of currents generated at several beads must summate at some point further along the axon until their combined effect is sufficient to generate a propagated impulse. This mechanism would help to account for the fact that the discharge from many sense organs consists of approximately equally spaced impulses in spite of the subdivision of the axon into a number of branches at the sensory terminal.

THE MAMMALIAN MUSCLE-SPINDLE

The muscle-spindles found in mammals are more complex than those of the frog. The general layout is similar to that in the frog, but the intrafusal muscle-fibres are more clearly differentiated from the extrafusal fibres, in their diameters, in the arrangement of their myofibrils, and in the position of their nuclei. Instead of the nuclei being spread out along the length of the muscle-fibre and displaced to lie close under the sarcolemma, as is usual for extrafusal fibres, the nuclei of the intrafusal muscle-fibres are more centrally placed in the cross-section, and they are grouped together near the region of the spindle that is surrounded by the lymph-space and which contains the sensory receptors (Figure 8.5).

Two types of intrafusal muscle-fibre may be distinguished by the

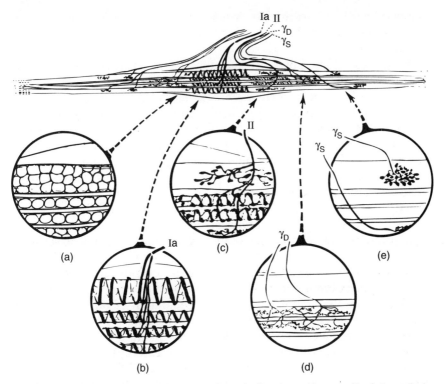

Figure 8.5 Typical mammalian muscle-spindle. Less than half of the whole length is shown and the transverse dimensions have been exaggerated to show some of the details. The ends of the nuclear chain fibres would be just out of this picture (typical length 4 mm). The nuclear bag fibres extend a further 2 mm or so at each end (say 8 mm overall). (a) Arrangement of nuclei in the central region of the intrafusal muscle-fibres as seen after all the nervous elements have been allowed to degenerate: (from above downwards) capsule; lymph space; nuclear bag fibre; two nuclear chain fibres; part of a nuclear bag fibre (in a typical spindle there will be two nuclear bag fibres and four nuclear chain fibres). (b) Primary sensory receptor connected to group Ia afferent (there is always one and only one of these to each spindle). (c) Secondary sensory receptor connected to a group II afferent (there may be up to five secondary endings, some on each side of the primary ending). (d) Trail ending of a static gamma fusimotor fibre. (e) Plate ending of a dynamic gamma fusimotor fibre. In some situations plate endings are more commonly associated with nuclear bag fibres and trail endings with nuclear chain fibres; in other places both types of ending occur on both types of intrafusal muscle-fibre. (Based on Boyd, 1962.)

arrangement of their nuclei. In one type there is a linear arrangement of nuclei, and these fibres are called 'nuclear chain fibres'. In the other type the nuclei are bunched together so that several can be seen in the same transverse section. The latter are called 'nuclear bag fibres'. This 'bag' of nuclei within a single intrafusal muscle-fibre should not be confused with the connective-tissue 'capsule' which contains the lymph-space and which surrounds the whole bundle of intrafusal fibres (Figure 8.5(a)).

The nuclear chain fibres are usually, but not always, considerably shorter than the nuclear bag fibres. Typically there may be two nuclear bag fibres and four nuclear chain fibres in each spindle, though there is a good deal of variation from spindle to spindle. Both polar regions of all the intrafusal muscle-fibres receive motor innervation, often from several different axons (7–25), and one particular axon may innervate several intrafusal muscle-fibres, sometimes involving more than one spindle.

The sensory endings in mammalian muscle-spindles are of two types, called primary and secondary. Each spindle has one, and only one, primary sensory ending. This lies in the middle of the lymph-space region of the spindle, and embraces all the intrafusal muscle-fibres. Each intrafusal fibre has its own branch of the parent axon. The sensory termination takes the form of a ribbon of nerve wound several times around the muscle-fibre to form an irregular cylindrical spiral (Figure 8.5(b)). In electronmicrographs it is seen that the nerve and muscle membranes lie very close together at a separation of only 150 Å, and that there are often flaps of muscle-cell membrane wrapped over the edges of the ribbon of nerve as though to ensure a particularly firm anchorage. The nerve branch connecting the ending to the stem axon usually comes off about the middle of the spiral. All the spirals lie close together giving, in most preparations, a very complicated appearance. Sometimes there are small sprays attached to one or other end of one of the spirals.

The secondary sensory endings may be in the form of spirals, similar to those of the primary ending, or they may form sprays of beaded nerve strands, or they may contain both spirals and sprays (see Figure 8.5(c)). They are associated principally, but not exclusively, with the nuclear chain fibres, and there may be from zero to five secondary endings in any particular spindle. The secondary endings lie close to the primary ending and to one or both sides of it. At one time the primary ending was referred to as 'annulospiral' and the secondary as 'flower-spray'. These names do not, however, provide a satisfactory guide to identification and they are now falling into disuse.

DISTINCTIONS BETWEEN THE INTRAFUSAL MUSCLE-FIBRES

The grouping of the cell nuclei into the central, 'equatorial', region of the intrafusal muscle-fibres is in some way related to the presence in that region of the terminations of the sensory nerve-fibres. After the afferent nerves have been cut and allowed to degenerate, the clustering of the nuclei becomes less marked. In addition to the classification as 'nuclear bag' or 'nuclear chain', there are other differences, both anatomical and functional (Table 8.1).

In the striation pattern of the nuclear chain fibres, the Z-lines appear thinner than in some nuclear bag fibres and there is an additional line, the M-line, that can be distinguished in the centre of the comparatively

Table 8.1 Distinctions between intrafusal muscle-fibres

	Dynamic bag$_1$	Static bag$_2$	Chain
Number in spindle	One, sometimes two	One	Three to five
Equatorial nuclei	Nuclear bag	Nuclear bag	Nuclear chain
Length	Intermediate (8 mm)	Long (9 mm)	Short (4 mm)
Diameter	Large (20 µm)	Large (25 µm)	Small (12 µm)
Rate of atrophy when denervated	Slow	Slow	Fast
ATP activity (alkaline pre-incubation)	Low	Medium/high	High
Glycogen content	Low/medium	Medium	High
Elastic fibres at poles	Scarce	Prominent	Present
Distinct single M-line in electronmicroscopy	Absent except extracapsular region	Present except equatorial region	Present
Development	Second formed	First formed	Last formed
Motor innervation	Dynamic gamma (or beta)	Static gamma	Static gamma (or beta)
Contraction when axon stimulated at 10 Hz	Smooth, barely visible	Small, smooth	Oscillatory
Stimulation frequency for maximum contraction	75–100 Hz	100 Hz	150–200 Hz
Time to tetanic contraction	1.0 s	0.6 s	0.4 s
Amplitude of movement	Small	Large	Large
Maximum extension	2–8%	12–30%	15–20%
Creep back in spirals following stretch of active fibre	20–30%	Usually absent	Absent
Electrical response at motor nerve-ending	Local response non-propagated	Local response non-propagated	Propagated action-potential
Response to topically applied acetylcholine	Contraction (most sensitive)	Contraction (less sensitive)	No contraction (neuromuscular block)

clear zone, the H-zone, between the ends of the two sets of thin filaments in each sarcomere. One of the nuclear bag fibres in each spindle has relatively thick Z-lines but no M-lines, in sharp contrast to the nuclear chain fibres. Other nuclear bag fibres, however, show a striation pattern more like that of the nuclear chain fibres.

The subdivision of nuclear bag fibres into two types can be seen also in several histochemical procedures. The staining reaction of one of the nuclear bag fibres is usually readily distinguishable from that of the nuclear chain fibres. The other nuclear bag fibre, however, either resembles the nuclear chain fibres in staining behaviour or reacts in an intermediate fashion. Yet another distinction is made on the basis that one only of the nuclear bag muscle-fibres has a surrounding coat of elastic fibres; in this respect it resembles the nuclear chain fibres.

When we come to study the electrical activity of the intrafusal muscle-fibres either with intracellular or with extracellular microelectrodes, problems of interpretation arise because of the difficulty in deciding which muscle-fibre is contributing to the observed responses. It appears that the trail endings on the nuclear chain muscle-fibres produce junctional potentials rather like the end-plate potentials of extrafusal muscle-fibres. The time-constant of decay of these junction potentials is about 3 ms. Some summation occurs on repetitive activation but the individual peaks remain separate even at frequencies of stimulation as high as 225 Hz. Sometimes the junction potential at a trail ending generates a full action-potential which then propagates outwards towards the end of the muscle-fibre. The two poles of the intrafusal muscle-fibres behave independently, and action-potentials do not propagate across the equatorial region from one pole to the other.

Activation of a plate ending on a nuclear bag muscle-fibre also produces a junctional potential, but with a longer time-constant of decay, around 15 ms. These junction potentials summate during repetitive activation but do not generate full action-potentials. This is somewhat surprising in view of the fact that some plate endings are the terminations of beta fibres which presumably generate propagated action-potentials at their anatomically rather similar terminations on extrafusal muscle-fibres.

The mechanical events associated with activity in intrafusal muscle-fibres are deduced from the movements of striations and other markers, as seen or filmed under the microscope in spindles isolated by dissection except for their blood supply and neural connections. The movements of nuclear chain muscle-fibres are characteristically brisk and twitch-like. The extent of the observed movement increases with increasing frequency of repetitive activation to attain a maximum at around 150 Hz. The two nuclear bag fibres differ from one another in their behaviour so that they can be labelled 'slow' and 'fast' respectively. Very little response can be seen to follow single shocks. Repetitive activation at 10 Hz already produces smooth contractions in both kinds of nuclear bag fibres, whereas the nuclear chain fibres show marked oscillations at this frequency. The onset of the movement in the slow nuclear bag fibre is characterized by a long latency and a slow initial velocity, whereas the latency and the initial velocity of the response in the fast nuclear bag fibres are not very different from those seen in nuclear chain fibres. The two types of nuclear bag fibre also differ in the speed of relaxation at the end of a period of activation.

The most noticeable difference of all, however, is the occurrence in the slow nuclear bag fibre, but not in the fast nuclear bag fibre, of the phenomenon of 'creep'. The different regions along the length of a slow nuclear bag fibre change their mechanical properties with different time-courses. In consequence, a change in the loading, such as that produced by an applied stretch, is followed by a period of readjustment during which one part that was at first more resistant to extension becomes pulled out by a region that was at first more compliant. The readjustment shows as a slow longitudinal creep of parts of the muscle-fibre, continuing for about two seconds after the end of the applied stretch.

The tensions developed by intrafusal muscle-fibres are very small compared with those developed by the extrafusal muscle-fibres. The combined activity of all the intrafusal muscle-fibres in a single spindle can develop no more than about 5 mg of active tension, whereas a spindle can bear about 4–5 g of passive tension just before breaking. In extrafusal muscle-fibres the stresses developed in activity can approach and occasionally even exceed the point at which the tissues rupture.

THE SENSORY DISCHARGE FROM THE SPINDLE

Let us turn back now to consider the operation of the spindle as a sense organ. As has already been mentioned, the receptors in the spindle generate streams of impulses in their afferent nerve-fibres when the central part of the spindle is put on the stretch. Because of the concentration of nuclei within the intrafusal muscle-fibres in this central region, there is not much room left there for myofibrillar material such as forms the contractile apparatus of all muscle-fibres. In consequence, it is reasonable to regard this part of the spindle as relatively inert. It will, of course, have compliance, that is to say, it will stretch when the tension applied to it increases. It is presumably this stretching which in some way leads to the generation of the impulses in the sensory nerve-fibres.

The mammalian muscle-spindle thus resembles, in principle, the simpler spindles of the frog described earlier. However, the complexity of the intrafusal apparatus in the mammalian spindle makes it even more unrealistic to regard this sense organ as a simple length-detector.

The main 'polar' parts of the intrafusal muscle-fibres, on either side of the central region, contain fewer nuclei and plenty of myofibrillar material. One of the characteristic properties of this contractile apparatus of muscles is its viscosity, that is to say, the fact that a change in length is opposed by a force related to the rate-of-change of length. It is this property which gives rise to the shape of the tension–length relationship for muscle (described in Chapter 4) where, during shortening, the tension transmitted to the tendon is less than the isometric tension by an amount which increases with increasing speed of shortening. Similarly, the tension needed to extend the muscle must exceed the isometric tension by an amount related to the speed of lengthening. It is clear that the relationships of the viscous forces in muscle to the velocities of shortening and of lengthening are neither of them linear, but these nonlinearities do not affect the present argument.

Let us consider, now, what happens when the overall length of a spindle is increased from one value to another, by a device which moves at a constant speed. Unless the spindle is slack to start with, this stretching will produce an increase in the tension in the spindle. The central region is in series with the rest, so this part also will undergo an increase in tension, with a corresponding increase in the degree of its stretching. When the central part of the spindle is on the stretch, the receptors generate impulses at a repetition-frequency which depends on the degree of stretch in this particular region. Thus the firing-frequency in the afferent nerve-fibres will be higher after the stretch than it was before.

During the actual stretching the polar parts of the intrafusal muscle-fibres, by virtue of the viscosity of their myofibrils, will show an extra resistance to extension depending in amount on the velocity of stretching. The central part of the spindle, with proportionally less myofibrillar material, will not show this effect to the same extent. Correspondingly, the central region will be more stretched during the movement at each particular value of tension than it would be at the same tension in the absence of movement.

The peculiar mechanical properties of the slow nuclear bag muscle-fibres introduce further complications because the central receptor-bearing region of the spindle will be affected by the adjustments of tension that accompany the 'creep' seen in the isolated spindle. When the spindle is being stretched, the polar parts of the slow nuclear bag fibres resist extension, so that the central region of these fibres has to 'give' to a correspondingly greater extent. At the end of the imposed movement, the polar parts relax slowly and give in their turn, allowing the central part to creep back to a less extended condition.

Because the firing-frequency of the afferent discharge depends on the degree of stretching of the central region, the effects of the viscosity of the polar parts of the spindle will be reflected in the time-course of the impulse-frequency in the afferent discharge. It will, in fact, be possible to distinguish two components in the response to stretch: a static component whose magnitude depends only on the spindle tension, and a dynamic component dependent on the rate-of-change of tension (Figure 8.6). At the beginning of a constant-speed stretch, the dynamic component in afferent discharge-frequency does not jump immediately to the appropriate new value, but rises towards it with an approximately exponential time-course. Similarly, at the end of the movement, there is an approximately exponential decay.

One effect of the dynamic component is that if the spindle tension is allowed to fall, there is a dramatic drop in the afferent firing-frequency. This is because, in these conditions, the dynamic component, related to the rate-of-change of tension, is of opposite sign to, and is consequently deducted from, the static component. Even quite small fluctuations in tension can have large effects if they take place sufficiently rapidly.

MODELLING THE DYNAMIC COMPONENT

The dynamic component in the response can, in principle, be described mathematically as a relationship between firing-frequency and spindle tension using the following procedure. We suppose that, when the conditions of stimulation are changing, a fractional component of response is generated at each moment whose magnitude is proportional to the rate-of-change in the conditions at that moment. This fractional component then decays with time, its remnant adding its effect to that of the remnants of similar fractional components generated at other times. Many situations are encountered, in physics, in chemistry, and in engineering, where leakage from some store occurs at a rate dependent on the driving pressure. In these cases the driving pressure decays exponentially with time. It is therefore natural to attempt to fit exponentials to the time-course of the exaggerated responses to change of stimulus in sense organs.

To derive the necessary numerical values for the parameters, it is convenient to use 'ramp stimuli', that is to say, tests in which conditions are altered, from one value to another, at a constant rate-of-change of value. An example is shown in Figure 8.6, where a cat muscle-spindle has been stretched, at constant speed, from one length to another. A dynamic component of response, formulated as described above, follows a time-course like that shown in Figure 8.6(c). Its magnitude does not jump up immediately at the onset of change as does the rate-

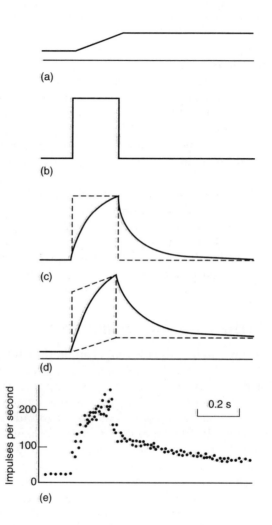

(a)

(b)

(c)

(d)

(e)

Figure 8.6 Scheme to indicate the relationships of the static and dynamic components in the discharge from a muscle-spindle in response to stretch. (a) Time-course of spindle tension during a change from one state to another. (b) Time-course of the rate-of-change of tension. (c) Time-course of an event which shows a sluggish response to rate-of-change of tension. (d) The sum of two components related respectively to (a) and to (c) above. (e) Experimental record obtained from a muscle-spindle. For each point the abscissa is the time of occurrence of an impulse in the afferent nerve and the ordinate is the reciprocal of the interval elapsed since the previous impulse. Note the resemblance between (d) and (e). ((e) is from Bessou *et al.*, 1965, by courtesy of *J. Physiol.*) (From Roberts and Murray-Smith, 1970, by courtesy of AGARD, NATO.)

of-change itself (Figure 8.6(b)), but gradually rises so long as the rate-of-change continues to generate further fractional contributions. The dynamic response gradually decays at the end of the movement. These features indicate that, to some extent at least, our mathematical model successfully simulates the target behaviour. To obtain a good fit to the observed time-course of the discharge from this spindle, it is necessary to combine three velocity-dependent components, each decaying with a different time-constant. Figure 8.7 shows the degree of goodness of fit that can be achieved by modelling on these lines.

At least seven parameters are required – three sensitivities and three time-constants for the dynamic component, in addition to a representation of the static component. In many cases the static component of response does not vary linearly with the imposed stimulus, and it may take different values according as the current stimulus intensity is approached by an increase from below or by a decrease from above. This feature of the static component can, however, be adequately dealt with using a plot of experimental values.

It may be argued that such a multiplicity of parameters is undesirable. Against this view may be set the fact that the physical situation being

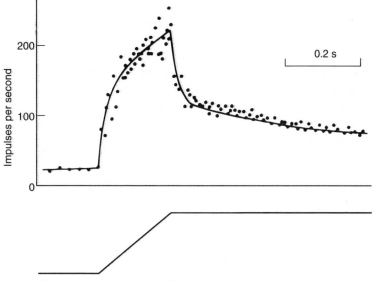

Figure 8.7 Computer simulation of the response of a spindle primary receptor compared with the experimental record. An analogue computer performs the necessary transformations using manually adjusted parameters. The experimental record is that illustrated in Figure 8.6. (From Roberts and Murray-Smith, 1970, by courtesy of AGARD, NATO.)

modelled is itself far from simple. In practice, a set of parameters derived from a single ramp test serves to fit the responses to a whole family of ramps. The formulation is less successful for repetitive changes in conditions, such as by a cyclic change in length, and it may be necessary to use different parameters for shortening from those used for stretching.

This technique of modelling has been applied to joint receptors, to tendon organs, and to frog muscle-spindles, but further study of the mammalian muscle-spindles on these lines has not been pursued because of the complications introduced by the effects of the activity of the intrafusal muscle-fibres.

EFFECTS OF THE ACTIVATION OF INTRAFUSAL MUSCLE-FIBRES

The motor innervation of the intrafusal muscle-fibres is provided mainly by axons of the gamma group, in the classification by conduction-velocity, while the motor axons serving the extrafusal muscle-fibres come in the alpha group. In addition, some spindles also receive an axon, referred to as a 'beta axon', which branches to serve some intrafusal muscle-fibres as well as some extrafusal muscle-fibres. The alpha, beta and gamma groups of motor axons are subdivisions of the same A group in the overall system of alphabetical classification of nerve-fibres. In contrast with this system for motor axons, sensory axons are classified according to a numerical scheme. Afferents from the primary sensory receptors in the spindles come in group Ia in this scheme, and those from secondary endings in group II. (The afferents from tendon organs come in group Ib.)

The effects of fusimotor activity on the sensory discharges from the spindles depend on which intrafusal muscle-fibres are being activated. Figure 8.8 shows the discharge recorded from a Ia primary spindle afferent in response to a standard ramp stretch, a) without gamma activation and, b) and c), with repetitive stimulation, at 100 shocks per second in each case, of each of two different gamma axons. Two different types of fusimotor effect can be distinguished here. In Figure 8.8(b) it is the static component of the afferent discharge that is affected, the unit firing at a higher frequency both before and after the stretch, without any marked effect on the dynamic component associated with the movement. In Figure 8.8(c), on the other hand, the dynamic component is very much enhanced while, at the same time, the static component is also increased to some extent. This type of experiment leads to a subdivision of fusimotor axons into 'static gammas' and 'dynamic gammas'. The static gammas can be further subdivided because some of them produce marked effects on the discharge of

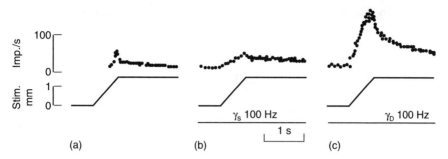

Figure 8.8 Effects of static and dynamic gammas on the discharge of a primary spindle receptor to stretch. The upper traces show the time-course of the discharge of impulses in a single group Ia primary afferent fibre, using reciprocal pulse-interval display. (a) No gamma stimulation: the receptor is at first silent, then starts to fire part way through the stretch. (b) With stimulation of a single static gamma axon at 100 shocks per second. (c) With stimulation of a single dynamic gamma axon, again at 100 shocks per second. (From McWilliam, 1975.)

secondary afferents and comparatively little effect on the responses of primary afferents.

A summary scheme of the different types of interaction between fusimotor activation and ramp stretches is shown in Figure 8.9, which also shows (under the heading 'static bag$_2$ fibre') the effect of static gammas which innervate the fast nuclear bag fibre as well as the chain fibres. Dynamic gammas innervate the slow nuclear bag fibres (also called 'bag$_1$ fibres') with marked effect on the exaggerated response of the primary afferents during stretching (Figure 8.9(a)), and comparatively little effect on the discharge in secondary afferents (d). Some static gammas innervate the fast nuclear bag fibres ('bag$_2$') which contract rapidly but with a high fusion frequency. The static component in the response of the primary afferent is markedly increased (b) and may partially occlude the dynamic component of the response to stretch. Other static gammas preferentially innervate chain muscle-fibres. Activation of these fusimotor axons increases the static component in the discharges of both primary (c) and secondary (f) afferents with little effect on the dynamic responses of either.

In the organization of its balancing behaviour, an animal needs to have information about the relative disposition of the body segments. It also needs to know whether each segment is playing its appropriate part in contributing to supporting the weight with a stiffness, maintained by suitable activation of muscles, that is adequate to prevent collapse. When the body is in motion, appropriate values of torque have to be exerted at various joints, both in generating the required momentum of movement and in absorbing such momentum as

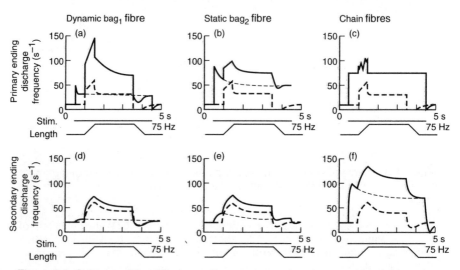

Figure 8.9 Scheme of the effects, on the responses to a 'ramp and hold' length-change, of a primary (above) and of a secondary (below) sensory ending in an isolated mammalian muscle-spindle, produced by repetitive stimulation (75 Hz) of fusimotor axons of different types. (The broken line indicates the response in the absence of fusimotor activation.) Note that in no case does the time-course of the afferent discharge reflect the time-course of the stimulus with any precision. (From Boyd, 1980, by courtesy of *Trends in Neuroscience.*)

inevitably develops in undesired directions as a result of naturally-occurring fluctuations in muscle force. Attempts have been made to describe this behaviour in engineering terms with servomechanical models operating on 'physicist's variables' such as muscle lengths and tensions, and the angles at joints. However, from the accounts given here of the nature of the sensory performance of joint-receptors, tendon organs and muscle-spindles, it must by now be abundantly clear that the task of recovering such parameters as muscle length, tension, or joint angle from mathematical manipulation of the sensory discharge patterns is very far from being the trivial matter that proposers of servo-mechanistic models apparently take it to be. A corresponding set of problems arises in interpreting the signals generated by the sense organs in the labyrinth.

THE BALANCING ORGAN IN THE INNER EAR

An important contribution to the avoidance of overbalancing, both at rest and during locomotion, is provided by the balancing organs in the inner ears on the two sides of the head. The inner ear itself is an elaborate system of tubes and sacs, called the 'membranous labyrinth' from its confusing shape (Figure 8.10). It is filled with fluid, the 'endo-lymph', and suspended, by fine trabeculae, within a set of matching passages and cavities, the 'bony labyrinth', lying deep inside the thick-ness of the dense (stony) 'petrous temporal' bone of the skull. The space between the membranous labyrinth and its containing bony labyrinth is filled with another fluid, the 'perilymph', which is nowhere confluent with the endolymph.

One part of this system, which takes the form of a conical spiral, the 'cochlea', is concerned with hearing. The rest of the organ is concerned with equilibrium. It is referred to as the 'vestibular' part because it forms, as it were, a sort of entrance hall through part of which sound has to travel to pass from the oval window to the hearing organ in the

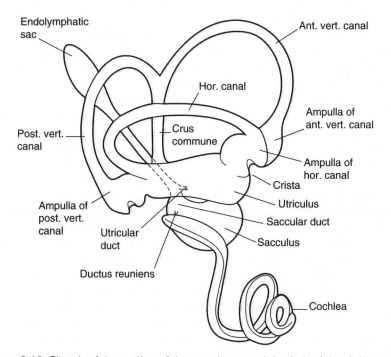

Figure 8.10 Sketch of the outline of the membranous labyrinth of the right ear of a guinea-pig, seen from a little below and slightly behind the interaural line. Note the indentation of the wall of the ampullae at the region of the cristae. The endolymph cavity of the scala media of the cochlea communicates with the cavity of the sacculus by the ductus reuniens. Sacculus and endolymphatic sac in turn communicate with the utriculus, which also receives all the openings of the semicircular canals. The endolymph cavities of the whole labyrinth thus form a continuous closed system of bags and tubes. (Sketch based on com-parisons of photographs given by Lindeman (1969) with earlier illustrations by Retzius (1884) and by Gray (1907).)

cochlea. Within the vestibular portion of the labyrinth one may distinguish the tubes of the semicircular canals and the sacs of the otolith organs.

The receptors of the labyrinth are specialized cells called 'neuromasts'. They form part of the epithelial lining of the membranous labyrinth and they have long hair-like processes which project into the endolymph space. The neuromasts are grouped into patches, the 'maculae' of the sacculus and utriculus, the 'cristae' of the canals, and the organ of Corti in the cochlea.

The endolymph surrounding the hairs of the neuromasts is of a jelly-like consistency; elsewhere it is liquid. The jelly over the maculae in the utriculus and sacculus is loaded with crystals, or concretions, of calcareous material. In the bony fishes there is so much of this material, and it is so compacted together, as to form the so-called 'ear stones' or true otoliths. The absence of the calcareous concretions from the semicircular canals and from the cochlea makes it possible to subdivide the labyrinth into three sections, the canals, the otolith organs and the cochlea. This subdivision also corresponds fairly well to the separation of physiological function between the parts.

In each of the sensory parts of the labyrinth a similar mechanism is involved in generating the discharge of impulses in the afferent nerve. The auxiliary structures are, in each case, so arranged as to produce, in the appropriate conditions of mechanical stimulation, some small relative movement of the jelly overlying the hairs of the neuromast cells. This shearing movement bends or displaces the hairs and thus alters the electrical characteristics of the hair-bearing part of the cell membrane of the neuromasts. Because of the asymmetries in the fine structure of the neuromast cell, a local circuit current flows between the hair-bearing part of the cell membrane and the regions bearing the synaptic contacts with the afferent nerve-fibres. A change in the intensity of this local circuit current, occurring as a consequence of the displacement of the hairs, alters the rate of liberation of transmitter at the synaptic region and thus changes the frequency at which impulses are generated in the nerve. It is usual for the afferent nerve-fibres to show a continuous repetitive discharge of impulses when the sense organ is at rest. Deflection of the hairs in one direction increases the frequency of the afferent discharge, while deflection of the hairs in the opposite direction decreases it.

In addition to the afferent nerve-fibres which carry the sensory messages, the neuromasts are furnished with efferent nerve-fibres through which they receive impulses from the central nervous system. The synapses of these efferent nerve-fibres are cholinergic. When active, they produce hyperpolarizing postsynaptic potentials in the neuromast cells themselves. The effect of the efferent discharge is thus to stabilize the membrane potential of the neuromast so that the local circuit currents, generated by the bending of the hairs, become less effective in liberating transmitter to excite the sensory nerve-fibres.

Recordings from the efferent nerves indicate that they are active when the animal is moving about. One may thus conclude that the function of the efferent nerve supply to the labyrinth is to reduce the intensity of the sensory signals when the head is being moved voluntarily by the animal.

Each of the semicircular canals opens at both ends into the same sac, the utriculus. The individual canals thus form a set of complete rings, closed through the common utricular space. Disregarding minor irregularities, the three rings of the canals on each side of the head lie in mutually perpendicular planes, one horizontal and two vertical, each of these being angled at 45° to the midline. The plane of the anterior vertical canal of one side is parallel to the plane of the posterior vertical canal of the opposite side (Figure 8.11). Each canal swells out at one point to form an 'ampulla' (Figure 8.12) which encloses the sensory apparatus of the canal. The wall of the ampulla is partially invaginated at one side and thickened into a ridge, the 'crista', which bears the sensory neuromast cells together with the nerve-fibres serving them. The hair-like processes of the neuromasts of the crista project into the endolymph space within the ampulla, where they are embedded in a jelly-like mass, called the 'cupula'. The cupula, mounted on the crista, completely blocks the lumen of the ampulla.

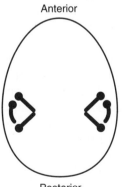

Figure 8.11 Schematic plan view of the head of a mammal to show the disposition of the planes of the vertical semicircular canals.

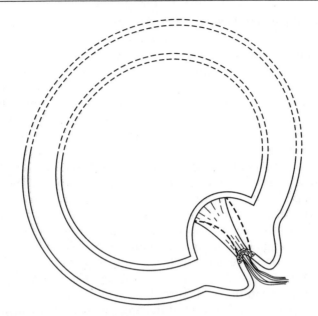

Figure 8.12 Mechanism of action of a semicircular canal. The canal, with its ampulla, is represented as forming a complete circle. In most cases part of the circle is shared with other canals. In clockwise angular acceleration of the skull in the plane of the diagram, the force to accelerate the endolymph is provided by the cupula. This accordingly suffers elastic deformation as indicated by the dotted lines.

THE MECHANICS OF THE SEMICIRCULAR CANAL

The elecronmicroscope reveals that the 'hairs' of a neuromast each consist of a bundle of cilia closely packed together side by side in an orderly hexagonal array (Figure 8.13). In each bundle of cilia there is a single kinocilium whose fine structure resembles that of a motile flagellum. The other cilia are all of another kind called stereocilia. The kinocilium usually lies to one side of the bundle and the stereocilia are of orderly increasing length, the longest being adjacent to the kinocilium. The arrangement is indicated diagrammatically in Figure 8.13. Each hair bundle thus shows a morphological polarization, and it is possible to map out the orientation of the hairs in different parts of the sensory epithelium in each of the receptor areas in the labyrinth. A correlation of this information with the results of electrophysiological experiments indicates that the afferent nerve-fibre shows an increase in discharge frequency when the hairs of its neuromasts are deflected towards the kinocilium and *vice versa*.

The deflection of the hairs of the neuromasts is a manifestation of the

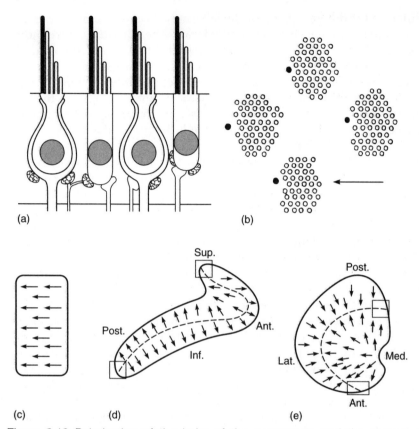

Figure 8.13 Polarization of the hairs of the neuromasts and the pattern of polarization in the sensory epithelia of the labyrinth. The morphological polarization vector of the neuromasts (arrow) is determined by the position of the kinocilium (dark) in relation to the stereocilia. (a) Section perpendicular to the epithelial surface; note increasing length of the stereocilia towards the kinocilium. (b) Section parallel to the surface. ● = kinocilium; ○ = stereocilium. (c) The neuromasts of the cristae of the semicircular canals are all polarized in the same direction. (d) Macula sacculi and (e) macula utriculi, in each case divided by an arbitrary curved line into two areas, internal and external, with opposite morphological polarization in each. In the sacculus the neuromasts are polarized away from the dividing line; in the utriculus towards the line. In the peripheral areas at each end of the lines (rectangles) the pattern is irregular. (From Lindeman, 1969, by courtesy of *Ergeb. Anat. Entwickl.-Gesch.*)

strain occurring within the structure of the sensory apparatus. Because the endolymph filling the cavities of the labyrinth is fluid and not rigidly coupled to the skull, some relative movement can occur. The conditions for producing relative movement of the endolymph are different for different parts of the labyrinth. In the case of the semicircular canals, the mechanism is as follows. The jelly-mass surrounding the hairs of the crista extends right across the lumen of the ampulla, forming a complete plug across the canal. When the head is moved about, the force needed to accelerate the endolymph within the labyrinth is, for most movements, provided by pressure against the containing wall. An exception to this arises in the canals when angular accelerations occur about an axis through the plane of a canal.

The ring of endolymph contained in a canal has a certain inertia and, if it is to be set into angular motion about an axis through the centre of the ring, the only structure available to exert the necessary accelerating force is the jelly-mass of the cupula blocking the lumen of the ampulla. An angular acceleration of the skull about any axis through the plane of the canal will therefore lead to elastic deformation of the cupula. This deformation deflects the hairs of the neuromasts and consequently generates a sensory signal in the afferent nerve-fibres.

It is a general property of neuromasts that, even when apparently at rest and not being affected by any external perturbation, they generate a continuous stream of impulses in the sensory nerve. It may be that, in the course of development in the embryo and during subsequent growth, the individual hairs become distorted in some way and this may be the origin of the 'resting discharge'. An important consequence of this feature of neuromast behaviour is that they can signal changes in imposed strain in two directions: an increase in discharge frequency occurring when the hairs are displaced towards the kinocilium and a decrease in discharge when the displacement is in the opposite direction.

The amount of the preset deformation in the neuromasts of the cristae in the canals varies from one neuromast to another. Whereas the majority are firing steadily in conditions of no angular acceleration, there are some neuromasts which are silent when the skull is at rest and which only begin to fire when the angular acceleration exceeds a certain value. Other neuromasts, on the other hand, are found to be discharging at a comparatively high frequency which is little affected by small accelerations in either direction. The frequency of discharge from neuromasts of this type can, however, be decreased by imposing a sufficiently large angular acceleration in the appropriate direction.

A plot of firing-frequency against cupula-deflection gives an S-shaped curve. The typical neuromast has this curve so positioned that the steep and approximately linear central part of the curve occurs near the rest position of the cupula. The types of response differing from the most usual type in the two extreme ways mentioned above would then correspond to neuromasts whose response-curves were displaced to the right and to the left respectively along the deflection axis. This arrangement, with the majority of the receptors preset into the middle of the most useful region of their response-curves, ensures a maximum sensitivity for the organ as a whole, together with the absence of any dead zone such as might occur if the stimulus had to exceed a threshold strength before it was effective in producing a response.

The degree of deflection of the cupula in a semicircular canal, and hence the magnitude of the stimulus to the neuromasts, is very much dependent on the dynamics of the relative motion of the endolymph. Three factors have to be taken into account:

1. the mass of the column of endolymph that is to move;
2. the spring-stiffness of the cupula in resisting displacements;
3. the viscous damping arising from movement of a column of liquid along a narrow tube.

The equation of motion of the system is the same as that for a heavily damped torsion pendulum, taking the moment of inertia as that of a ring of endolymph and the restoring torque as the product of the elastic force produced by deformation of the cupula multiplied by the distance from the cupula to the centre of the ring. The equation involves three parameters, related respectively to inertia, stiffness and damping. In the case of the canals both the inertia effect and the damping effect are relatively large compared with the effect of the force restoring the cupula to its rest position after a deflection. The system is heavily overdamped. This means that, after a perturbation, the system will take some time to recover from deflections produced during the perturbation. This leads to a convenient routine for studying the dynamics.

In an experimental study it is inconvenient to have to follow effects which are present only while the skull is in motion. The problems of recording are simplified if we adopt the procedure indicated in Figure 8.14. The skull is first subjected to a moderate angular acceleration in one direction. After a suitable angular velocity has been attained, the accelerating force is removed and the rotation is allowed to continue for some time at constant speed. During this period, the cupula gradually moves back to its rest position, in spite of continued rotation. The top three traces in the figure show the time-courses of the applied acceleration, the angular velocity, and the orientation of the skull. The rotation is about a vertical axis.

After a suitable interval the rotation is stopped by the brisk application of an angular deceleration, e.g. by putting on the brakes. The same deceleration must also be applied to the endolymph, because otherwise it would continue to rotate by virtue of its inertia. The momentum of the endolymph thus produces a cupula-deflection in a sense opposite to that brought about by the initial angular acceleration. Because of the damping, this deflection takes some time to die away after the decelerating force has been removed. A period of several seconds is thus available, during which we may study the effects of the persisting cupula-deflection with the skull completely at rest.

The precise time-course of the deceleration is immaterial provided that it is all over within a period which is short compared with the time-constants of the cupula movement. The reason for this is that, for short-lasting accelerations, the magnitude of the cupula-deflection maintains a very close proportionality to the time-integral of the acceleration; that is to say, it is related to the achieved change in angular velocity. Now, if we are decelerating to rest from a fixed starting value of angular velocity, the total change in velocity will be the same for any value of the deceleration. Larger decelerations will produce the required change in velocity in a shorter time, but in each case the product of the magnitude of the deceleration multiplied by the duration of its action will come to the same value. Thus any pattern of deceleration which brings the skull to rest from the same starting value of angular velocity will produce the same cupula-deflection at the moment of stopping.

This is the basis of the 'impulsive deceleration' method of testing the functioning of the canals. It is called 'impulsive' because the word 'impulse' is used in mechanics to mean the product of the magnitude of a force multiplied by the duration of the period during which it acts, particularly if the duration is short. During the post-deceleration phase the effects of the remaining cupula-deflection can be studied with the skull at rest. The time-course of the decay of these effects (bottom trace in Figure 8.14) depends on the ratios of the parameters of the equation of motion, which can then be deduced from the observed shape of the decay curve. The resulting equation can then be used to predict the responses to other routines of stimulation.

It is inadvisable to use too brisk a deceleration in this procedure because, if excessive peak force is applied to the cupula, it may become detached from the wall of the ampulla opposite to the crista. Later angular accelerations will then cause the cupula to be deflected like a swing door, instead of simply bulging. In consequence, the sensitivity of the detector apparatus will be much reduced, until sufficient time has been allowed to elapse for the detachment to heal up.

Figure 8.15 shows what happens during the initial acceleration phase. At the point A, a constant angular acceleration, about a vertical axis, is applied suddenly, the skull having been at rest up to this point. Under the influence of the applied acceleration, the skull will begin to rotate at a steadily increasing angular velocity. The orientation, i.e. the direction in which the skull is pointing, changes at first slowly, and then progressively faster and faster. The plot of orientation against time should have a parabolic form, but in our diagram this has been broken into segments to correspond to the successive full circles of rotation.

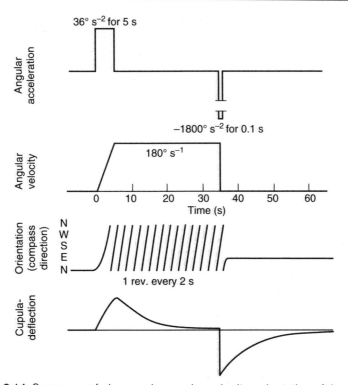

Figure 8.14 Sequence of changes in angular velocity, orientation of the skull in space, and cupula-deflection, during the procedure for imposing an impulsive deceleration. Note that the cupula-deflection persists after the skull has been brought to rest. Note also that, if the deceleration were spread over 1 s, instead of occupying only 0.1 s, the force needed would be reduced to one tenth, yet the cupula-deflection reached in the rest position would have the same value as that shown here.

The broken line corresponding to cupula-deflection indicates the deflection that would be expected if the cupula followed the imposed angular acceleration exactly. Because of the damping, the actual deflection of the cupula follows a different time-course, indicated by the full line. After a step in the broken line, the full line moves more slowly and approaches exponentially towards the new steady value indicated by the broken line. The time-constant of this exponential has been found experimentally to be about 10 s for man.

At the point B, the driving force is removed and the angular acceleration falls to zero. The angular velocity thereafter remains constant at the value which it has achieved during the acceleration phase. The skull continues to rotate steadily at constant speed. The cupula-deflection gradually declines to zero as the restoring forces generated

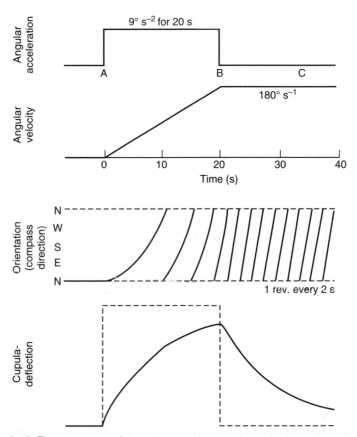

Figure 8.15 Time-courses of the changes in angular velocity, orientation, and cupula-deflection, arising from the application of a constant angular acceleration during the period from A to B.

in the cupula act against the viscous friction and gradually push the endolymph back into place. The time-constant for the decline in cupula-deflection is the same as for the increase in deflection at the onset of the applied acceleration.

The diagram brings out two features of the behaviour of the canals. In the first place the effect of the damping during the early stages of the applied angular acceleration is to alter the time-course of the cupula-deflection until it approximately resembles the time-course of the angular velocity rather than that of the angular acceleration itself.

This effect has been the source of considerable confusion, particularly as the subjective sensations which are presumably derived from the canals are usually interpreted in terms of 'speed of turning', whereas the physics of the canal itself indicates that the adequate stimulus must be angular acceleration. The distinction is emphasized by the second feature shown in the diagram. When, at C and after, some time has been allowed to elapse after the acceleration has come to an end, the cupula-deflection correctly indicates that the skull is no longer being subjected to angular acceleration. Correspondingly, there are no sub-jective sensations of turning. Nevertheless, the skull is still continuing to turn round and round at constant angular velocity.

The conditions illustrated in Figure 8.15 are not often encountered except in the experimental laboratory. The skull is seldom exposed to a prolonged period of constant angular acceleration followed by a pro-longed period of rotation at constant speed. A more usual sequence is the one illustrated in Figure 8.16. The skull is subjected to an angular acceleration which waxes and wanes fairly smoothly and which is followed, after only a very short interval, by a deceleration, i.e. by an angular acceleration in the opposite direction, which waxes and wanes in its turn. The angular velocity rises in an S-shaped curve to a maximum and then declines again with another S-shaped curve. The orientation

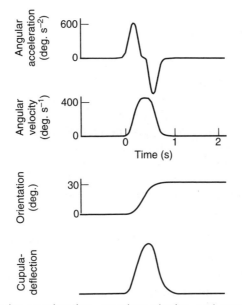

Figure 8.16 Angular acceleration, angular velocity, and cupula-deflection, to be expected during a naturally-occurring movement. The curve for acceleration (generated electronically) was chosen to give (by double integration) a time-course of displacement which closely matched an experimental record from a human subject. The cupula-deflection (y) is computed from the angular acceleration (x) of the skull, using the equation, $\ddot{y} + 10\dot{y} + y = kx$, and an analogue computer.

of the skull changes smoothly from one position to another. The time-course of the deflections of the cupula may be predicted from the time-course of the angular accelerations using an analogue computer, programmed according to the known equation of motion of the canal dynamics, to take account of the exponential lag. The result is shown by the last line in Figure 8.16.

It will be seen that the phase of deceleration occurs so soon after the initial acceleration that the cupula is still deflected in the one direction when the time comes for it to begin to move the opposite way. In consequence, the effect of the deceleration is all used up in restoring the cupula to the rest position and there is nothing left over to produce a deflection in the opposite sense. It is evident from this diagram how it comes about that, in many physiological movements, and even in clinical tests, such a good correlation is found between the sensation of turning and the angular velocity. This resolves the old controversy between clinicians who held that the canals gave rise to the sensation of turning (angular velocity) and physiologists who concluded, from the anatomy of the canals, that these must function as detectors of angular acceleration, rather than of angular velocity.

THE OTOLITH ORGANS

The expression 'otolith organs' refers to the two sacs, the utriculus and the sacculus, shown in the middle of Figure 8.10. The utriculus receives the openings of the semicircular canals, while the sacculus connects to the cochlea and to the endolymphatic duct, a narrow tube ending blindly in a small sac lying inside the cranial cavity, between the dura and the surface of the temporal bone. (The endolymphatic duct and sac have a secretory function concerned with maintaining the differences in composition between the endolymph and the perilymph.) An additional small duct connects sacculus and utriculus. Both sacculus and utriculus have maculae, i.e. patches of sensory epithelium containing neuromasts.

The structure of the otolith organs enables them to function as differential-density accelerometers. Each is an irregularly-shaped sac with somewhat rounded outline, completely filled with fluid. In the neighbourhood of the sensory epithelium of the macula the fluid is stiffened by mucopolysaccharides to form a gel containing a network of fibrils tethered to the underlying macula. The gel is loaded with calcite crystals, the 'otoconia', which appear to be trapped in the fibrillar matrix of the gel, so that the region containing the otoconia has a greater mean density than the rest of the endolymph.

Under the influence of the supporting forces that normally prevent the skull from falling to the ground under the action of gravity, the contents of the sac tend to form a density-gradient, like the contents of a centrifuge tube. The jelly mass tends to slide round to place the denser part at the bottom of the cavity. This movement is prevented by the fibrils that tether the gel to the macula, but any relative movement that does take place will bend the hairs of the neuromasts and generate a sensory signal.

Because of the morphological polarization of the hair bundles (Figure 8.13), the signal from the afferent nerve-fibres will reflect the magnitude of the resolved component of shear along the direction of polarization. A full circle rotation of the skull about a stationary horizontal axis will thus produce a sinusoidal change in the stimulus, the amplitude of this change depending on the orientation of the polarization vector to the plane of the rotation, where the expression 'polarization vector' indicates that direction in which the shearing motion of the otolith mass is most effective in generating afferent impulses in the unit under consideration. The vector for an individual neuromast lies in a plane tangential to the epithelial surface in which that neuromast lies, and it passes through the centre of the bundle of stereocilia in the direction of the kinocilium.

Because the stimulus to the neuromasts is a consequence of the application of stress forces to the skull, the effective shear at a particular neuromast will be at a maximum when the resultant supporting force applied to the skull is aligned with, but opposite in direction to, the polarization vector for that neuromast. The receptors themselves are fixed in the skull so that a particular polarization vector may be characterized as a direction relative to landmarks on the skull. When speaking of a sensory unit, in which a single afferent neuron receives influences from a number of neuromasts, we select that direction, relative to the skull, in which a particular direction of support force produces the maximum discharge. This is most easily done by having the skull fastened to a stationary tilting apparatus. The resultant of the supporting forces will then be exactly opposed in direction to that of the pull of gravity, and we may use the earth's horizon as a reference plane.

The responses of individual sensory units in the otolith organs during changes in the orientation of the skull have been studied electrophysiologically by Lowenstein and Roberts. They used the labyrinth of an elasmobranch fish – the ray – chosen partly for the size of the labyrinth, and partly for the ease in dissection afforded by the fact that the skull of the elasmobranch is almost entirely cartilaginous. They were able to dissect small twigs from the nerves to the various otolith organs and to record the discharge of impulses from single sensory units, both with the skull in different positions and while the skull was being tilted in various directions. The receptors recorded from did not all behave in the same way.

Some of the receptors found seem to be admirably suited to the role of position indicators. They give rise to a steady stream of nerve-impulses at a repetition-frequency which depends only on the position of the skull in relation to the vertical. When the skull is slowly rotated about a horizontal axis, the discharge from a receptor of this type gradually waxes and wanes according to the angle of tilt. When a particular position is reached on the second time round, the corresponding discharge-frequency is the same as it was on the first occasion. If the tilting is carried out in the opposite direction, the sequence of changes in discharge-frequency is reversed also (Figure 8.17). If the skull is left stationary in one particular position, the discharge remains at the appropriate frequency for a prolonged period. Each angle of tilt corresponds to a particular impulse-frequency, and *vice versa*, with the single ambiguity inevitable in a cyclic relation of this type. That is to say, a particular impulse-frequency is passed through twice during the full-circle tilt: once during the phase of rising impulse-frequency and once during the declining phase.

Localization is not very precise near the positions corresponding to the discharges at the maximum and minimum of the frequency range. However, the various receptors differ among themselves in the precise positions in which they develop their maximum frequencies of discharge. Thus, if we take the information from several receptors together, we not only eliminate the ambiguities, we also improve the discrimination over the whole range.

Various horizontal axes were used in the tilting experiments. For purposes of classification it is convenient to confine our attention to the effects of rotations about two fixed axes: the fore-and-aft and the transverse horizontal axes. Some units gave their maximum discharges on side-up tilting and also on nose-up tilting, others showed maxima on side-up tilting and also on nose-down tilting. Presumably for each individual receptor there is a particular horizontal axis which will give the widest range of discharge-frequencies, and thus the greatest discrimination of degree of tilting. It is clear that sufficient information is available from all the receptors taken together to enable the central nervous system to deduce not only the angle of tilt, but also the axis of rotation about which the tilt has taken place.

Special position-receptors were found in the lagena. (This is a pouch of the sacculus found in some lower animals which do not possess a cochlea. It is not present in mammals.) The general character of the response of these receptors was similar to that already described, i.e. there was a definite relationship between skull-position and impulse-frequency, with waxing and waning of the discharge during the course

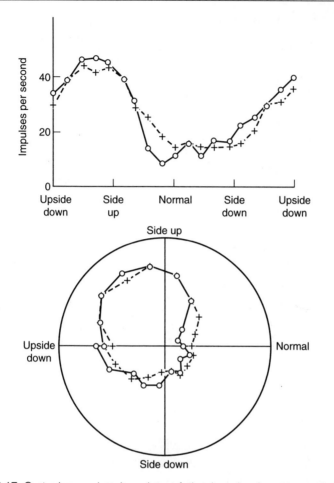

Figure 8.17 Cartesian and polar plots of the impulse-frequency of the discharge from a single unit in the utriculus of the ray during two full-circle tilts in opposite directions. The continuous curves are to be read from left to right and clockwise, the dotted curves from right to left and anticlockwise. Receptors with responses of this type are suited to function as position-detectors. (From Lowenstein and Roberts, 1949, by courtesy of *J. Physiol.*)

of a full-circle tilt. In this case, however, the whole range of variation in impulse-frequency occurred over a comparatively small range of angles of tilt (Figure 8.18). A sharp maximum in the discharge occurs in the neighbourhood of the normal position, and the impulse-frequency falls off sharply on either side, within about 45° of tilting. During a full-circle tilt, receptors of this type are relatively quiescent during most of the tilting, and then suddenly burst into high-frequency activity as the normal position is approached. When the tilting is continued beyond

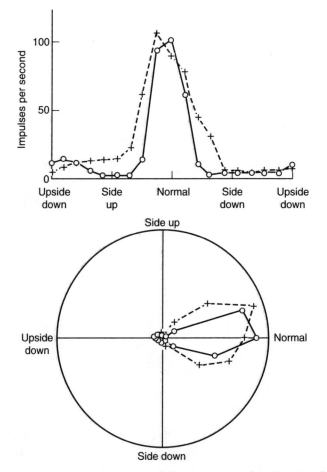

Figure 8.18 (Compare with Figure 8.17) The response of an 'into-level' receptor in the lagena (a diverticulum of the utriculus) of the ray, during two full-circle lateral tilts in opposite directions. The continuous curves are to be read from left to right and clockwise, the dotted curves from right to left and anticlockwise. (From Lowenstein and Roberts, 1949, by courtesy of *J. Physiol.*)

the normal position, the discharge declines, over a few degrees of tilting, just as suddenly as it began. Receptors of this type were nick-named 'into-level receptors'.

Other receptors, whose afferent fibres were lying side by side with those from the position-receptors described above, were found to respond to tilting in a rather different way (Figure 8.19). They seemed more responsive to the motion of tilting, and were less concerned with the actual position attained. If the skull was held stationary in any position, the discharge from these endings tended to adapt towards

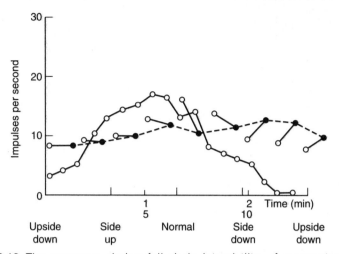

Figure 8.19 The response, during full-circle lateral tilts, of a receptor in the utriculus of the ray which showed a predominantly 'dynamic' type of response, with adaptation. The continuous line shows the response during a continuous rotation occupying about 2.5 min. Superposed are readings taken during an interrupted tilt in the same direction, occupying in all about 13 min. The time-scales have been adjusted to bring the positions of the skull into correspondence for a comparison of the two tilts. ○ = frequency on reaching a particular position; ● = frequency after 1 min rest in that position. The broken line connects the values of the 'adapted' discharges. (From Lowenstein and Roberts, 1949, by courtesy of *J. Physiol.*)

some standard value which was sometimes only slightly different in different positions.

In some of these cases of dynamic responses to tilting, the organ gave the same type of response, i.e. a decrease in its discharge, when the tilting was started in either direction. This was followed, as in the other cases, by cyclic waxing and waning in impulse-frequency during continued tilting through several complete revolutions (Figure 8.20).

Yet another type of receptor was indifferent to the position of the skull and indifferent to the motion of smooth tilting in any direction but, at the same time, was exquisitely sensitive to any vibrations occurring in, or conducted to, the preparation-holder. The presence of these vibration-receptors accounts for the ability of the otolith organs of the fish to act as a primitive hearing organ.

The range of responses encountered in these neuromasts of the otolith organs may be considered in terms of static and dynamic responses, as in the discussion of deformation-receptors earlier in this chapter. The true position-receptors and the 'into-level' receptors show a preponderance of the static component of the response to deformation, with little sign of a dynamic component. The next type, with

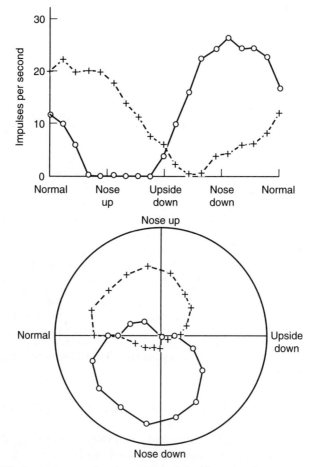

Figure 8.20 Cartesian and polar plots of the impulse-frequency of the discharge from a single unit in the utriculus of a ray during two full-circle fore-and-aft tilts in opposite directions. The continuous curves are to be read from left to right and clockwise, the dotted curves from right to left and anticlockwise. Compare with Figure 8.17. Receptors with responses of this type are unsuited to the signalling of position. Their discharge can be interpreted only as an indication that a movement of some sort is taking place. (From Lowenstein and Roberts, 1949, by courtesy of *J. Physiol.*)

its marked adaptation in discharge-frequency after the skull has been brought to rest in any position, shows the dynamic component of the response to deformation, with only a comparatively small static component. The third type, responding to movement, but without discrimination as to the direction of movement, provides a link, of considerable theoretical importance, between the directional deformation-receptors and the last type, the receptors for vibration.

It has already been pointed out that the receptors in the otolith organs are sensitive to the stress-gradients associated with linear accelerations of the skull, as well as those associated with supporting the skull against the action of gravity. Now the oscillatory motions, of which vibrations are composed, involve alternating accelerations and decelerations. It is therefore not surprising to find that specific receptors for the detection of vibrations have evolved alongside the receptors for detecting linear acceleration. Where the accelerations are fluctuating rather than steady, it is advantageous to emphasize the dynamic component of the response at the expense of the static component. Indeed, the static component may be dispensed with altogether in a receptor adapted particularly for the detection of vibration.

The next transition in the evolution of the receptors for hearing has been to dissociate the impulse-frequency in the afferent nerve from the repetition-frequency of the mechanical oscillations. In the early stages, as represented by the position-receptors, the movements involved in the adequate stimulus are very slow, compared with the firing-frequency of the impulses in the nerve. In these conditions, impulse-frequency can be used to signal the magnitude of the excursion in each movement as it occurs. When more and more rapid movements are encountered, the afferent impulses come in a succession of bursts until we reach a stage where the repetition-frequency of the movements falls in the same range as the repetition-frequency of the nerve-impulses. What often happens at this point in the experimental stimulation of a deformation-receptor is that the nerve-impulses become synchronized with the imposed vibrations, each cycle of deformation giving rise to a single impulse.

There is now the possibility of confusion between changes in the frequency of the stimulating vibration and changes in its intensity. If the central nervous system receives an increased frequency of discharge, how is this to be interpreted? The confusion is avoided if the receptor signals the mean amplitude of the imposed vibrations rather than the amplitude of the excursion in one particular direction. Discrimination as to frequency of imposed oscillation can be provided by having different receptors specialized to respond preferentially to particular ranges of frequency of vibration. The neuromasts in the organ of Corti in the cochlea of the mammals are specialized to respond in this way. It is interesting to see that the disregard of the direction of deformation, which is a necessary prerequisite for the full development of the hearing organ, already begins to show itself in the responses of the movement-receptors in the otolith organs of the cartilaginous fishes.

The full list of types of receptor found in the otolith organs is:

- wide-range position-receptors with static response;
- 'into-level' position-receptors;

- position-receptors with predominantly dynamic response;
- movement-receptors;
- vibration-receptors.

The 'into-level' receptors were found only in the lagena. Part of the sacculus contained only vibration-receptors. With these exceptions, the different types were distributed over all three otolith organs.

Later studies on the cat and on the squirrel monkey have yielded discharge patterns somewhat similar in form to those illustrated here for the ray. However, when recording from a microelectrode in the eighth nerve, it is not always an easy matter to determine where the receptors contributing to the observed discharge are actually situated within the labyrinth. Even when the direction of the polarization vector has been precisely located by comparing the effectiveness of tilts about various axes, this still does not define the location of the receptors themselves. Suppose, for the moment, that the otolith organ is roughly spherical, and that we have found a sensory unit whose polarization vector points to one pole of the sphere: neuromasts with parallel polarization vectors may still lie anywhere around the equator of the

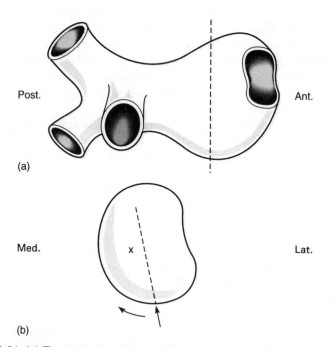

Post.

Ant.

(a)

Med.

x

Lat.

(b)

Figure 8.21 (a) The utriculus of the right side, with canals removed (detail from Figure 8.10). (b) Diagrammatic transverse section in the plane indicated by the broken line in the drawing above, viewed from the left in that figure.

sphere. The otolith membrane actually covers only a part of the inside surface of the organ (see Figure 8.21, which shows a section through the utriculus). The macula bearing the hair cells is, however, curved in two directions, with unequal curvatures. The same principles apply as to a sphere. A thrust directed along the broken line in Figure 8.21 will produce a similar shearing action between otolith membrane and macula to that of a side-down rotation of the skull, as indicated by the curved arrow.

It is interesting to note that one group of investigators found that, for the whole of their population of recorded units, the polarization vectors lay near to the plane of the horizontal canal, although within this plane they were distributed right round the compass. This suggests that the system as a whole is particularly well-suited to reporting tilts in any direction in the immediate neighbourhood of the normal head pose of the animal.

We have now concluded our survey of the manoeuvres that an animal performs in the course of maintaining its balance and of carrying out acts of locomotion. We have also examined the nature of the sensory messages that are available to it as a basis for formulating the patterns of motor command by which these manoeuvres are executed. We now need to consider how the sensory information is processed within the central nervous system. In the next chapter we start by considering some of the stages in central co-ordination about which we have relevant information. In the later part of the chapter I present a scheme which could account for the co-ordinating processes themselves.

Central processing 9

In the context of the present book it is not appropriate to examine whatever relationship may exist between nervous activity and conscious experience. We confine our attention to the processes involved in generating the command signals needed to control the musculature in a manner appropriate to the messages received from the sense organs. These sensory messages are conveyed by the impulse traffic in a large number of separate and independent sensory neurons. The motor output also involves an equally large number of separate neurons.

Conventional views of the operation of the central nervous system tend to be unduly influenced by accounts of what goes on in the jerk reflexes. The concept of reflex activity depends on the idea that messages of some kind are initiated at peripheral sites and are passed, along nerves, to the central nervous system which, by some process not usually specified, generates other messages which pass out, again along nerves, to the peripheral effectors. For a particular type of reflex response to occur it is necessary that the stimulating conditions at the appropriate sensory area should conform to a particular pattern, referred to as the 'adequate stimulus' for producing that response. No further details of the mechanism of reflex activity were specified when the idea was first launched.

This omission has had the unfortunate effect that generalizations about other aspects of central nervous behaviour have been based on what has since been learned about the details of jerk reflexes. When the stretch reflex was first discovered, the differences between it and the jerk reflexes were clearly set out. In later years, however, these differences came to be ignored in favour of the seductive simplicity of the concept of 'stretch', which was held to be the common adequate stimulus for each of these two reflexes. This confusion does not take account of the complexity of the distribution of stresses and strains through the tissues of muscles and tendons.

THE 'ADEQUATE STIMULUS' FOR THE JERK REFLEX

When the physician taps a patient's tendon, a shock wave of transitorily increased tension spreads from the point of impact throughout the combined length of tendon and attached muscle. Deformation-receptors of various kinds are affected. Especially important is the effect on the primary receptors in the muscle-spindles of the affected muscles. Because these show a dynamic component in their response to local stretch, the shock wave causes many of these primary receptors to activate their sensory nerve-fibres more or less at the same time. In consequence, a set of synchronized impulses passes in a number of fibres of the afferent nerve trunk, and these impulses arrive at their destinations in the spinal cord at much the same time as one another. This pattern of afferent bombardment of the spinal cord can be imitated, fairly closely, by applying an electric shock to the nerve trunk, a technique that lends itself to precise recording of the timing.

As a result of the arrival at the spinal cord of a set of synchronized impulses in the nerve serving a particular muscle, another set of synchronized impulses appears in the motor nerve-fibres running to that same muscle. It is this synchronized volley of motor impulses that is responsible for the form of the jerk response, since the motor units served by the active motor nerve-fibres all develop their mechanical activity at the same time, to produce the sudden increase in muscle force that is manifested as the jerk response.

Synchronized volleys of nerve-impulses are easily timed, and it is found that the outgoing impulses in this situation follow the incoming volley with a delay which cannot be entirely accounted for as the time of conduction along the nerve-fibres running between the stimulating and the recording electrodes. Recordings from microelectrodes inserted into motoneurons tell us that this small but irreducible residual delay can be accounted for as the excitation time for activating a single cell. This delay time has come to be spoken of as 'synaptic delay'. Where the residual time between stimulus and response (called the 'latency') in a particular pathway, after taking account of the time needed for conduction along the nerve-fibres concerned, turns out to involve only a delay of this small duration, the transmission pathway is referred to as 'monosynaptic'. One should avoid the temptation to infer that only a single synapse is involved. Before any response can be observed it is necessary that the strength of the stimulating shock be great enough to excite a number of nerve-fibres. Large fibres are more readily excited by electric shocks than smaller fibres so that it can be arranged, by using a suitably small shock, that only the largest fibres will be activated. The largest afferent fibres in a muscle nerve are the Ia axons connected to primary receptors in the muscle-spindles.

SYNAPTIC TRANSMISSION

The central terminations of the primary afferents branch extensively in the grey matter of the spinal cord (Figure 9.1). Each of the fine terminal branches of the afferents carries several blob-like expansions called 'end-knobs' which are the sites of communication with other cells. Each of the motoneurons has an extensive dendritic arborization (Figure 9.2). There is a considerable overlap between the region that can be influenced from a single afferent axon and the region from which a motoneuron can receive synaptic influences. Histological examination of the spinal cord reveals a dense interlacing of nerve-fibres surrounding the motoneurons, and electronmicrographs show many sites of

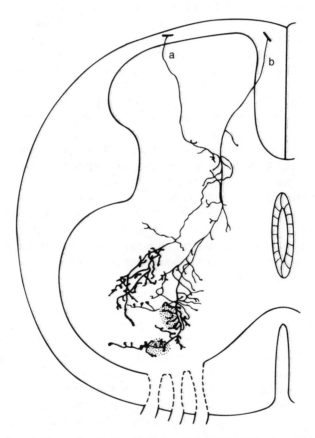

Figure 9.1 Terminal ramifications of two Ia afferents (a, b) in the grey matter of the spinal cord of a newborn kitten. The cell bodies of two motoneurons are indicated by stippling. Those nerve branches that lie within the motor nucleus are coarser than the others. Golgi rapid procedure. (From Szentágothai, 1967, by courtesy of Elsevier.)

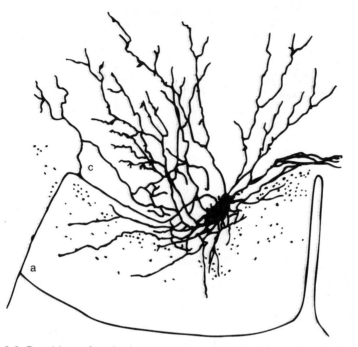

Figure 9.2 Dendrites of a single motoneuron ramifying through a thick slab of tissue. A recurrent collateral, c, can be seen branching off the axon, a. Golgi stain. (From Cajal, 1952, by courtesy of the Instituto Ramon y Cajal.)

specialized intercell contact in each field of view. Each motoneuron dendrite is closely encrusted with end-knobs which are derived from axons reaching the region from many different sources and not from muscle afferents alone. The indications are that each motoneuron receives functional connections from several, possibly several hundred, other nerve cells. This is an important difference from the situation obtaining at a neuromuscular junction, where a single nerve cell innervates a number of skeletal muscle cells, and each muscle cell commonly receives only one motor nerve-fibre.

In electronmicrographs of the ventral grey matter of the spinal cord, the two cells forming a synapse are seen to be closely apposed to one another over a restricted area, at a spacing of 200–300 Å. Elsewhere the cell membranes are further apart, often with portions of other cells interposed. The precise details of the synaptic morphology differ from one site to another, as may be seen from the examples illustrated in Figure 9.3. Because messages are transmitted across a synapse in one direction only, we may speak of one cell as 'presynaptic' and of the other as 'postsynaptic'. A number of 'synaptic vesicles', each about

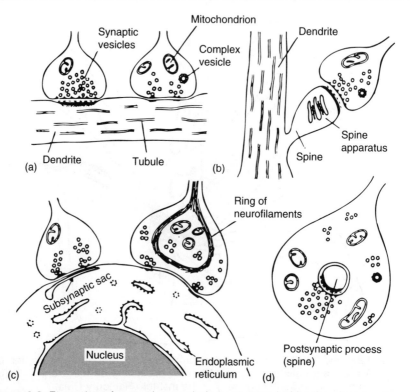

Figure 9.3 Examples of synaptic morphology as revealed by the electronmicroscope. (a) Two types of axodendritic synapse; (b) synapse involving a spiny process on a dendrite; (c) two types of axosomatic synapse; (d) synapse in which an invagination of the presynaptic terminal surrounds the postsynaptic spine. (From Whittaker and Gray, 1962, by courtesy of *Brit. Med. Bull.*)

400 Å in diameter, can be seen in the cytoplasm of the end-knob of the presynaptic cell near the junctional region. These vesicles contain packets of the chemical substance that will act as a transmitter at the synaptic junction.

Each of the end-knobs, when active, releases packets of transmitter into the specialized 'synaptic cleft' which is the effective contact region with the postsynaptic cell. The result is a local change in membrane permeability, and consequently a change in dendritic membrane potential, leading to local circuit currents which affect the cell membrane of the cell body. At the root of the axon of a motoneuron there is a specialized region called the 'axon hillock' which is continuous with the unmyelinated initial portion of the axon. The rest of the axon, down to its termination on the muscle cells it serves, is covered by a myelin sheath, interrupted only by nodes of Ranvier. The axon hillock

is devoid of end-knobs so that, in common with the bare initial segment of the axon, it is readily depolarized by local circuit currents. If
these are of sufficient intensity, they initiate action-potentials that propagate outwards along the length of the axon, and sometimes also
backwards over the surface of the cell body.

The detailed mechanics of synaptic transmission are quite complicated. In some features they resemble those responsible for transmission across neuromuscular junctions. The transmitter substance is
synthesized in the presynaptic cell and stored in the synaptic vesicles,
which accumulate in close proximity to the junctional area. Small
amounts of transmitter escape spontaneously from time to time
into the synaptic cleft to produce local changes in the membrane
permeability of the postsynaptic cell. The electrical consequences of
these changes in permeability depend on the nature of the transmitter,
and some 40 different chemical substances have so far been identified
as active as transmitters in various parts of the central nervous system.
We return to this topic in more detail later in this chapter.

The large cell bodies of the motoneurons in the spinal cord can be
penetrated with saline-filled micropipettes from which the electrical
effects on the cell membrane can be recorded. The usual inside-negative
membrane potential appears at the moment of penetration. Superposed
on it may be seen a number of small irregular variations which are
referred to as 'synaptic noise'. These fluctuations are usually taken to
be the result of sporadic casual impulses in individual end-knobs
arising from interneurons of various kinds, among which there is
always a certain amount of background activity. Some of the noise is
also attributable to the effects of leakage of transmitter from end-knobs.

POSTSYNAPTIC POTENTIALS

When the presynaptic cell at the synaptic region becomes depolarized
during the invasion by an impulse, the liberation of transmitter is
much enhanced. A number of postsynaptic miniature effects occur
simultaneously, to produce a substantial 'postsynaptic potential', recordable through the micropipette. The time-course of the postsynaptic
potential shows a sudden onset followed by a much slower decay. This
decay corresponds to the gradual reduction in concentration of transmitter produced partly by simple diffusion into surrounding tissue
spaces and partly by enzymatic decomposition of the transmitter
molecules to render them ineffective. The component fragments resulting from this decomposition are taken up by the presynaptic cell
and used in synthesizing further transmitter molecules.

The nature of the changes in permeability produced by each of the
various transmitters can be deduced from the changes they cause in

the membrane potential of the postsynaptic cell when this is deliberately shifted from its normal value by passing electric currents through the second barrel of a twin-bore micropipette. In the resting state, the membrane potential of a motoneuron is usually about 10 mV or so below the equilibrium potential for potassium ions. Successful penetration of a cell is accordingly indicated by a sharp change that occurs in the recorded voltage while the micropipette is being cautiously advanced through the grey matter. The cell can be identified as a motoneuron if it can be made to respond promptly, with a single action-potential, to a shock applied to a muscle nerve. Since the action-potential is the electrical sign of an impulse propagated antidromically up the motor axon, all the delay between stimulus and response can here be accounted for as conduction time. The procedure also identifies which muscle it is that contains the motor unit served by the impaled motoneuron.

A group of interneurons, called 'Renshaw cells', are also excitable by antidromic impulses in muscle nerves because these impulses also travel into recurrent collateral branches of the motor axons ('c' in Figure 9.2). Activation of a Renshaw cell involves a synaptic delay, and the response is usually a train of impulses in rapid succession, rather than a single spike. Furthermore, while the antidromic activation of a motoneuron depends on an impulse in the single axon belonging to the impaled cell, the synaptic activation of a Renshaw cell requires the convergence of collaterals from several motor axons.

ACTION OF SYNAPTIC TRANSMITTERS

The voltage attained at the peak of the action-potential in a motoneuron approaches the equilibrium potential for the sodium ions. This indicates that the mechanism for propagation of the nerve impulse involves a temporary increase in permeability preferentially to sodium ions. As already mentioned, when a motoneuron is activated reflexly, by stimulating the Ia afferents from the appropriate muscle, the action-potential develops after a synaptic delay. By using a smaller shock as the stimulus, so that fewer afferents are effectively stimulated, the response in the motoneuron, instead of being a fully-fledged action-potential, appears as a much smaller deflection, referred to as an 'excitatory postsynaptic potential' (EPSP). The size of the EPSP can be varied, both by grading the shock strength, to alter the number of afferents contributing to the effect, or by shifting the membrane potential by passing electric current through the second barrel of the micropipette. Experiments of this type show that the excitatory transmitter increases the permeability of the postsynaptic membrane to all ions indiscriminately, with an effect equivalent to that of a short circuit of the 'membrane batteries'.

After identifying which muscle is served by a particular motoneuron, the afferents from an antagonist muscle can be stimulated. A different form of postsynaptic potential now appears. In this case the residual delay, after taking account of the conduction time, is found to be about twice as long as for afferents from the motoneuron's own muscle. Impulses along this pathway have an inhibitory effect, reducing the excitability of the jerk reflex. The equilibrium potential at the peak of the 'inhibitory postsynaptic potential' (IPSP) is found by exploring the effects on it of changing the membrane potential by passing current through the second barrel of the micropipette as before. It turns out to be near the equilibrium potential for chloride ions, which is somewhat lower than that for potassium ions. The inhibitory action depends on the fact that, because of the changed permeability produced by the inhibitory transmitter, the cell membrane is less easily depolarized by the local circuit currents associated with activity at excitatory end-knobs.

The inhibitory process just described affects the response of the postsynaptic cell to all its inputs. If enough inhibitory end-knobs are active, and if they are suitably distributed over the surface of the postsynaptic cell, onward propagation can be completely blocked. Another, more selective, inhibitory system depends on the fact that some end-knobs have their synaptic contacts located on other end-knobs rather than on dendrites. The mechanism of transmission at the synaptic patches of these terminals on end-knobs resembles the mechanisms found at excitatory and at inhibitory synapses on motoneurons, but the nature of the permeability change induced in the end-knob by this transmitter lies somewhere between the changes seen in the other two cases. It has been estimated that the equilibrium potential here lies in the neighbourhood of 30 mV (inside negative), but precise measurement is technically difficult as the end-knobs themselves are too small to be penetrated by a micropipette.

When these synaptic patches are active, the subsynaptic membrane of the end-knob is stabilized at this equilibrium potential. This means that when an incoming impulse starts to invade the end-knob, some of its local circuit current can be provided by the already depolarized active synaptic patches, instead of by normal resting membrane. There will be less current available to depolarize the rest of the cell membrane and the affected end-knob will fail to release enough transmitter to excite the postsynaptic cell. The size of the EPSP seen by a micro-electrode in the motoneuron will be much reduced. The process is referred to as 'presynaptic inhibition', to distinguish it from the 'postsynaptic inhibition' produced by inhibitory synapses located directly on the motoneurons. Presynaptic inhibition can block particular pathways while leaving the motoneurons still susceptible to activation through other pathways.

Activation of the axon hillock depends on the intensity of the combined effects of all the local circuit currents generated at end-knobs all over the dendritic tree. There is thus great scope for summation processes based both on the convergence of afferents and on changes in the repetition-frequency of the activations at individual end-knobs. The axon hillock acts as a kind of sense organ, generating a stream of impulses in the axon, at a repetition-frequency that depends on the prevailing intensity of the local circuit current contributed to by all the various end-knobs located on the surface of the cell body or on that of its dendrites. As these end-knobs are derived from many different sources, some with inhibitory and some with excitatory effects, it is possible, by altering the pattern of bombardment, to make considerable changes in the output of the motoneuron.

Because of the anatomical complexity of the arrangement of connections, it is clear that the so-called monosynaptic response in the jerk reflex must involve an interaction between the dispersal of influences from individual afferent nerve-fibres (one to many) and the convergence of influences from several sources (many to one) onto each individual motoneuron. A large number of individual synapses must be activated in near synchrony to produce the synchronized volley of outgoing motor impulses needed for the jerk response. The variation observed in the intensity of the jerk response to a standardized tap on a tendon in certain clinical conditions can be accounted for in terms of the converging effect on the motoneurons of the end-knobs derived from fibres originating in other parts of the central nervous system.

VARIATIONS IN STRETCH-REFLEX SENSITIVITY

The synchronized afferent firing associated with a tendon tap does not occur during sustained stretch of a muscle. In these conditions it is not only the primary spindle receptors that are active. Secondary spindle receptors and tendon organs are also active, their afferent impulses passing, respectively, in group II and group Ib nerve-fibres. The impulses set up by different endings are not synchronized with one another; they are propagated at different speeds; and they influence interneurons in the spinal cord as well as the motoneurons themselves. In turn, the interneurons influence other interneurons as well as motoneurons.

The 'Renshaw cells', which are interneurons receiving impulses in collateral branches of the axons of motoneurons, exert an inhibitory influence on other motoneurons that happen to lie in close proximity to the parent motoneuron. This arrangement resembles the 'negative feedback loops' familiar in the treatment of servomechanisms in engineering. It has been argued that negative feedback over the Renshaw cell circuit may be responsible for the fact that, in many postural contexts, the firing-frequency observed in individual motor units is restricted to a very narrow range, say 8 to 12 impulses per second.

Variation in muscle force is achieved by altering the number of motor units recruited into activity, each of the units either firing at a frequency within this preferred range or not at all. The point of this arrangement is that there are disadvantages in using other frequencies. At lower frequencies, the mechanical responses of the muscle cells do not fuse, and the resulting series of twitches would introduce undesirable tremor. At higher frequencies, the mechanical responses fuse into a smooth tetanus and further increments in firing-frequency achieve no increment in tension. At the same time, another effect of the sustained mechanical activity of the muscle cells is to occlude the blood supply to the active muscles, thus impairing their efficiency. At the preferred firing-frequency, the mechanical response is a partially fused tetanus which includes moments of slightly reduced tension during which blood flow can take place, thus reducing the liability to fatigue.

Another feature that contributes to reducing the liability to fatigue is the way the individual muscle cells making up a single motor unit are scattered through the main mass of the muscle (Figure 9.4). They lie well separated from one another with numbers of muscle cells belonging to other motor units in between. This arrangement reduces competition between the cells of a single unit for the available blood supply.

The variations in the tension developed by individual motor units will not, in general, be synchronized with one another; while the tension in one unit is declining, that in another is likely to be increasing. Since many units transmit their force to a common tendon, some mechanical smoothing takes place, and the fluctuations in the overall tension at the tendon are much less than those in the tensions generated by individual units.

Where the tension required is less than the maximum that the muscle is capable of exerting, some of the motor units in that muscle will be resting while others are being activated to provide the necessary tension. From time to time some of the active units stop firing and other units are then brought into play to maintain the total force at its previous value. This rotation of units serves to share out the work and to distribute the liability to fatigue.

Activity in stretch reflexes is sometimes considered in terms of the

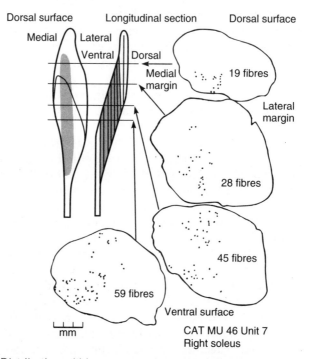

Figure 9.4 Distribution within an anatomical muscle (cat soleus) of the muscle-fibres making up a single motor unit. The muscle-fibres are connected at each end to tendinous sheets (aponeuroses) on the dorsal and ventral aspects of the muscle, as indicated (top left) in dorsal view and in longitudinal section. The thin parallel lines in the longitudinal section represent the arrangement of the fascicles of muscle-fibres. A single motor axon has been stimulated repeatedly so that the muscle-fibres in its motor unit could thereafter be distinguished histologically by the depletion of their glycogen content. This unit consists of some 80 fibres distributed as shown in the sections and by the shading. The muscle contains about 150 motor units in all, with from 50 to 400 muscle-fibres in each. Total number of muscle-fibres: 22 000 to 30 000. (From Burke *et al.*, 1974, by courtesy of *J. Physiol.*)

grading of stimulus and response on the supposition that a continuous variable is involved in each case. It is also supposed that some form of mathematical relationship can be devised to describe the transformation from input signal to output signal. This view is influenced by the idea that muscle control in some respects resembles the operation of a servomechanism, where the magnitude of some output variable is regulated by feedback signals in such a way as to minimize departures from a preset or desired control value. Various features have been put forward as candidates for the role of controlled variable. This is the variable that has to be monitored by the detector part of the servomechanism. The possibilities include joint angle, muscle length, muscle tension, and the stiffness with which muscle extension is resisted, together with the rates-of-change of each of these measures.

The literature contains a number of reports of experimental studies aimed at characterizing the responses in afferent nerve-fibres to a variety of stimuli. As may be seen from the accounts in the previous chapter, it is by no means clear how the patterns of observed discharge are to be related to the physical features of the stimulus, because of the interacting effects of dynamic and static components in the responses, adaptation, hysteresis, and, in relation to the spindles, the consequences of intrafusal activations. Nevertheless, it is often claimed that the ensemble of messages in the totality of afferent nerve-fibres 'conveys enough information' for the central nervous system to be able to deduce the values of the relevant features of the stimulus, such as displacement or force, as a basis for regulating the force to be developed by the muscles. No suggestions are offered, however, as to how the desired measures and their rates-of-change are to be separately recovered from the pattern of the impulse traffic.

DEFICIENCIES IN THE FOLLOW-UP LENGTH SERVO HYPOTHESIS

One of the servo theories put forward at one time was based on the discovery that, with a few exceptions, the innervation of the intrafusal muscle-fibres in the spindles is separate from the innervation of the extrafusal muscle-fibres, while it is these that are responsible for by far the major part of the force developed by the muscle as a whole. Since the intrafusal muscle-fibres lie in parallel with the extrafusal fibres, it was supposed that the reflex activation of the extrafusal fibres in response to afferent impulses from the spindles might serve to reduce any discrepancy arising between the lengths of the two sets of muscle-fibres, as in a 'follow-up length servo' like those used in engineering. If the intrafusal muscle-fibres were caused to contract, by fusimotor activity, this would activate the spindle discharge and thus reflexly activate the extrafusal muscle-fibres. If they contract to the same degree as the intrafusal muscle-fibres, this would remove the stimulus to the spindles, as in an error-correcting servo. Changes in muscle length would then follow the changes produced in the intrafusal muscle-fibres by the fusimotor signal. Any departure from the desired change in length would be automatically corrected by the reflex recruitment of extrafusal muscle-fibres.

There are many objections to this scheme, one of which is that when a movement is to be initiated, the scheme predicts that the fusimotor axons should be active before those serving the extrafusal muscle-fibres. This expectation is not borne out by recordings from the motor nerves. In fact, the alpha motoneurons serving the extrafusal muscle-fibres are often the first to show relevant activity. There are also serious problems with the idea that muscle activity can control overall muscle length directly. In many muscles the distance between the origin and the insertion includes a significant length of tendon in addition to the muscle cells. This is particularly true of the many pinnate muscles, where the muscle cells run obliquely between parallel tendinous sheets, called 'aponeuroses', one of which forms the connection to bone at the muscle origin while the other is continuous with the tendon running to the point of insertion. In such muscles, the length of tendon in series with the contractile material may be several times the length of the muscle cells themselves. Since both tendon and muscle are extensible, the overall length is greatly influenced by the conditions of loading, as well as by the degree of activation of the muscle cells. A mechanism that stabilizes the length of the contractile part of the muscle will therefore not be particularly effective in stabilizing the overall length from origin to insertion, which is what would be required for the stabilization and control of joint angle.

PROBLEMS OF CODING

The difficulties in deciding which variable is to be regarded as signalled by the afferent discharge have already been pointed out. Further difficulties arise from the way the afferent messages are conveyed. Since the character of an individual nerve-impulse is entirely determined by the membrane properties of that portion of a nerve cell which is engaged in the activity cycle of which the impulse is a manifestation, the only way a nerve-fibre can convey information is by being either active or not active at a particular time. Variations in the intensity of the signal are conveyed by the intervals at which successive impulses follow one another. The idea of 'impulse-frequency', considered earlier in relation to the transducer action of the sensory receptors, is really appropriate only to reasonably regular streams of impulses. In practice, many afferent nerve-fibres fire very irregularly and measures such as 'mean frequency', i.e. the number of impulses recordable in unit time, may not correspond to the physiological efficacy of the signal when it reaches the synapses where the message is to be passed on to another cell. This is because of the marked temporal summation effect arising when two impulses follow one another in rapid succession.

The mechanics of synaptic transmission, taken together with the anatomical complexity of the convergence onto each motoneuron, indicate that, even if some rational form of coding can be devised to describe the pattern of the discharge in single afferent nerve-fibres, such coding is most unlikely to survive in the firing pattern of the postsynaptic cell. There may be advantages in this insofar as the grading of signal intensity on the afferent side is conveyed as a grading of the repetition-frequency of firing, while the grading of the intensity of force-development is achieved by variation in the number of motor units that are currently being activated, where each unit either fires at its preferred firing-frequency or not at all. In many muscles, the motor units outnumber the afferent nerve-fibres by about three or four to one, and we have no information about how the discharges in these two sets of nerve-fibres are linked.

FRAMES OF REFERENCE

The management of the stretch-reflex sensitivity of individual muscles is only one part of the overall task of controlling the disposition of the limb segments and the deployment of muscle forces in a way appropriate to postural behaviour and locomotion. We have, in addition, to consider the problems of orientation. It is here that the sense organs of the labyrinth play an important role. In considering the way the labyrinth influences the body musculature we encounter yet another set of problems in addition to those already discussed in this chapter. These are concerned with the transfer of information from one frame of reference to another.

The aiming of the limbs has to be regulated in relation to the trunk, but the body of an animal is not a rigid structure. We need, therefore, a separate frame of reference for each limb, and another for the head, with a non-constant relationship between these different frames. On close scrutiny we find we need separate frames of reference for each joint, and perhaps also for each individual sensory receptor, insofar as each has its own individual polarization vector, governed by its anatomical relations to the rest of the tissue in which it is embedded.

In regard to the semicircular canals, the differences between the directions of the polarization vectors of the individual neuromasts in a particular crista, in relation to the plane of that canal, are reflected in differences between the sensitivities of individual units to specific deformations of the cupula. It may be supposed, therefore, that all the afferents from a single ampulla are reporting, in their various ways, a version of the angular acceleration of the skull in the plane of that canal. The information provided by these afferents should not, however, be taken to imply that the axis of rotation of the movement of the skull is at right angles to the plane of that canal. Any angular movement of the skull will have some component in the plane of the canal unless that plane actually contains the axis of rotation itself. This leads to the conclusion that a decision as to which is the direction of the axis of angular acceleration of the skull must depend upon a process of assessment based on a comparison between the combined signals received from each of the six canals.

One of the functions of the semicircular canals is to regulate the movements of the eyeballs in the skull. This is usually arranged in such a way that the direction of gaze is not altered when the head moves, as you can verify by moving your head while continuing to read the page before you. Eye movements are controlled by three pairs of muscles for each eye: one pair for vertical movements, one pair for horizontal movements, and one pair for rotations of the eyeball around the visual axis. The planes of operation of these three pairs of muscles for each eye do not correspond with the planes of the semicircular canals, so each eye-socket has its own frame of reference, which is not the same as that for the skull as a whole. Yet another frame of reference is required for description of the location of visual images on the retina.

The direction of gaze is relevant to the maintenance of balance because of the contribution made by movement detectors in the peripheral retina to the indication of whether or not the head is moving relative to the environment, as it might do at the moment of overbalancing. If the indication is that the head is not moving, other cues about the imminence of overbalancing may fail to initiate corrective actions. This is what happens when a subject, standing on a restricted base, is overbalanced by surreptitiously moving the whole of his visual field, as in the moving-room experiment described earlier.

In determining the direction to be adopted as the behavioural vertical, account has to be taken of signals from the labyrinth that indicate the direction of the stress-gradient in the skull arising from the supporting forces. This signal is derived from the neuromasts in the otolith apparatus in the utriculus and sacculus. The polarization vectors of the neuromasts in these otolith organs cannot be simply characterized into three planes of space, like those in the ampullae of the canals. Each neuromast is affected by shear between the epithelial surface and the overlying jelly-mass of the otolith membrane. Both utriculus and sacculus are sac-like organs, so that the surface of shear is curved (Figure 8.21). The discharge from an individual neuromast will therefore depend, not only on the way the plane of shear for that neuromast is inclined to the direction of the stress-gradient in the skull, but also on the orientation of the polarization vector of the neuromast within the plane of shear. In the afferent discharge, a similar change in firing-frequency can be produced either by altering the direction of the stress-gradient, relative to the skull, or by altering its intensity. The direction is altered by tilting the head; the intensity changes with the upthrust effort, as during the different phases of locomotion as well as in special environments such as moving vehicles and the like. In addition to the differences between the polarization vectors of individual neuromasts, some of the variation between the response patterns found among the different afferents from the otolith apparatus may be accounted for by the fact that each afferent may be influenced by more than one neuromast.

Whatever signal is derivable from the otolith apparatus, it will reflect a mixture of many interacting factors. Even supposing that the brain can identify the direction of the stress-gradient relative to skull landmarks after disentangling this from its intensity and from the history of the rates-of-change both of direction and of intensity, we are still a long way from determining the direction of the thrust exerted against the supports. Forces in the neck muscles and elsewhere, together with the thrust transmitted to the skull through the vertebral column, all intervene between the stresses on the skull and those prevailing at the supports. Furthermore, the direction of the thrust currently being exerted is not necessarily the best direction in which to push in order to avoid falling over, since the thrust may be one intended to initiate locomotion rather than to arrest it. The mechanics of the sensory apparatus in the labyrinth can produce misleading impressions of movement in certain conditions. Attempts to correct these false indications can lead to loss of balance, sometimes with unfortunate results. These factors make it a far from simple matter to attribute the values chosen for the vector representing the behavioural vertical to a specific transform of the pattern of discharge in a named set of afferents.

MOVING VEHICLES

Special problems arise if the supports available to the body are themselves moving. The direction and point of application of the thrust against the supports then have to be regulated in different ways according to the extent of the imposed movements. For example, the short-lasting accelerations of a vehicle travelling over rough ground can be absorbed by suitably supple reactions in the limbs, allowing the supporting surface to move under the body without much movement of the body itself. On the other hand, the body has to retain its mean position relative to the vehicle in order not to be left behind. In principle, the variations in force that are required are of similar character to those involved in locomotion, with the important difference that the forces deployed in locomotion are initiated by the animal, whereas those arising from movement of the vehicle generally involve reaction to unexpected perturbations. Locomotion in a moving vehicle involves adjustments of both types.

ORBITING SPACECRAFT

Locomotion on the ground makes use of the fact that, after the body has been thrown upwards and forwards for a step, the action of gravity brings the body back into contact with the ground, ready for the next step. This sequence is not available to astronauts in an orbiting spacecraft. After all the adjustments following the initial launch have been completed and the rocket motors have been switched off, the spacecraft and all its contents go into free fall. In this situation, if an astronaut takes a step, he is not automatically returned to the floor because the floor of the spacecraft falls, under gravity, in the same way as the astronaut himself. Because the astronaut is left drifting, until he collides with the ceiling or some other part of the vehicle wall, the condition has come to be known as 'weightlessness'. Any loose objects that are accidentally displaced in the spacecraft also tend to drift free.

A ROTATING ENVIRONMENT

It has been proposed that any large future space station should be caused to rotate in order to avoid the inconvenience of uncontrolled drifting in the weightless state and to restore some normality to locomotion. This suggestion is based on the mistaken belief that 'centrifugal force' can act as a subsititute for the action of gravity. As part of the exploratory programme in preparation for this plan, a 'slow rotating room' was constructed at the US Naval Aerospace Research Institute in Pensacola, Florida. The room is about 15 feet in diameter and it can be rotated smoothly at chosen constant speeds up to about $10\,\mathrm{rev\,min^{-1}}$. The room was initially furnished, for long-stay occupation, with laboratory equipment, seats, refrigerator, sink, cooking facilities, toilet and sleeping accommodation for four persons. Subjects stayed in the room continuously for periods lasting from a few minutes up to about 12 days. Many difficulties were encountered, including severe motion sickness.

One type of difficulty is highlighted in attempts to throw a ball into a basket. The task appears simple; the ball is aimed at an apparently stationary target, but it appears to curve sharply in its flight and consequently completely misses its target. This is because the basket, unlike the freely-moving ball, is continually accelerated towards the centre of rotation by stress forces against the structure of the room. While the ball is in flight, the basket moves from the position it was in when the ball was thrown. It proves very difficult, but not impossible, to train oneself to make the necessary adjustments in aiming.

Although there was not much room to move about, because of the presence of the furniture, the subjects reported some difficulty in locomotion. When I visited the facility in 1967 the furniture had been cleared away, leaving the full area of the floor unencumbered. Quite marked difficulties in locomotion were now evident. One had no sensation of movement so long as one was standing still in the rotating room, but on any attempt to take a few steps one felt strongly thrown to one side. The reason for this is that, during the steady rotation of the room, objects at a particular distance from the centre of rotation have a linear velocity along a tangent to the curved path, this velocity being dependent on the speed of rotation and on the length of the radius of curvature of the path. The different parts of the floor of the room are moving at different tangential velocities. When one starts to walk, this usually involves changing the distance to the axis of rotation. Because linear momentum is conserved, one now finds oneself on a part of the floor that is moving at a different speed from one's body. One feels as though about to be swept off one's feet. The effect is unexpected, and contrasts so strongly with the impression that the room is not moving that it is hard to make the necessary adjustments. The process of determining the direction of the behavioural vertical is apparently grossly disturbed during walking.

THE CORIOLIS EFFECT

The consequence of movements that change the distance from the centre of rotation is called the 'Coriolis effect'. It is sometimes attributed to a 'Coriolis force'. However, 'Coriolis forces', just like 'centrifugal forces', are not Newtonian forces in the sense of rates-of-change of momentum; the effects are, in contrast, entirely attributable to the conservation of momentum.

The true nature of the phenomenon can be demonstrated with a weight hung on a string. The string is passed through a ring held in one hand, while the other hand holds the free end. With the hands together, the weight is swung in a circle. After the circular movement is well established, the ring is held still while the string is drawn through it with the other hand. As the distance from the ring to the weight is gradually shortened, the weight is seen to go round faster and faster, slowing again when the string is let out. While the weight is moving in a curved path it will have a certain momentum, given by the product of its mass multiplied by its velocity. The force to maintain the curved path is directed towards the centre of rotation. It is to provide this horizontal force, as well as a vertical supporting force, that the line of the string is inclined to the vertical. The radius of the circular path of the weight will be rotating with a certain angular velocity. When the string is shortened, to bring the weight nearer to the centre of rotation, the linear momentum of the weight will be unchanged, because there is no force acting on the weight in the direction of the tangent to the path. However, if the same tangential velocity is maintained at a smaller radius, this implies an increase in the angular velocity of rotation of the radius. If we wish to keep the angular velocity constant, as during a walk in the rotating room, we need to exert a tangential force. It is the absence of such a force that gives rise to the sensation that one is being swept off one's feet when the speed of the floor does not correspond with that of the body.

A more familiar example of this Coriolis effect is seen when we remove the plug from the outlet of a bath or washbasin. Removing the plug reduces the upthrust and the water moves into the wastepipe under the action of gravity. Horizontal movement is needed to reach the orifice. The horizontal plane is inclined to the axis of the earth's rotation, except at the equator. Horizontal movement towards the equator thus involves an increase in the distance from the axis of rotation of the earth, and the water tends to lag behind the earth, or is seen to move westwards, while water moving away from the equator moves ahead of the earth, or eastwards. In consequence, the water approaching the outlet comes to rotate counterclockwise in the northern hemisphere or clockwise in the southern hemisphere. Similar rotation is seen in the wind pattern surrounding a depression.

MISLEADING SIGNALS FROM THE LABYRINTH

In an aircraft moving in a curved path, the force for inward acceleration along the radius of curvature of the path is provided by banking the wings over. This means that, at the onset of the turn, the aircraft and its contained passengers must be rotated about an axis aligned with the flight path. This rotation in roll will affect the vertical semicircular canals, but if the manoeuvre is carried out correctly, the support vector will remain at right angles to the plane of the wings. The otolith organs will thus experience a change in the magnitude of the support force, but no change in its direction, just as they might in an elevator at the start of an ascent. The aircraft passengers feel an increase in the pressure against the seat.

If the information from the canals corresponds to the impressions from the changing visual field, a passenger who is looking out of the window at the onset of the turn will be aware of the banking manoeuvre. However, there will be a conflict between the conclusion, based on canal and visual information, that the body has performed a roll, and the conclusion, based on the otolith signal, that the body is still upright. If the turn continues without further messages from the canals, the interpretation of the visual experience gradually changes to correspond with the otolith signal, and the ground comes to appear tilted.

The roll manoeuvre at the start of the turn involves angular acceleration followed by angular deceleration in roll in a pattern similar to that of Figure 8.16, with little residual effect. However, the turn itself involves angular acceleration in one direction only, in a sequence of changes in the horizontal plane like those shown in Figure 8.15, although this time the vertical canals as well as the horizontal canals will be affected. At first the impression is that the aircraft is circling over the ground but, as the canal signals decay, the impression changes until, during a sufficiently prolonged turn, the ground appears to be rotating as well as tilted, and the aircraft feels as though it is in level flight.

If visual cues are absent, as they might be when flying through cloud, similar comforting sensations associated with level flight might be present when the aircraft is in fact in the course of spinning into the ground. If the pilot detects the spin and straightens out, there will be a corresponding angular deceleration which, by the mechanisms indicated in Figure 8.14, will generate sensations associated with spinning in the opposite direction. The pilot must learn not to respond to this sensation. If he does so, his attempt to avoid overcorrection for the first spin will have the effect of generating another spin in the same direction as the first, a manoeuvre known as the 'graveyard spin'.

Another spurious sense of rotation with possibly dangerous consequences can arise from the otolith organs. If a pilot coming in to land decides that he is going to overshoot the runway, he will open the throttle to accelerate away for another attempt. During the acceleration, the resultant support vector tilts forwards. The pilot, as usual interpreting the direction of the support vector as vertical, feels that his body is tilting backwards, as it might be at the start of a steep climb. Anxious not to stall his aircraft when near to the ground, the pilot is tempted to push the stick forward to correct the apparent nose-up attitude. The effect will be to produce a dive that may well prove fatal.

Many discrepancies can arise between the motion of an aircraft and the pilot's sense of orientation based on the signals from his labyrinth. This makes it essential that the pilots of modern high-speed aircraft should be carefully trained to respond to the indications of their flight instruments and to disregard their subjective impressions of the attitude and motion of the aircraft.

The sense of rotation is primarily dependent upon the sensory messages from the semicircular canals, but it is only within a restricted range of conditions that the canal signals correspond to the actual motion of the skull. Special complications arise from Coriolis effects in those movements that involve a change in the orientation of the head relative to the axis of rotation.

EFFECTS ON THE CANALS

In the Pensacola slow rotating room already mentioned, and indeed in any rotating environment, the Coriolis effect has serious consequences in the semicircular canals when the head is tilted about an axis that is not exactly parallel to the axis of rotation of the room. Such a tilt will bring some parts of the ring of endolymph in a canal nearer to the axis of rotation while other parts of the ring are carried further from the axis. Because of the conservation of linear momentum, the endolymph in those parts of the canal that are brought nearer to the axis will tend to move ahead, while endolymph carried away from the axis will lag behind. This endolymph displacement within the canal is the same as that associated with angular acceleration of the skull about an axis that is at right angles both to the axis of the original rotation and to the axis of the tilt. The consequent sensation and reflex movements have prolonged time-courses like the post-rotatory effects following impulsive deceleration (Figure 8.14) and can consequently be profoundly disturbing.

Suppose that a pilot is flying in a circle, turning steadily to the left, and is looking out over the wing to face along the radius of the flight path. Now suppose that, for some reason, he has to look down into the cockpit to attend to some instrument, tilting his head towards nose-down, but still facing along the radius. The Coriolis effect on the canals in these conditions corresponds to that of an angular acceleration of the head in left-side down roll. As the pilot is already looking to his left, this sensation may be interpreted as an upward pitch of the aircraft. Correcting this spurious sensation by a nose-down pitch of the aircraft, he may fly into the ground.

The Coriolis effects on the canals produced by head-tilting during a rotation do not correspond either with the movements of the visual field or with the information from the otolith apparatus. It is perhaps this extreme discrepancy between sensory cues that makes the resulting sensations so profoundly distressing and leads so often to the syndrome of motion sickness.

MOTION SICKNESS

The characteristic symptoms of motion sickness are: drowsiness, pallor, cold sweating, hyperventilation, malaise, yawning, nausea, and vomiting. There may also be some decline in motor skills but this may be masked by strongly motivated concentration. There seem to be several different ways in which motion sickness can be induced. Most, but not all, involve discordant sensory information related to balance. Different subjects differ in susceptibility and quite small changes in the pattern of sensory cues can produce marked differences in the responses. A small-boat sailor may happily tolerate the quite violent movements of his own boat and yet become very sick in a large ship. In some subjects motion sickness can be induced by visual cues alone, such as by a seascape filmed from a boat. Considerable changes in susceptibility may be produced by training.

The motion of a boat in a rough sea is made up of several fluctuating components, each affecting the labyrinths of the passengers in a different way. There will be yawing and pitching movements as well as the more prominent rolling. The boat rises and falls and also, because of the rotary component in the wave motion of the water, the boat will undergo fluctuating horizontal accelerations. In consequence, the resultant support vector acting on the skull varies in magnitude and swings about in direction. The rotary motion of the vector acting on the otolith organs does not correspond with the rotations signalled by the semicircular canals. If the subject is below decks and cannot see the sea, the only apparent movements of his visual field will be those produced by eye movements induced reflexly from the labyrinth. Each sensory system – canals, otolith organs, vision, and proprioception – contributes to the subjective impression of the relationship between the body and its environment, but in the conditions of complex motion occurring on shipboard in a rough sea the various contributions do not agree among themselves. It appears to be this discord between sensory cues that is in some way responsible for the motion sickness.

The movements that produce motion sickness in automobile passengers have similarities with those of a boat in a rough sea. Vertical accelerations are produced by unevennesses in the road surface, acting through the springing of the vehicle and its upholstery. Horizontal accelerations occur at bends in the road and as a result of differences in level between the surfaces under the various wheels. It is commonly observed that the passengers in the vehicle are more susceptible to motion sickness than the driver. The explanation for this difference in susceptibility lies in the difference in acceleration pattern that is imposed on the skull. When the vehicle is steered to one side or the other, a horizontal force is exerted through the wheels. The support vector is accordingly tilted inwards on the corners. However, the effect of the reflex-changes in the musculature of the passengers is to tend to roll the body outwards on the corners, relative to the vehicle. The canals signal this outward roll, while the otolith organs indicate the inward tilt of the support vector. In contrast, the driver, who has initiated the change of course by moving the steering wheel, tends to lean inwards on the corners, just as he would when running on foot or when riding a bicycle. His canals accordingly signal an inward roll, and this corresponds with the tilt of the support vector signalled by his otolith apparatus. The labyrinths of the driver and the passengers thus receive different patterns of stimulation. The pattern for the passengers is such as to induce motion sickness, while that for the driver is not. It is interesting to note that bus conductors come to acquire motor behaviour similar to that of the driver and consequently turn out to be less susceptible to motion sickness than their passengers.

It is the Coriolis effect on the canals that is responsible for the most serious effects on the occupants of the slow rotating room. Any casual movements of the head generate Coriolis effects on the canals, with the exception only of movements consisting entirely of rotations about an axis parallel to the axis of rotation of the room. The canal signals arising from the Coriolis effects are in conflict both with otolith signals and with movements of the visual field over the retina. The result is a severe, and often totally incapacitating, motion sickness.

PATHWAYS IN THE CENTRAL NERVOUS SYSTEM

The disturbances of balancing behaviour that arise when the labyrinth is exposed to unusual conditions of stimulation reinforce the belief that normal balancing is heavily dependent on the messages received from the sense organs. An immense amount of effort has been deployed in working out the destinations within the central nervous system of the messages from sense organs of different kinds, using a variety of different techniques. Gross dissection and inferences from localized lesions produced by accident or disease, including surgery for focal epilepsy, provide evidence of rather crude localization. More detail comes from recording the electrical activity in one location that follows stimulation applied elsewhere. However, any anatomical pathway that is identified by electrical stimulation depends on the simultaneous activation of numbers of nerve-fibres, a situation most unlikely to occur outside the laboratory of the electrophysiologist. Recognition of this fact must not be taken to imply a denial of the existence of the connections; it just raises a question as to the probability of such pathways being in regular use. In this context it is relevant to recall that the firing-frequencies encountered in afferent nerves are often very different from those seen in motor nerves. There must be some quite complicated transformation processes intervening between input and output.

Neuroscience is advancing very rapidly on several fronts at the present time. In giving an account of the resulting network of emerging new concepts we shall find we come upon certain topics more than once as the exploration of each mesh in the network throws more light on a different aspect of a nodal point in the overall system.

Important discoveries about the fine detail of the interconnections between individual neurons have come from refined histological techniques for tracing the branches of cells undergoing degeneration after local damage, or in which enzymes (such as horseradish peroxidase) have been injected into single cells. These enzymes are transported into all parts of the injected cell, so that even the finest branches can later be traced, after suitable histochemical stains have been allowed to react with the enzymes. Transmitter agents and their synthesizing enzymes can also be labelled and their active locations visualized by fluorescent microscopy. In some cases, it is possible to associate specific transmitters with recognizable types of synaptic structure, such as the shape of postsynaptic spines.

An inescapable conclusion from a study of detailed microanatomy is that the layout of the interconnections between individual cells is massively complicated. It is therefore extremely unlikely that any simple scheme of relations between input and output can represent the true state of affairs. In spite of the evidence for complexity, much of the interpretation of findings about identifiable pathways has been based on the supposition that the messages from the sense organs convey into the nervous system some coded version of the quantitative measures that an experimenter might use to characterize the stimulus situation, such as the location of the sites of stimulation and the intensity of the activation at those sites. The accounts in the previous chapter of the patterns of discharge generated by the proprioceptors argue strongly against the plausibility of this supposition, and we should now look for some alternative approach.

FEATURE EXTRACTORS IN THE CENTRAL NERVOUS SYSTEM

Studies of the visual system have provided indications of a possible principle of organization. The neurons in the cerebral cortex, especially those that receive directly or indirectly from the retina, turn out to be arranged in clusters, forming columns of cells at right angles to the cortical surface, with about a hundred cells to a column. Within each column the individual cells are elaborately interconnected, in marked contrast to the much lower density of connections to neighbouring columns. There is some evidence that each column is surrounded by a 'wall' of inhibitory connections that provides a degree of insulation between adjacent columns and makes independence possible.

Each column has its own pattern of input and output connections. Electrical recording reveals that each column reacts to a different aspect of the signals from a specific location on the retina, such as to the presence of an edge oriented in a specific direction, or to the motion of an image in a certain direction. Columns in the primary visual area pass their messages to columns of cells in secondary areas, where more complex attributes of the stimulus are picked up. Features such as the colour of a stimulus, the form of an object, its movement, its relative depth, and the disparity between the images in the two eyes, all appear to be processed in separate areas of the cortex.

These conclusions from electrical recording are supported by evidence of localized increases in activity in the relevant regions on appropriate stimulation of the retina. Increased activity involves increased uptake of glucose and increased blood flow. The location of this increased activity can be visualized by Positron Emission Tomography (PET) after injecting into the bloodstream a quantity of glucose labelled with a short-lived radioisotope. When the isotope decays it emits a positron which travels only a very short distance before encountering an electron. The collision produces a pair of photons of gamma radiation, emitted in opposite directions. The radiation is picked up by an array of detectors arranged around the subject's head. Simultaneous responses from a pair of detectors, one on each side of the head, define the line of the track of radiation through the skull. The detectors feed a computer that determines the origin of the gamma radiation from the intersection of its tracks and displays the result as a map of a section through the subject's skull. Differences in the intensity of radiation from different areas are displayed as false colours on the map. The spatial resolution of the method is about 1–2 ml, and it takes several tens of seconds to produce each map. The confirmation of the locations of specific feature extractors does not, however, tell us anything about how the signals are being processed in those areas.

The organization into columns of cells is found in all areas of the cerebral cortex. Some columns in the auditory cortex are sensitive to interaural delay, which is the basis for the localization of heard sounds. In the motor cortex, individual columns drive the motoneuron pools controlling single muscles, each column receiving afferents from the tissues in and around the joint at which the relevant muscle operates. The parietal cortex contains columns with specific but more complex functions, such as the aiming of a limb, a specific manipulation, visual fixation and tracking, visually evoked saccadic or pursuit movements of the eyes, detection of the sudden appearance of objects in the peripheral visual field, and so on.

Afferents reach the cerebral cortex from the specific nuclei of the dorsal thalamus, from other cortical areas of the same hemisphere, and from corresponding areas of the opposite hemisphere. All of these pathways have point-to-point connections, each separable location at one end of the pathway being connected to a discretely localized region at the other end. Such a pathway is said to be 'somatotopically organized'. More diffusely distributed afferents come from the generalized thalamic nuclei, from the basilar forebrain, and from the brainstem. The output from the cortical grey matter is carried exclusively by pyramidal cells whose axons run to other areas of the same or of the opposite hemisphere, to the basal ganglia, to the midbrain, to the cerebellum by way of the pons, and to the spinal cord. Connection from the afferent input to the pyramidal output is effected by complex networks of interneurons, some being excitatory and some inhibitory in their influences.

Within some parts of the central nervous system, and particularly in regions of closely-packed interneurons, the conduction distances between cells are relatively short, so that intercell communication can be effected without the need for propagated action-potentials. In some cases the communication is electrical, by the electrotonic spread of local circuit currents. In other cases, short-range diffusion of transmitter substances affects groups of cells all at the same time. Where chemical transmission of this kind occurs, there is a special susceptibility to widespread influences from substances carried in the bloodstream, such as the mood-changing drugs, hallucinogens, endorphins, and the like.

THE CEREBELLUM

The cellular organization found in the cerebellum is arranged in a different pattern from that in the cerebrum. The cerebellar cortex forms a series of parallel folds, called 'folia', running transversely across the midline, with a fairly uniform cellular pattern throughout. A set of large cells of characteristic shape, called 'Purkinje cells', lie side by side to form a thin sheet parallel to the cortical surface. The dendritic trees of the Purkinje cells are each confined to a thin flat slab of tissue, so that all their dendritic trees lie parallel to one another, across the axis of the folium. All the other neurons in the cerebellar cortex are of only four different types, labelled 'granule', 'basket', 'Golgi' and 'stellate' cells respectively, each with its own characteristic distribution of connections (Figure 9.5).

Afferents to the cerebellum are of two types, called 'mossy fibres' and 'climbing fibres' respectively. The mossy fibres are derived from a number of different sources:

- the cerebral cortex;
- the basal ganglia;
- the superior colliculi and peri-aqueductal grey matter in connection with eye-movements and fixation reflexes;

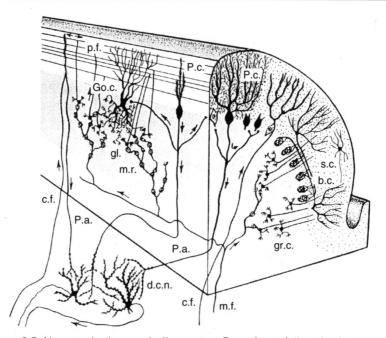

Figure 9.5 Neurons in the cerebellar cortex. Part of one folium is shown cut in two planes. To the left, along the folium (i.e. across the animal); to the right, acoss the folium, in a rostro-caudal plane. The dendrites of Purkinje cells (P.c.), basket cells (b.c.), and stellate cells (s.c.) are confined to slabs of tissue oriented in rostro-caudal planes. The dendrites of Golgi cells (Go.c.) ramify in all directions. Incoming mossy fibres (m.f.) carry many rosettes (m.r.) forming glomeruli (gl.) with the dendrites of granule cells (gr.c.) and with axonal terminations of the Golgi cells. Axons of the granule cells form parallel fibres (p.f.) running in the superficial molecular layer of the cortex in a direction at right angles to the planes occupied by the dendrites of individual Purkinje cells. Climbing fibres (c.f.) from the inferior olives closely invest the Purkinje cell dendrites (stippled). In addition to running to the deep cerebellar nuclei (d.c.n.), the axons of Purkinje cells form collaterals running to other Purkinje cells, to basket cells, and to Golgi cells. The arrows indicate the direction of impulse traffic. (From Crosby, Humphrey and Lauer, 1962, by courtesy of Macmillan.)

- the inferior colliculi and superior olives in connection with acoustic localization;
- the labyrinth and vestibular nuclei in connection with balance;
- the spinal cord.

In each case two different types of connection may be distinguished: 'point-to-point' and 'convergent'. By virtue of the somatotopic connections we distinguish a 'forelimb area', a 'hindlimb area', a 'face area' and so on, but with some degree of overlapping. These point-to-point projections to the cerebellum are nowhere so circumscribed as those to be found in some parts of the cerebral cortex.

The pathways here referred to as 'convergent' correspond to the 'pathways of diffuse projection' to be found in anatomical texts. Where one peripheral location sends afferents which are distributed over an area of cerebellar cortex, it follows that each particular area of cortex must receive convergent afferents from a variety of different sources. A further classification of afferent pathways can be made in terms of whether the connections are crossed, uncrossed, or bilateral, giving a combination of six types of connection from six types of source. Some of the connections are fairly direct, some relay in the nuclei of the pons, some relay in the reticular formation and some in the inferior olive.

Each mossy fibre branches to serve several areas of the cerebellar cortex, there to branch again into 20–30 small lobulated enlargements, called 'rosettes', each of which is surrounded by the dendrites of about 20 granule cells to form a 'glomerulus'. Thus each branch of an afferent fibre influences some 600 or so granule cells. Axons from the granule cells pass radially towards the cortical surface and there bifurcate at a T-junction to form long fibres running, parallel to one another, along the line of the folium. The direction of the parallel fibres is thus at right angles to the planes of the dendritic trees of the Purkinje cells, so that each granule cell can make contact with about 60 Purkinje cells. Each Purkinje cell dendritic tree is traversed by some 250 000 parallel fibres. Excitatory synaptic connections occur in enormous numbers between small swellings on the parallel fibres and the spiny branchlets of the Purkinje dendrites. All the neurons of the cerebellar cortex apart from the granule cells have inhibitory effects at their terminations.

The dendritic trees of the basket cells are arranged, like those of the Purkinje cells, each in a single thin slab of tissue. Their axons form a number of branches, all in the same plane as the dendritic tree, and each of these branches surrounds the cell body of a single Purkinje cell with a basket-like network of fine fibres. The action at these terminations is strongly inhibitory. The stellate cells have similar connections to those of the basket cells, but with a more restricted range, and with no baskets. The dendritic trees of the Golgi cells are not confined to thin slabs of tissue but ramify extensively among the parallel fibres. They also receive direct connections from side-branches of some mossy fibres. The axons of the Golgi cells run each to a number of the glomeruli that lie on the afferent pathway into the cerebellum. The climbing fibres all originate in the inferior and accessory olives in the brainstem. Each terminates in a complex arborization that closely invests all the dendrites of a single Purkinje cell, like ivy climbing up a tree, forming a multiple synapse with powerfully excitatory action.

The number of cells in the olive is only about a quarter of the number of Purkinje cells, so each olivary cell must give rise to several climbing fibres, all of which serve Purkinje cells lying in roughly the same plane. Climbing fibres also have a few side-branches running to Golgi cells, and also to basket cells. The output from the cerebellar cortex is carried entirely by the axons of the Purkinje cells, which run to the deep nuclei within the cerebellum and to the vestibular nuclei of the brainstem. Purkinje cell axons also have extensive collaterals running to Golgi cells, to basket cells, and probably to other Purkinje cells also, in an arrangement reminiscent of the pattern, seen in the spinal cord, of the connections of collaterals from motor axons onto the Renshaw cells.

The high degree of regularity in the network of connections in the cerebellar cortex prompts speculation about its function. Each mossy fibre makes excitatory connection with a number of granule cells, and each granule cell receives from several mossy fibres. Transmission from mossy fibre to granule cell is not guaranteed, indeed it may be inhibited at the glomeruli by the action of Golgi cells. The firing of the granule cells must therefore be supposed to be intermittent and to be dependent on the pattern of impulses arriving along the mossy fibres. Thus the occurrence of an impulse in a granule cell may be taken as an indication that a specific group of mossy fibres have all been active together within the immediate past. This does not imply that a coincidence of inputs is necessary for granule cell activation, because spontaneous firing can be observed after the mossy fibres have been cut and allowed to degenerate. The probability that a granule cell will fire in a particular interval of time can be taken as enhanced if the appropriate set of mossy fibres has very recently been active.

The dendritic tree of a single Purkinje cell receives the excitatory action of a very large number of parallel fibres, each of which reports the activity of a single granule cell. If we visualize the activity at an excitatory synapse as a flash of light, each parallel fibre behaving like a twinkling star, then the information presented to a single Purkinje cell resembles that displayed, moment to moment, on the screen of a domestic television receiver, where each parallel fibre synapse corresponds to a single resolvable dot on the television screen.

For a television picture to be recognizable there are two conditions that must be satisfied by the signal controlling the display screen. The overall intensity has to be adequate to produce illumination of the 'spot' without being excessive, and the range of intensities providing the picture information has to be great enough for differences in brightness to be discernible. Adjustment of these two aspects of the signal intensity are provided by the controls for 'brightness' and for 'contrast'. Comparable problems are involved in any recognition process. In the case of the pathway from the mossy fibres to Purkinje cells, the equivalant of brightness control is provided by the negative feedback by way of the Golgi cells. They receive activation from the parallel fibres and distribute inhibitory influences widely to the glomeruli. Contrast control is provided by the stellate cells which also sample the excitatory activity of the parallel fibres, but whose inhibitory influence is on the Purkinje dendrites exposed to the same field of parallel fibres.

We may suppose each Purkinje cell to be tuned to a specific pattern of excitatory input, as to a snapshot of a specific television picture, so that whenever this particular pattern appears, this event is reflected in the excitatory state of that cell. Some uncertainty is permitted, and presumably a less precise match leads to a less well-marked change in the cell. There will also be some ambiguity, because it is likely that there may be several patterns of interacting excitatory and inhibitory influences distributed over the surface of a single dendrite that can give rise to identical patterns of change in the local circuit currents contributed by that dendrite to the soma of the cell. An arrangement of this sort is particularly well suited to playing a part in a mechanism for pattern-recognition.

Activity in a particular Purkinje cell amounts to a 'claim to have seen' some specified pattern of parallel fibre activity, but the firing pattern of the cell will convey no information leading to a discrimination between alternative inputs that generate similar local circuit currents at the trigger zone. The basket cells provide what amounts to a second opinion. They also receive their input from the parallel fibres. If they are 'satisfied' as to the pattern of their input, they respond by inhibiting the output of 'rival' Purkinje cells lying to either side. The discrimination between the votes of an array of Purkinje cells is thus enhanced by the competition between neighbouring basket cells, each favouring its own candidate, so to speak.

The rest of the nervous system does not 'attend' continually to the whole of the Purkinje cell output from the cerebellar cortex. Relevant parts of the record are scrutinized, from time to time and as occasion demands, by impulses in the climbing fibres. The collaterals from the climbing fibres to the deep nuclei indicate which part of the cerebellar cortical record is being consulted. The response of the corresponding Purkinje cells shows whether or not the pattern sought has been found to be present in the mossy fibre input. We must suppose large numbers of such 'consultations' to be continuously in progress on a moment-to-moment basis. While this outline gives a plausible view of the functioning of the neuronal circuitry, we must remember that the cerebellar cortex normally operates in conjunction with a number of other structures, especially the brainstem nuclei and the basal ganglia.

The cerebellum has been shown to be involved in the learned

modification of motor responses to a variety of stimuli, including both classical conditioning and the development of anticipatory pre-emptive actions.

Localized damage to the cerebellar cortex results in disturbances of motor coordination. Movements that involve several joints are normally performed smoothly, with suitably coordinated action of the muscles controlling the various joints. After cerebellar injury, the relative timing of the activity in the individual muscles becomes more haphazard and the limb consequently moves in a jerky fashion, and may overshoot its target. This finding has led to the view that the cerebellum plays a part in the learning of the motor coordination needed to perform skilled tasks. We have already seen that the triggering of certain components of balancing behaviour depends upon the recognition of a gestalt signalling the appropriateness of the current moment for the initiation of a specific motor act. We may now suppose the cerebellum to be concerned in some way in such recognition tasks.

MOTOR PATTERNS

As well as the 'motor area' in the cerebral cortex there are several cell groups in the brainstem that are involved in motor control. The list includes:

- the basal ganglia and subthalamic nucleus;
- the reticular formation, the red nucleus and the pontine nuclei;
- the vestibular nuclei and the periaqueductal grey matter;
- the motor nuclei of the cranial nerves.

A general feature of all these cell groups is that they have profuse interconnections, with one another, with many parts of the cerebral cortex, and with the deep nuclei of the cerebellum. There is little evidence of localized specialization of function, except perhaps in the basal ganglia.

THE BASAL GANGLIA

Localized damage to parts of the basal ganglia occurs in certain diseases. Disabilities of various kinds follow. These are grouped into named syndromes such as Parkinson's disease, Wilson's disease, Huntington's chorea, and so on. The extent of the damage varies from patient to patient, so that each shows his own pattern of symptoms, which may not necessarily include the tremor, rigidity and indistinctness of speech that characterizes the rest of the group.

Two types of disability can be distinguished. Both are related to voluntary movement. There are some actions that the patients are unable to perform, and there are certain other actions or movements that are executed by the patients' bodies without either any deliberate intent or any ability to refrain. There may also be disturbances in the time scale for the execution of certain actions, which may be performed either very slowly, with long pauses, or may be carried through with quite extraordinary rapidity, as in speaking at four times the normal word-rate.

The performance of any voluntary action involves the regulation of the activity of many muscles throughout the body. For example, if one hand is engaged in writing, adjustments are needed in the trunk muscles to alter the distribution of support forces as the hand moves over the paper. The head moves on the neck as the eyes follow the line of writing, and so on. Whenever we deliberately move any one part of our body, we involuntarily also make compensatory and auxiliary adjustments elsewhere in the body. These adjustments almost always occur without our being conscious of them. We do not know we have initiated them, and we do not know whether or not they have been carried out, unless they fail in some respect. It is in these background activities, essential for the support of voluntary movement, that the disorders associated with basal ganglion disease manifest themselves. In each case the disturbance may take the form either of an inadequacy or of an excess in the actions of certain muscles. The effects are usually widespread and not confined to a specific group of muscles. Where a particular action fails, this is not usually the result of a paralysis or of muscular weakness. Thus a patient whose head tends to droop forwards when his eyes are closed can sometimes raise his head quite strongly against an observer's hand. The positive symptoms, shown by affected individuals but not by normals, must be 'release phenomena', since a positive symptom cannot be generated by a structure that has been destroyed by disease. These symptoms must be generated by some undamaged structure whose activity is normally held in check.

On the basis of the negative symptoms, the normal functions of the basal ganglia may be classified under the following headings:

1. postural fixation and equilibrium;
2. righting;
3. locomotion;
4. phonation and articulation;
5. various.

This last is a heterogeneous group of functions which, if disturbed, lead to the symptoms referred to as 'akinesia', or failure to react. It includes some control of facial musculature, of chewing and swallowing, and of defecation and micturition.

Under the heading of postural fixation are included those actions of controlling the musculature that are needed to maintain one part of the body in a suitable posture to support the activity of another part: keeping the head upright on the neck, keeping the trunk upright on the pelvis, holding the arm up at the shoulder while doing something with the fingers, and so on. It is characteristic of patients with basal ganglion disease that they tend to droop. The head and sometimes the trunk also will sag forwards as soon as the eyes are closed. If the patient is asked to touch alternately the tips of the examiner's two fingers held about a foot apart at the level of the patient's shoulder and at about arm's length from him, he may perform quite well with his eyes open, but on closing his eyes the patient's hand almost immediately falls away and the movements cease.

Postural fixation is intimately bound up with equilibrium because a failure to maintain a suitable attitude may lead to a loss of balance. Several different stages may be distinguished in the normal actions that maintain the equilibrium of the body. In the first place there are the stabilizing actions, initiated from receptors in the labyrinth and in the neck, and including responses to angular acceleration initiated from the canals, and responses attributable to the otolith organs. Then there are the compensatory adjustments by which the centre of gravity is suitably positioned over the points of support when these happen to be displaced from symmetry with respect to the supporting upthrust from the ground. These have already been described above in the context of reactions to tilting. Finally there are the rescue reactions initiated at the point of overbalancing: staggering, sweeping and fall-breaking.

In basal ganglion disease the actions of stabilizing and compensation, and the rescue reactions of staggering, sweeping and fall-breaking, may all be separately affected to different extents. There may also be disturbances of the 'righting reactions', which are those movements by which a subject restores himself to the upright position after being displaced from it either voluntarily or after a fall. A subject with such a disability may not be able to rise from a chair or from the ground, and he may have difficulty in turning over in bed. Some patients who are unable to rise from the floor may be quite mobile after being helped to their feet, whereas others who may be able to get up without help are unable to walk or to control their gait once they have risen to their feet.

Successful locomotion is achieved by strategies of successive reduction and enhancement, in appropriate sequence, of various of the reactions used to maintain balance. It is thus not surprising to find that patients who have disturbances in the functions that maintain their equilibrium also have difficulties with locomotion.

The complex and highly coordinated movements used in speech depend on processes of muscular organization which have some features in common with locomotor activity, such as the need for accurate control of timing and of force, developed over long periods of training. Speech disturbances in basal ganglion disease may take the form either of indistinctness and block, or alternatively of accelerating rushes finishing in an incomprehensible jumble of syllables. Such headlong rushes are referred to as 'festination'. Similar disturbances of both kinds may occur in locomotion. Some patients have difficulty in making any of the preparatory displacements of the centre of gravity that are essential before one foot can be raised from the ground to make a step. They stand frozen to the ground, unable to move. Others, after a casual disturbance of their precarious balance, walk and run forwards with accelerating small steps until they crash into an obstacle.

Disturbances also occur in the movements of the facial muscles used to generate the facial signals that indicate mood and express interest and attention, and which contribute so much to the communication of personality. A common characteristic in basal ganglion disease is a mask-like, immobile countenance, showing no reaction to surrounding events. This immobility is often associated with continuous tensing of the facial muscles, like that responsible for the rigidity of the limbs. In other cases the facial muscles may produce grotesque grimaces, or continuous mastication. There is often profuse salivation and the skin is excessively oily. The eye muscles may also be affected, the gaze being forced in one direction or another for prolonged periods. These episodes are called 'oculogyric crises'.

The rigidity which is a characteristic positive symptom in basal ganglion disease may affect the limbs, trunk, neck or facial muscles. It differs from the rigidity of decerebration in that the force with which a displacement is resisted does not depend much on the speed of the displacement. In decerebrate rigidity the enhanced stretch reflexes generate much more force to oppose a more rapid displacement. If the imposed force is large enough, the response changes over suddenly into a yielding, in the clasp-knife reaction. The rigidity of basal ganglion disease resembles more closely that of a lead pipe, which can be forcibly bent to a new position, which it then maintains with the same stiffness as before. The clasp-knife reaction does not occur. Instead the resistance to forced movement of the limb fluctuates in jerky fashion, giving rise to the description as 'cogwheel rigidity'. In some cases the muscular activity responsible for the rigidity can be reduced by voluntary effort, to give a short-lasting relaxation, during which the patient may successfully execute a brief voluntary movement such as to catch a ball thrown to him. In one famous case a drowning man was saved by a Parkinsonian patient who leapt from his wheelchair into the breakers. Most of the time, however, the patient is, as it were, 'imprisoned in his own reflexes' and may remain practically motionless for several years at a stretch. Sometimes the rigidity is loosened if the patient is suspended in water or swimming.

Another common symptom is tremor, which has given to Parkinson's disease the name of 'paralysis agitans' or the 'shaking palsy'. This tremor is often confined to the hand, where the fingers work against the thumb in a characteristic 'pill-rolling' motion. The tremor is increased by nervousness or fatigue and disappears in sleep. It may be completely absent when the subject is concentrating on some skilled task. The tremor of basal ganglion disease is characteristically a tremor of rest, as opposed to the 'intention tremors' of cerebellar disease and of multiple sclerosis, where the tremor is associated with voluntary movement, and increases in intensity as the hand approaches its target.

More dramatic involuntary movements occur in other syndromes known as the 'choreas', in some of which there is damage to parts of the cerebral cortex as well as to the basal ganglia. In these conditions, extensive well-coordinated but purposeless movements occur, involving the whole of one or more limbs, to give an impression of dancing or swaggering. Some of the postural adjustments normally associated with voluntary actions may become greatly exaggerated, as though exceptional effort were required. A patient asked to lift a small object may use both hands and adjust his posture as though to lift a heavy weight.

Most of the disabilities associated with basal ganglion disease develop rather slowly. There may be a lapse of several years between the acute stage of encephalitis and the first appearance of motor disturbances. These thereafter progress gradually over a number of years. An exception is 'hemichorea of sudden onset', or 'hemiballismus'. The precipitating cause is a vascular accident affecting the subthalamic nucleus. Accordingly the symptoms develop fully within the course of a few hours. The limbs of one side only of the body undergo a ceaseless succession of extremely violent, flail-like movements of wide amplitude. The arm is usually more severely affected than the leg, and one side of the face may also be involved. Because of the anatomical linkages between the head and the shoulders through the trapezius and cleidomastoid muscles, the violent movements of the arms are communicated to the head. The head movements excite the labyrinth and generate more limb movements in positive feedback. If the head is held still by an assistant, the involuntary movements subside, particularly in the arms. Some movement may persist in the legs. All the movements of hemiballismus cease when the subject is asleep.

TILTING REACTIONS IN BASAL GANGLION DISEASE

In all cases of basal ganglion involvement there is some disturbance of the mechanisms for maintaining postural equilibrium. The deficiencies can be demonstrated with a tilting apparatus. This is a cushioned platform that can be tilted about a horizontal axis. The subject to be tested may sit astride the tilt axis with his legs dangling free of the ground, or he may be placed in the all-fours position and tilted either laterally or in the fore-and-aft direction. Tests are carried out with the subject blindfolded.

On the tilting apparatus the normal subject maintains the attitude of his head in spite of the tilted support (Figure 6.34). When he is tilted laterally in the seated position, his neck and trunk show compensatory lateral flexions to take up the difference in tilt between the pelvis and the head. The legs, which are hanging free, show a lateral sweep by rotation of the femur in the same sense as the rotation of the tilt table. The normal subject is not easily overbalanced, so that rescue reactions of the arms are seldom seen. When tilted laterally in the all-fours position the limbs show compensatory extension on the downhill side.

A subject with total absence of labyrinth function, either as a result of disease or after bilateral surgical interruption of the eighth nerves, shows no stabilization of the head or trunk, but tilts over passively with the platform (Figure 6.35). At the moment of overbalancing he shows the rescue reactions of sweeping with the legs, and with the arm on the upper side, while the arm on the lower side shows a vigorous fall-breaking reaction (Figure 6.36). The subject is easily overbalanced, and while righting himself afterwards he may overcompensate and fall again to the opposite side.

All subjects with basal ganglion disease are very deficient in stabilization and in compensation, although their labyrinths appear to be functioning normally, according to the usual clinical tests with rotational or caloric stimulation. There may be some transitory stabilization against slow tilts, but after a few moments the subject falls over. The rescue reactions of sweeping with the free limbs and fall-breaking on the downhill side are much delayed and often of reduced intensity. Some subjects show transitory stabilization in the lateral direction when seated, provided that the tilt is fairly rapid. However they soon fall over if the tilt is maintained. These subjects often show no stabilization at all in the all-fours position. The differences between the responses to slow and to rapid tilts may be related to the separate roles of the semicircular canals and of the otolith organs.

It is only in the case of hemiballismus that we have a clear-cut correlation between specific symptoms and a strictly localized lesion in the basal ganglia. The condition has been reproduced in monkeys by stereotaxic lesions confined to the subthalamic nucleus. Other correlations are relatively less well established, partly because of the long delays, often amounting to several years, between the onset of symptoms and the opportunity for post-mortem examination of the brain, and partly because the lesions, when they have been located, turn out to have involved several structures in varying degree. However, the following indications seem to be emerging.

Patients in whom the lesions are confined to the pallidum or in whom this structure and the substantia nigra are the ones most severely affected, particularly if the damage is bilateral, show marked deficiencies in postural fixation. The head tends to droop forwards and to be followed by a forward droop of the trunk. The head may sometimes be held up for a time by visual cues, as when the patient is watching television, but it at once droops forwards again as soon as the eyes are closed.

In the all-fours position these patients are unable to keep their heads up for more than a few moments even with their eyes open. The head slowly droops forwards until the subject comes to rest with the top of his head on the floor, as though about to perform a somersault. This 'somersault posture' has been seen in monkeys with bilateral lesions of the pallidum. When raised to his feet by an assistant, the patient can support his weight but his balance is precarious. His head and trunk slowly droop forwards until he is standing with the knees bent and the head bent right over.

The buttressing reactions, by which a normal subject resists being pushed over, are absent and there are no staggering reactions. The subject cannot carry out the adjustments in buttressing that are needed to get the weight onto one foot in preparation for walking, but if an assistant rocks his body for him from side to side he can often execute a series of steps quite well. Some subjects can make use of visual cues to initiate stepping. They can step over a series of chalk lines on the floor but come to a standstill when they run out of cues. Some have learned to carry a supply of paper pellets so that when they are stuck they can drop one or two of these to provide visual cues to help them to get going again.

There is no deficiency in the support forces in the limbs. The defect is in the organization of the transfer of weight, both in the sway reaction to resist applied forces and in the voluntary sway needed to initiate locomotion. In some cases the deficiency may be more marked in one direction than in another. A patient may have relatively good lateral stability, and may even be able to stand on one leg, and yet may be easily overbalanced backwards. The difficulties in turning over in bed, in rising from a chair, and in righting generally, are consequences of the deficiency in the transfer of weight. In attempting to turn over, the patient does not use the swing of the arm over the body that a normal subject would use to initiate the roll. In rising from a chair the patient may fail to make the usual preparatory movement of drawing the feet well back under the weight.

The slow forward droop of the head characteristic of Parkinson's disease results from a failure to transfer the weight into a suitably balanced position over the supports. In a normal subject the head and trunk continually sway slightly, and the muscular forces needed to keep them upright fluctuate around a position of minimum total effort. The patients with damage in the pallidum have lost the mechanism for transferring the weight to restore the posture to the minimum-effort position. Increasing deviation from this position calls for increasing muscular activity. In the absence of correcting reactions, the working muscles gradually lengthen and allow the head and trunk to droop, usually forwards.

The association of the defects of postural fixation with lesions in the pallidum is derived from a study of patients with post-encephalitic Parkinsonism. It receives some confirmation from the results of stereotactic lesions in the pallidum in monkeys. The patients, however, all showed degeneration in the substantia nigra as well as in the pallidum. Experimental lesions confined to the substantia nigra in animals have not so far provided indications of its function.

The defects in postural fixation and in weight transfer are negative symptoms giving information about the normal function of the structure that is damaged. Hemiballismus, on the other hand, is a positive symptom, and we need to work out what function has been interfered with to release this behaviour. The feedback between arm movements and head movements suggests that the damaged structure may normally be concerned in computing the line of thrust relative to the body from a comparison of labyrinth signals with those from the neck. When this computation is interfered with, casual movements of the head are treated as threats to overbalance the body, and excessive corrective movements in the limbs are elicited, because inadequate account has been taken of the change in neck posture. When patients with hemiballismus are placed on the tilt table, they show exaggerated reactions on the affected side.

The putamen and the caudate nucleus together form a single functional entity conveniently referred to as the 'striatum'. This is the part of the basal ganglia most closely associated with the cerebral cortex and which is therefore most likely to be concerned with organizing the background activity to support voluntary movements. Damage to the striatum is followed by inappropriate weight transfer. Patients with damage in this region tend to fall in one direction or another. The falling initiates stepping as though to regain balance, but this is ineffective in maintaining the centre of gravity over the area of support. Accordingly the stepping accelerates into the headlong rush of festination. It may occur either forwards or backwards. A patient with a tendency to fall backwards may be enabled to stand and to walk forwards if he carries a heavy object, such as a chair, in front of him.

Other patients who can stand without falling, but who are rather unstable, may be precipitated into festination when they are given a chair to hold up in front of them. Locomotor festination of this kind is associated with bilateral degeneration in the caudate nuclei, but there is usually other damage elsewhere also. The behaviour following damage to the striatum corresponds to the effect to be expected from an incorrect judgement as to the direction of the behavioural vertical. Festination has been produced in animals by bilateral lesions in the caudate nuclei. A unilateral lesion produces marked lateral curvature of the spine and forced circling towards the side of the lesion.

In Huntington's chorea there is usually rather widespread brain damage. Often the striatum is greatly shrunken. Patients with Huntington's chorea do not show festination, but the other involuntary movements of the limbs, trunk and face are markedly increased during locomotion – so much so that running is practically impossible. The involuntary movements often diminish in amplitude when the subject sits on a table with his feet off the ground. The pathology in this syndrome is very variable. The involuntary movements may be seen as supporting reactions released in inappropriate context.

Inappropriate postural fixation may manifest itself as rigidity, in which a part of the body is maintained by muscular activity in a fixed attitude even when this is not needed to support any voluntary actions. Patients with severe rigidity show marked cell-loss in the putamen, while the pallidum is relatively much less affected. It appears therefore that the rigidity of Parkinsonism is a result of the release of inappropriate postural fixation generated in the pallidum in the absence of the coordination normally provided by the putamen.

Many of the positive symptoms of basal ganglion disease can be relieved by interrupting the outflow from the pallidum. Surgeons differ in their choice of the ideal site in which to place the lesion. Some attempt to interrupt the fibres as they leave the globus pallidus, others prefer to aim for them as they run through the ventrolateral part of the thalamus. The operation is performed under local anaesthesia and in a successful case one may witness the abrupt cessation of the tremor of the fingers when the current is switched on to make the lesion.

Some degeneration of the substantia nigra is usually present in cases of post-encephalitic Parkinsonism. The substantia nigra is particularly rich in dopamine. As well as being an intermediate in the formation of the melanin that gives the substantia nigra its black colour, this substance is also a neural transmitter whose presence has been demonstrated at the terminals in the striatum of nerve-fibres originating in the substantia nigra. This discovery suggested that the symptoms of Parkinsonism might be attributable to a deficiency of dopamine.

EFFECT OF L-DOPA ON LONG-TERM
PARKINSONIAN PATIENTS

Dopamine itself does not pass through the blood–brain barrier, but the levels of dopamine in the brain can be raised by administering a related substance, laevo-dihydroxyphenylalanine, or L-Dopa, which can be given by mouth. The effects of administering L-Dopa to patients who have been immobilized for years with Parkinson's disease turns out to be spectacular and astounding. An impressive account is given in the book *Awakenings*, by Oliver Sacks.

The drug was administered in gradually increasing doses over a number of days. In a typical case there was very little change for the first few days. Then, quite suddenly, a patient who has been immobile for over forty years, and totally mute for twenty, jumps up and starts to sing and dance with joyous exuberance and animation. A number of similar case-histories are given, each with the same general pattern but with minor variations. From the reports of these patients after their 'awakening' it is clear that their intellectual faculties had been in no way affected by their disease. The change from drooping, drooling immobility to alert, charming vivacity is most strikingly conveyed in the book.

Unfortunately, the cells lost from the basal ganglia are not replaced by the drug, and although the functioning of the surviving cells can be reinforced by administering L-Dopa, the effect is not permanent. After a short period of a few days or weeks other troubles appear. There may be wild fluctuations in mood, from frenzy to deep depression, with overpowering hallucinations. Sudden uncontrolled movements, 'tics', appear, often recurring with great frequency. When the dosage of L-Dopa is reduced, the patient may revert suddenly to deep immobility. Some patients can be awakened again, and can thereafter continue to oscillate in almost all-or-none fashion between immobility and vivacity. There appears to be no middle course corresponding to a specific dose level of the drug. Perhaps this is because the level of requirement fluctuates from hour to hour or from moment to moment during the day.

Not the least remarkable of the consequences of the administration of L-Dopa to Parkinsonian patients has been the recovery of the power of speech and of the communication of feelings by facial expression, often after many years of silent, mask-like immobility. Patients recall their feelings before they received the drug, describe their reactions to the awakening itself, and then their turmoil of emotions during the subsequent phase of difficult readjustments while seeking for the knife-edge balance between the appearance of new disabilities and the recrudescence of the old. Some of the suddenly acquired appetites and behavioural drives exhibited by patients awakened by L-Dopa may be related to the neuronal connections between the basal ganglia and the hypothalamus. In some cases the results are pleasant and gratifying; in others the effects are heart-rendingly devastating.

When the administration of L-Dopa to an immobile patient restores to him the ability to perform certain motor acts, this implies that the neural mechanisms for the necessary motor control must have survived the disease. The ability to walk unaided was restored in about half of the cases reported by Sacks. All of these had shown positive symptoms of rigidity with or without tremor or festination, and we may accordingly conclude that at least part of the pallidum must have been spared. One patient who had lost the power of postural fixation, and whose pallidum may consequently be presumed to have been damaged by the disease, in other respects made a good recovery under L-Dopa but could achieve only a few steps and for this needed the constant support of a handrail.

It is interesting to compare the effects of L-Dopa on immobile Parkinsonian patients with the locomotor effects produced by L-Dopa in decerebrate and spinal animals. In each case the effects are presumably attributable to generalized changes in the level of excitability at synapses of a certain chemical type, rather than to any form of structured command that might specify the performance of particular movements. In the behaviour of patients it is clear that effects in the cerebral cortex are involved, because the involuntary tics and mannerisms that develop in some cases after administration of the drug resemble those attributable in other patients to cortical damage.

RHYTHM GENERATORS FOR LOCOMOTION

Attempts have been made from time to time to locate within the nervous system 'centres' for the control of specific patterns of motor behaviour. For example, groups of cells have been sought that show some form of cyclic activity that can be related to the cyclic movements of locomotion. Such kinds of rhythmic activity have been found at a number of sites. In many cases the activity turns out to be related to the sensory messages from the limbs, so that the rhythm has to be regarded as a passive result of limb movement, rather than as a contribution to its cause. The distinction is not clear-cut, since localized lesions at the sites in question may lead to disturbances in the pattern of the locomotor movements, or in the precision with which the feet are placed on the available supports, as when a cat is induced to walk along the rungs of a horizontal ladder. Accurate placing is dependent on the integrity of the motor area of the cerebral cortex and, since much of the experimental work on locomotor rhythms in the central nervous system has been carried out on reduced preparations, the experimenters have had to content themselves with somewhat imperfect precision in the performance of the locomotor movements.

The involvement of sensory messages from the limbs can be eliminated either by denervation or by physical restraint on the limb movements. In this way sites have been discovered in the midbrain that show rhythmic activity that is not dependent on rhythmic sensory input, and which persists even if the animal is paralysed with curare. This finding has encouraged the belief that locomotion is driven by some central 'pattern generator'. Further sites with similar neural behaviour are uncovered when the general level of excitability of the neurons has been raised by administering such agents as amphetamine, a drug whose action may involve the liberation of dopamine, thus enhancing the effectiveness of naturally occurring synaptic transmitters. It has already been argued, in Chapter 7, that rhythmic activity revealed in these special experimental conditions may be attributable to the interplay of the various local reflexes that link the behaviour of single limbs to the conditions prevailing in other limbs. One has also to take account of the processes, largely unanalysed as yet, by which the activity of different parts of the axial musculature is coordinated with the activity of the limbs. Reliance on pattern generators is not appropriate to the real-life situation where the aiming of the limbs at each step has to take account of irregularities in the terrain.

Another approach to the analysis of motor control has been to suppose that the various muscles in a limb are organized into 'synergies', that is to say, into sets of muscles that are invariably active in co-operation, as in resisting flexion at different joints when the limb is loaded in compression, or in furling the limb for a step. Although such synergies would appear to be advantageous for some tasks, electrical recordings of motor unit activity do not support the idea of this being a general principle of motor organization.

The overall task of the central nervous system that we are concerned with in relation to balancing behaviour and locomotion consists in the formulation of appropriate patterns of control signals to regulate the forces exerted by the individual motor units. We need to remember that the task involves **all** the motor units in the body, including those in the large numbers of small muscles linking the individual vertebrae. In the face of this complexity, it is tempting to look for other simplifying strategies.

THE SIZE PRINCIPLE FOR THE RECRUITMENT OF MOTOR UNITS

One such strategy has come to be known as the 'size principle', according to which the motor units in a particular muscle are always recruited into activity in a fixed order, which is governed by the electrical excitabilities of the motoneurons. One advantage of such a scheme would be that it might reduce the uncertainties in the relation between tendon organ discharges and the overall tension exerted by the muscles which they serve. The muscle cells that make up a single motor unit are scattered through the substance of the muscle belly in which they lie, and the tendon organs are each influenced by a small group of muscle cells, each of which is likely to belong to a different motor unit. In such an arrangement, the tendon organ signal depends on which of its contributing motor units happens to be active. If the motor units are recruited in a fixed order during an increase in muscle tension, there will then be some consistency in the way the tendon organ signal changes with the activity of the muscle as a whole.

The measure of 'size' at first sight might seem ambiguous, as it might refer to the motoneuron cell body, to the diameter of its axon, or to the peak tension that the motor unit can develop. It is possible to assess the tension contribution made by individual motor units to the overall muscle tension by a special technique, known as 'spike-triggered averaging', that has proved useful in a number of other neurophysiological contexts also. The use of this technique depends on the fact that the activity cycles of the motor units in a particular muscle are not synchronized with one another in the reflex response to sustained stretch.

SPIKE-TRIGGERED AVERAGING

In this procedure, an electrical trigger pulse is first selected, in this case the action-potential of a single motor unit, recorded through suitably placed fine electrodes. The output signal being studied, in this case the tension in the tendon, is sampled repeatedly at intervals that are small compared with the time-course of the response that is being analysed. When each trigger pulse is detected, a set of sampled values of the output variable are added each to the appropriate member of an array of storage 'bins' in a computer, according to the time interval between the trigger pulse and the moment of sampling. Events that are not synchronized with the trigger contribute randomly distributed amounts to each store, so that their cumulative sum tends to zero. On the other hand, synchronized events contribute consistently similar amounts at each pass. After a number of passes, the accumulated totals are read out in sequential order to give the time-course and amplitude of the events that were consistently related in time to the moment of triggering. In this way, the force generated by a single motor unit can be separated out from the total. It is found that the largest peak forces are produced by motor units served by the largest motoneurons, and these are the ones with the largest axons, as determined by their conduction velocities. Thus the attribute 'large' applies to all three criteria without ambiguity.

In a great many muscles it turns out that the motor units are recruited, during progressively increasing stretch, at a sequence of thresholds that corresponds to the sequence of increasing sizes, in accordance with the size principle. Some instances have been found, however, where a pair of units in a particular muscle are recruited in a different order according to the task in which the muscle is engaged. Many joints are capable of movement in more than one plane, the direction of movement being governed by the relative degree of activity in the various muscles operating at that joint. For example, the first dorsal interosseus muscle in the human hand contributes to flexion as well as to abduction of the finger, and the order of recruiting of motor units may not be the same for abduction movements as it is for flexions. Recruitment according to the size principle does not take account of the need for rotation of units to reduce the liability to fatigue in muscles that are called upon to exert sustained tensions over long periods.

Since none of the simplifying assumptions that have so far been put forward has turned out to be of universal application, we are left with the conclusion that each motor unit requires the formulation of its own private pattern of activation, and that the initiation of each such pattern is dependent upon some local process of gestalt recognition. Even simple reflexes involve some mechanism for recognizing a gestalt made up of sensory messages from many sources that together indicate that the overall stimulus situation is one that can properly be regarded as an appropriate 'adequate stimulus' for the generation of that particular motor response.

RECOGNITION DEVICES

Until recently, the mechanics of recognition processes has remained obscure. Recent developments in computing with parallel distributed processors have now introduced fresh possibilities. This development in computing techniques was prompted by the realization that, in contrast to the strictly serial processing of information in a conventional digital computer, the nervous system handles information delivered simultaneously by a large number of afferent nerve-fibres and that it processes this information stream with a very large number of cells between which there are very extensive interconnections. Confusingly, computer research in this field has progressed in divergent streams. In one, where massive amounts of data are to be processed as in meteorology, the initial stages of processing are distributed between a number of separate conventional serial processors, each of which performs its own sequence of algorithms on aspects of the common data stream. These processors operate independently but simultaneously, in parallel, and pass their results to other conventional serial processors for later stages of computation. This is true 'parallel distributed processing'. Despite this name it has little to do with what goes on in the nervous system.

Another stream of development is concerned with artificial neural networks. Devices have now been constructed in which a number of computing elements are linked together in a 'neural net', each of the elements having properties reminiscent of actual neurons. Each element has a number of inputs and a number of outputs. Interconnections are arranged so that each element can be influenced by several others, and can in turn itself influence several others. The effectiveness of the influence to be exerted across a particular link, known as its 'weight', is adjustable, according to a certain routine, and by means of such adjustments of weighting, the behaviour of the whole network can become modified. The earliest such networks were composed of discrete interconnected items of hardware, but more recently the whole of each network has been simulated on a conventional serial computer using an appropriate high-level computer language. Further development in this direction concentrates interest on algorithms for regulating the adjustment of the weights of the linkages between elements of the net. This branch of computing science is now referred to as 'connectionism'.

Even some of the early artificial networks were capable of surprisingly complex tasks, such as to indicate the sex of the person portrayed in a photograph. More advanced devices perform such tasks as converting a printed text into a sequence of phonemes to drive a speech synthesizer, or controlling a complex chemical plant according to the continually changing qualities and quantities of the available raw materials. Devices of this sort perform 'recognitions' of a kind, in the sense that the production of a particular pattern of output is dependent on the presence, in the input data, of a specific trigger pattern, which has to be distinguished from other configurations of the input data. In the case of a controller, the output has to be varied in an appropriate fashion to suit variations in the input pattern.

The majority of the artificial neural networks studied in computing science are designed in terms of overall performance without much regard for the ways equivalent performances are achieved in animal or human brains. The fact that such devices perform so well on complex tasks like those performed by real brains, together with the lack of progress in accounting for neural behaviour in terms of the activity of individual neurons, has suggested that we should look at specific anatomical groupings of neurons which might prove to be interconnected in ways similar to those that work in artificial networks.

CONNECTIONISM

The artificial networks of most interest to neurophysiologists usually conform to the following layered plan. They contain a number of input units, forming one layer, a number of output units in another layer, and one or more layers of 'hidden units' in between. Each input unit is connected to several hidden units, each of which receives from many input units. Similarly, each output unit receives from several hidden units, each of which influences many output units. The hidden units are interconnected in ways that differ in different designs. Each link has associated with it a specific weight, which expresses the efficacy with which signals in that link affect the output of the receiving unit. The outgoing signal produced by an individual unit is related, sometimes in nonlinear fashion, to the weighted sum of all its input signals.

When the network is first set up, arbitrary values are assigned to each of the weights. There follows a 'training regime' during which the weights are adjusted according to a selected protocol. Many of the protocols currently in use require prior knowledge of what is to count as the desirable behaviour of the network in order to arrive at an assessment of how successful the training has been so far, and to determine what further adjustments are required at each stage. One procedure with these features is the 'back propagation algorithm'. A set of training examples is prepared in which possible input patterns in a chosen range are each paired with a specification of what is to be counted as a 'correct response' at the output. Taking one such practice pair at a time, the discrepancy between observed and desired output is measured as a basis for a round of weight adjustments in a sequence of steps. For every output unit, each of the weights on its incoming linkages is examined in turn to see what effect a change in that weight will have on the overall error of the network as a whole. That particular weight is then adjusted in such a direction as to reduce the error. The next linkage in turn is then modified by the same procedure until all the links to all the output units have been dealt with. The procedure is then repeated for the adjacent hidden units, and so on for the whole network, before passing on to another of the set of practice input patterns. Finally the whole procedure is run through again and again until the discrepancies for all the practice input patterns have been reduced to some preset tolerance level. Where many iterations are necessary, the burden of computation can be very considerable indeed, especially when there are more than a very few tens of hidden units.

David Robinson, with his colleagues in Baltimore, has set up artifical networks, with back propagation weight adjustments for error correction, to convert the signals from the semicircular canals into suitable command signals to control the eye muscles in the vestibulo-ocular reflex. The function of this reflex is to move the eyeballs in their sockets in such a way that the direction of gaze is unaffected by movements of the head. The six muscles acting on each eye are arranged in pairs which rotate the eyeball about mutually perpendicular axes. The canals are also arranged in three mutually perpendicular planes, but these planes do not correspond with the axes of the eyeball movements. A transformation of vectors is required.

An artificial network to perform the task of compensating for pitch and roll was made up of four input units, one for each vertical canal, and four output units, one each for the superior and inferior recti, and one each for the superior and inferior obliques of one eye, together with 40 hidden units. The system was trained on a number of combinations of pitch and roll, using a variety of horizontal axes. The network required only 500 iterations to generate an accurate vertical compensatory control signal in terms of eyeball velocity, the input signals being taken as representing skull velocities.

A complication in the real case is that the canal signals are related to head velocity, provided that the movement is brief, while the eye muscles are effectively position-activators. A separate network was constructed to handle the transformation from a velocity signal to a position signal, and to provide the necessary frequency-compensation to deal with the sudden changes in eyeball position called for in a saccade. This network was required to deal with pursuit movements and saccades as well as with vestibular compensatory movements, a task which it quickly learned to perform successfully.

When the hidden units in these artificial networks are examined, after training, they are found to have polarization vectors in a variety of directions, not corresponding closely either to the planes of the canals or to the axes of eyeball rotation produced by the individual opposed pairs of eye muscles. In this respect, their behaviour resembled that seen in individual neurons in the brain, where the scattering of polarization vectors could not otherwise be accounted for. This finding must not be taken to imply that the brain performs the necessary signal transformations in the same way as the artificial network does. Indeed, it has been found that, if a trained network was restarted from scratch, the arrangement of hidden units developed during training was different at each trial. Clearly there are alternative ways of arriving at a solution to the problem of producing correct responses to a range of inputs. The indications are, however, that it might well prove profitable to think of neural behaviour in terms of networks of some kind.

There are strong reasons for supposing that iterative procedures, such as those necessary for weight modification by the back propagation algorithm, are unlikely to have their counterpart in neural activity. It is also unlikely that the nervous system contains anything resembling a 'teacher' to provide advance knowledge of what is to count as a 'correct answer' to be used in error assessment as a basis for weight modification in training procedures. There are, however, other regimes available for training artificial neural networks in addition to the back propagation algorithm described above. The regimes not requiring external supervision include direct association learning and learning by reward. All such learning routines involve modifying the efficacy of the various linkages in a network.

The notion of adjustable weights, which is at the heart of the design of artificial neural networks, has its counterpart in the variation in synaptic efficacy that occurs at the end-knobs on the dendrites of neurons in the brain. There are various ways in which the transmission process at a single synapse can be modified. During repetitive activation, there is a tendency for synaptic vesicles to migrate towards the synapse so that, when presynaptic impulses arrive in rapid succession, the amount of transmitter released at each impulse may increase. A process of this kind is postulated to account for the phenomenon of temporal summation, where two stimuli in rapid succession lead to a greater total response than the sum of the responses to single stimuli. This mechanism cannot, however, be held to account for long-term changes in synaptic sensitivity.

ASSOCIATION LEARNING

In a connectionist version of weight adjustment in direct association learning, the correlation between the output of a unit with the messages in a particular link is used to modify the weight of that link. Effects of this kind occur in neurons in the brain. The density of synaptic connections between neurons is considerably greater in very early life than it is in adult animals. It is supposed that some synaptic connections disappear as a result of 'disuse atrophy'. A corollary of this idea is that individual synapses are maintained in functional condition by repeated use. It is known that all the molecules forming the structures of the body are from time to time broken down and replaced with fresh molecules, this process being essential to the growth and repair of all tissues. At an individual synapse, the process may lead to a change in the area of synaptic contact between the cells involved and also to a change in the form of the postsynaptic membrane surrounding the synaptic contact area itself. This change in form may affect the shape of the dendritic spine and thus the efficacy with which the permeability change at the active synapse affects the membrane potential of the rest of the postsynaptic cell. There are instances where a long burst of high-frequency pulses, say at 100 per second for 10 s, can lead to a repetitive discharge which may persist even for some weeks.

In the brief account of synaptic transmission given at the beginning of this chapter, it was mentioned that a considerable number of substances have been identified as serving some sort of transmitter function within the nervous system. We now need to look at the action of these substances in more detail. When a presynaptic end-knob is depolarized by the arrival of an impulse, the first effect is to open the membrane channels that permit the entry of calcium ions. These ions facilitate the binding of the envelope of the transmitter vesicles to the proteins of the cell membrane of the synaptic patch. The vesicles then rupture to deliver their contents into the synaptic cleft. The vesicles contain substances of two kinds. The neurotransmitters proper act on the postsynaptic membrane in the manner already described. This action has the very brief time-course outlined earlier and it can have either an excitatory or an inhibitory effect on the generation, by local circuit currents, of electrical activity in the postsynaptic cell, the outcome in each case depending on the nature of the receptors in the postsynaptic membrane. The other set of substances are more properly referred to as 'neuromodulators'. They act on the cell membranes of both pre- and postsynaptic cells, with a very much slower time-course than that of the 'transmitters'.

ACTION OF NEUROMODULATORS

The neuromodulators react with the glycoproteins of the cell membrane to release an intracellular enzyme, such as adenylate cyclase, which catalyses the formation of cyclic AMP from ATP and leads to the activation of a protein kinase. This in turn leads to phosphorylation of certain glycoproteins in the cell membrane of the synaptic patch to produce a short-term facilitatory effect. In addition, 'second messenger' molecules, which may be either a protein kinase or perhaps the calcium ions themselves, pass through the cytoplasm of the cell to the nucleus. Here they activate certain genes in the DNA that is held in the nucleus. These genes are then copied into RNA to initiate and regulate the synthesis of specific glycoproteins, which eventually, over a time-course of some hours, come to be incorporated into the cell membranes at the synaptic region, increasing the area of the synaptic patch and modifying the shape of the postsynaptic dendritic spines. This complex cascade of biochemical reactions produces long-term changes in the synaptic efficacy of those connections that happen to be repeatedly active, and thus provides a basis for association learning.

THE HIPPOCAMPUS AND RELATED STRUCTURES

It is understandably difficult to pinpoint changes of this kind when they occur in small-scale but widespread fashion, but there are localized sites in the brain where concentrations of significant changes can occur in certain learning situations. The effects of local lesions tell us that certain areas of the hippocampus in mammals are essential for the laying down of memories of certain kinds. After damage to the hippocampus during surgery for the relief of epilepsy, a patient was found to have lost the capacity to form long-term memories. His existing memories of the past were unaffected, and he remained able to perform intelligence tests of the type that do not rely substantially on memory, but he could not commit anything new to long-term memory. For example, he consistently failed to recognize people, such as close neighbours and family friends, whom he had got to know only after his operation. A corresponding condition has been produced by experimental lesions in the hippocampus in animals. In related studies it has been shown that the formation of long-term memories during training procedures can be interfered with by injecting an antibiotic of a kind known to inhibit protein synthesis. This suggests that the laying down of long-term memories depends on protein synthesis in the hippocampus. This hypothesis has been extensively studied with biochemical techniques.

Steven Rose has carried out parallel studies on very young chicks of the domestic hen. These animals are chosen for study because they perform prodigious learning tasks as soon as they emerge from the egg. They learn to distinguish the appearance of the mother hen, by a process known as 'imprinting' which involves such a rudimentary recognition act that the chick will follow, as if it were its own mother, any large object that moves in its field of view just after hatching. They also need to distinguish other objects in the environment, and to classify them as edible or inedible, threatening or indifferent, since the chicks are dependent on their own efforts for the food necessary for their survival.

The structure of the avian brain is rather different from that of the mammals. In place of the cerebral cortex of mammals the birds have a complex solid forebrain, referred to as the 'tectum'. Cell groups have been located in the chick tectum that have similar functions to those of the mammalian hippocampus. The procedure for this process of localization starts with the selection of a training routine that involves substantial learning in a very short time. Chicks were selected which had a propensity to peck freely at a proffered bead. They were then offered a bead dipped in a pungent bitter solution. After one peck at the bitter bead, a chick would shake its head vigorously, back away, and wipe its beak on the floor of the pen. Thereafter the chick would refuse to peck at a similar bead offered at any time from a few seconds to several days later. This is an example of one-trial passive avoidance learning.

Protein synthesis requires energy, which is supplied in the form of glucose in the bloodstream. A related substance, 2-deoxyglucose, labelled with a radioisotope and injected into the bloodstream, is taken up into the cells as though it were glucose, but it is not further metabolized and so it accumulates in the active cells. The location of the areas of high activity can then be found by autoradiography of frozen sections of the brain. The type of protein being synthesized in these conditions turns out to be a glycoprotein of the kind forming the cell membranes at the synaptic regions.

The timing of the process of protein synthesis in the course of training can be worked out because of the short time involved in developing the one-trial passive avoidance learning. There is a substance which specifically inhibits the synthesis of glycoproteins. If this substance is injected into the chick at around the time of the training session, the chick does not remember to avoid the proffered bead. Amnesia for the training session can also be induced by applying an electric shock across the bird's head shortly afterwards. The electric shock completely disrupts any electrical processes, such as impulse transmission, that may be going on in the brain at the time of the shock.

Three phases of memory formation can be recognized on the basis of these procedures. The earliest phase starts promptly, but lasts only a few minutes after the training incident. The second builds up over a few minutes but has fully declined again within an hour. The third phase builds up slowly over the course of an hour, after which it is no longer susceptible to inhibitors of protein synthesis. On histological examination 24 hours afterwards, the region in which protein synthesis took place shows, in neurons of a particular recognizable type, both an increase in the number of dendritic spines and changes in their shape. In electronmicrographs, changes can be seen in the lengths of the synaptic thickenings and in the numbers of vesicles of transmitter. Electrical recordings from these regions show sporadic bursts of firing during the learning phase.

Curiously, the cell groups that are active in protein synthesis during the formation of a memory do not appear to be involved in its recall, since amnesia for a trained response does not follow local ablation of those cells if this is carried out after a certain interval. In fact, different groups of cells appear to be involved at different stages in the development of long-term memory, and if one route is blocked by a local lesion, another can take its place. The location of the final version of the effective memory trace has not been discovered.

A corresponding set of processes to those found in the chick tectum have also been found in the mammalian hippocampus. In none of this work, however, can it be stated just what it is that is remembered, or why that feature of the afferent impulse stream should produce changes in those specific regions of the brain. It may well turn out that comparable changes may also be occurring in cells elsewhere in the brain and that these are less obvious because the cells involved are somewhat scattered, rather than being concentrated together as they are in the cell groups of the mammalian hippocampus or of the chick tectum.

REINFORCEMENT LEARNING

It is a common property of organisms that, if they associate some improvement in their situation with their performance of a specific behavioural act, they thereafter tend to perform that action more frequently. An experimenter can make use of this propensity in order to influence an animal's behaviour. The first step is that the experimenter must select some procedure by which he can affect the animal's environment in a way that is advantageous to the pupil. An obvious and much used such procedure in animal work is the presentation of a morsel of food. The experimenter then studies the pupil's apparently spontaneous behaviour to identify some particular action that can be used as a basis for a training routine. The next stage is to present a food morsel promptly every time the pupil performs the selected action. This procedure is known as 'positive reinforcement'. The technique can be extended by requiring that additional, previously spontaneous, actions are performed in conjunction with the act originally selected, thus 'shaping' the pupil's behavioural repertoire. By proceeding stepwise in this fashion it is possible to produce quite marked changes in the pupil's behaviour.

The training routine can be automated using a device that presents the reward mechanically when the pupil makes some move that triggers a suitable detector. This leads to a description of the training process as 'operant conditioning', where the 'operant' is the animal that performs the action to be rewarded (operates the lever or whatever), and whose behaviour is changed ('conditioned') by the reinforcement provided by consistent reward. The use of the word 'conditioning' can lead to confusion. The procedure is not the same as that used to set up 'conditioned reflex responses'. In 'classical conditioning', the experimenter's intervention (with the sound of a bell) has to precede the presentation of the adequate stimulus (meat juice in the dog's mouth) so that, after many repetitions, a response of the original form (salivation) is produced in response to the signal (bell) without the unconditioned stimulus (meat juice) being presented to the animal. The response in the conditioned reflex is the same as the response in the unconditioned reflex on which it is based. In operant conditioning on the other hand, the experimenter's intervention (reward) has to follow the action to be reinforced, which can be of any form and does not necessarily conform to the pattern of response that can be elicited in any reflex.

TRAINING TO A CUE

An animal can be trained to perform a specific action on command by a procedure based on positive reinforcement learning, and here the possible confusion with routines for establishing conditioned reflexes becomes particularly insidious. In training to a cue, positive reinforcement by reward is first established, as described in the previous section. The presentation of the rewards is now associated with some advance signal to which the animal would otherwise be indifferent. After a number of repetitions of the combination of signal and reward, the consistency of rewarding is altered. Instead of rewarding every instance of the animal's performance of the selected action, the reward is presented only on certain occasions, and then only in conjunction with the signal cue. After a time, the animal comes to associate the signal with the expectation of receiving a reward. The frequency with which it performs the selected act in the absence of the signal now declines, as such instances are no longer rewarded, and it comes to perform the action promptly on cue and not at other times.

The promptness of the response can sometimes be encouraged by 'negative reinforcement'. This term is used for routines in which, if the animal fails to perform the desired action promptly in response to the cue, some additional treatment is applied that the animal is to understand as a rebuke, or at any rate that puts it into a situation it would prefer to avoid.

Negative reinforcement routines, in the form of punitive sanctions of one kind or another, are very widely advocated as the preferred option for modifying undesirable human behaviour. The outcome, however, is all too often very far from what was intended. The reason for this is that the person whose behaviour we wish to change may discover alternative ways of escaping from the punishment situation. The resulting new behaviour may be just as undesirable, from our point of view, as the pattern we originally set out to alter, but this new pattern itself becomes reinforced by the rewarding effect of the escape from punishment. Further punishment just makes matters worse. Because of this inherent disadvantage of the negative reinforcement strategy, it is important not to neglect the proven efficacy of positive reward and to recall that in many cases a mild rebuke can be more effective than downright punishment.

Reinforcement learning does not appear to have lent itself readily to modelling with artificial neural networks. However, because learning by various kinds of reinforcement forms such an important part of the development of an animal's normal balancing behaviour, we need to examine by what mechanisms such learning can be achieved. For such a study we require first to set out such principles of the neuronal organization within the central nervous system as are known at this time.

NETWORKS WITHIN THE NERVOUS SYSTEM

An inescapable feature of the central nervous system of the mammals is that it contains a very large number of cells, with an even larger number of interconnections between them. In the cerebral cortex a form of systematic organization has been found. In the cortical columns referred to earlier, each column is relatively isolated from neighbouring cells by a barrier of inhibitory connections. It may be supposed that elsewhere in the nervous system also the neurons may be arranged in functionally separate groups, although the anatomical boundaries between the individual groups are not so readily discernible. Such groupings would make possible the construction of a general scheme for central nervous organization. In setting up such a scheme it is necessary to have regard to the nature of the functions that the nervous system has to serve, as well as how its anatomy came to be the way it is.

We may take the fertilized egg as the starting point, since much of development depends on what collocation of genes the egg happens to contain. To some extent the genes determine which parts of the embryo will form the nervous system, though there is some evidence, from experimental surgery on embryos, that even this determinism may not be entirely guaranteed. As the cells of the embryonic future nervous system multiply, their anatomical relations are not entirely random, since the space into which a nerve cell can advance a projecting fibre is constrained by the presence of other cells.

Certain types of neuron can be grown in tissue culture, where they develop elongated axons. The growing tip of the axon is swollen into a 'growth cone' from which protrude a number of very fine processes. By time-lapse photography it can be shown that the arrangement of these fine processes undergoes continual change. This enables the developing tip of the axon to locate the narrow spaces between other cells as possible pathways for future growth. The fine processes also serve to detect chemical gradients to guide the general direction which the axon will pursue, especially when the tip is approaching a suitable target cell with which it can make functional connection. Although some cells do migrate, the common pattern is that each cell has, as its close neighbours, cells with which it shares a common origin. This constraint accounts for such segregation as between hindlimb fibres and forelimb fibres in the long tracts within the central nervous system. It may also account for the somatotopic arrangement of certain projections from one area to another. The pattern of interconnections that eventually becomes established is the outcome of considerable multiple branching both of axons near their destinations and of dendrites. Presumably the localized branching itself is the result of chemotaxis of some kind. Functional contact with a target cell depends on the release by that cell of a 'neural growth factor' which encourages the maturation of the neural connection. Branches that fail to receive encouragement in this way tend to die off. The mechanism of reinforcing connections by the liberation of growth factor accounts for the rearrangement of projections that occurs when some of the target cells are experimentally removed from the developing embryo. It is not yet clear why some cells produce one kind of transmitter while other cells produce another, so that some connections come to be excitatory in function and others inhibitory.

On the functional side, we have to recall that it will not do to ignore signals in any one of the multitude of afferent nerve-fibres, since the one ignored may turn out to be what determines the distinction between safety and danger. It is essential to the survival of the animal that it can distinguish between 'the usual dull routine' and 'something unusual going on'. This distinction can be achieved by a repertoire of cell groups, with a certain type of interconnection between the individual groups. A group may be thought of as consisting of anything from about 50 to about 10 000 neurons having functional connections with one another together with a relative isolation from cells in neighbouring groups, but with discrete input and output pathways to and from the group as a whole.

Because of the constraints on the geometry of the branching of nerve cells, the interconnection patterns for different groups will tend to vary considerably, though not in a truly random fashion. The groups will also differ in the pattern of afferent nerve-fibres that make functional connections with the group, each afferent connecting to a number of neurons within the group, and each such input neuron receiving from a number of afferents. The total number of afferents feeding in information to the central nervous system is very large, and each carries its own fluctuating succession of impulses. The total input pattern is therefore not only very complicated but it is also changing all the time.

We suppose that, in the course of development, each cell group that is connected to the afferent nerve-fibres comes to be preferentially receptive to a particular general pattern in its input. If some approximately similar configuration is presented in the afferent impulse traffic, the group responds by emitting a specific output pattern, with a probability that depends on the closeness of the match between the pattern of impulses presented to it and the pattern preferred by its anatomical configuration of internal connections. If this output pattern is fed back to the input of the group, the inevitable delays in transmission make possible a comparison between successive states of the input pattern. Because so many afferent nerve-fibres are available to contribute to the input to a particular group, and because the temporal pattern of impulses in each is so variable, most of the comparisons performed by a particular cell group will fail to yield significant information. It can be expected, however, that the pattern of internal connections within a group will make that group more likely to produce consistent output for input patterns of one kind rather than of another. In this sense, that group comes to 'recognize' patterns of input activity. We must suppose there to be very large numbers of groups available so that the animal is not crucially dependent on any particular cell group, and that there are plenty of 'uncommitted' cell groups left over, so to speak, to develop new matches with patterns of input not previously encountered.

We now postulate another layer of cell groups which receive, as their inputs, the outputs from the primary layer, again with many-to-one and one-to-many connections. A similar feedback arrangement to that postulated for the primary layer now produces 'novelty detectors' which can signal that the overall pattern of sensory input is not what it was. Further feedback, coupled with modification of synaptic efficacy, results in fine tuning of certain of the cell groups in the primary layer so that they become more specifically associated with particular patterns of input. The general scheme can be built up further by adding more layers of cell groups, with various kinds of feedforward and feedback connections between the groups. This kind of plan corresponds to what has been discovered about 'feature extractors' in the visual system.

STAGES IN FEATURE EXTRACTION

The earliest stages of feature extraction occur within the substance of the retina itself, so that already at the ganglion cell level we find more complex patterns of response than those appropriate to primary receptor cells. The simplest pattern is the 'spatial opponent' type. When the retina is explored with a spot of light, these units respond to stimuli applied within a small, roughly circular, area of the retina with a burst of impulses. When the light is turned off they immediately fall silent. A similar stimulus applied to an annular area closely surrounding the first has the opposite effect. The unit is silent when the light is turned on and discharges when the light is extinguished. A spot of light applied further away from the centre of the area of positive response has no effect on the unit. Units of this type are called 'ON-centre, OFF-surround' units. Other units behave in the opposite way, responding to spots of light in an annular surround region with an 'ON' response and with an 'OFF' response to a spot applied in the central area.

A variation on this pattern of spatial-opponent responses is the group of colour-opponent units. Some of these, for example, respond positively to a red spot in the central part of their receptive field or to a green spot in the annular surround and give off-type responses to a green spot in the centre or to a red spot in the surround. They are unaffected by white light. Corresponding colour-opponent units react to other complementary pairs of colours.

The part of the visual cortex that receives visual messages directly from the relay in the lateral geniculate nuclei contains units with a slightly more complicated pattern of receptivity. The receptive field again consists of a central area and a surround with opposite effects from each, but the central area, instead of being roughly circular, is rather elongated. The whole of this bar-shaped area needs to be illuminated to give the maximum response. With this arrangement, the unit has a preference for a specific orientation of the bar.

It has been shown, by computer simulation, that contrast-sensitive units of the centre-surround and orientation-sensitive types can be formed spontaneously by artificial neural networks in which the connection weights are adjusted by association learning. In this work a succession of layers of units were connected with feedforward many-to-one and one-to-many links between the units of adjacent layers. Each layer contained 1000 units, each of which received up to 600 links from units in the previous layer, distributed in Gaussian fashion around a randomly assigned centre. At the onset, the links were randomly set to be either excitatory or inhibitory. A random input was provided, and the weight-adjusting algorithm was based on the correlation between input activity in a link and the overall output of the unit receiving that link. The modified weights were constrained to saturate at the limits of $+1$ for excitation and -1 for inhibition. After a number of iterations of the modifying algorithm most of the various adjusted connection strengths had saturated to the preset limits. When the output distribution in response to test inputs was plotted out, both centre-surround and orientation-sensitive units were found to have been formed, according to the values chosen for the parameters governing the rate of weight adjustment. The algorithm chosen for this weight adjustment is taken to be approximately equivalent in effect to the adjustment of synaptic efficacy occurring at synapses between neurons as a result of protein synthesis during and following repetitive activity, as described earlier in this chapter.

When cross-connections within a layer were added to the computer simulation it was found that the various orientation-sensitive units tended to aggregate into a mosaic of groups, where each member of the group preferred the same orientation of the input bar stimulus. This type of grouping corresponds to column formation in the cerebral cortex. Some of the orientation-sensitive units in the visual cortex, instead of having receptive fields consisting of a central excitatory zone with inhibitory zones on either side, have unsymmetrical receptive fields. Such units act as 'edge detectors'.

'COMPLEX CELLS' IN THE VISUAL PATHWAY

Further along the visual pathway, cells are encountered which do not respond to the stationary patterns of stimuli that excite the 'simple cells' described above, but react when the illuminating stimulus is moved over the retina. These are referred to as 'complex cells'. It is supposed that such movement-sensitive units are formed from sets of edge detectors each of which has the same orientation preference. Movement detectors thus have corresponding orientation preferences, responding to a bar stimulus moving at right angles to the bar. Some prefer movement in one direction, some prefer the opposite direction. Some units require that the bar be of a particular length, giving less vigorous responses if the bar is either longer or shorter than the preferred value. Some units prefer curved bars, of specific curvature and orientation. It is reasonable to suppose that the more complicated feature extractors are constructed from the repertoire of units with simpler response patterns such as those just described. It may also be supposed that other modalities of sensory transduction are built up in somewhat similar fashion to that set out for the visual system. It is the visual system on which the major part of the relevant research effort has so far been concentrated.

CONFUSIONS OF CATEGORIES

It is natural, in speaking of the visual system, to think of the stimuli in terms of spots of light at specific points on the retina. It may be argued, however, on philosophical grounds, that this practice in fact involves a confusion of categories. Strictly speaking, different realms of discourse are involved when we speak of neurophysiological events, of mental events, of events in the everyday world of common experience, or of events in the detailed and somewhat mathematical world of physics. The interactions between these four quite separate realms of discourse have puzzled philosophers for centuries without, so far, any universally acceptable solution being in sight. Spots of light belong in the realm of the everyday world. We know what we mean when we say we see such a spot. In neurophysiological terms, however, the activation of neurons in the retina does not distinguish between radiant energy and deformation as the stimulus, except in terms of intensity. The language that we all use has grown up in the context of the everyday world and, apart from a small number of technical terms, we use the same language when dealing with all realms of discourse. As a result many words inevitably come to have different meanings according to the context in which they are used. This practice, though common, is highly treacherous, as it can so easily lead us unwittingly into confusion of categories and thus tempt us to false conclusions.

A SCHEME FOR NEURAL DEVELOPMENT

In an attempt to keep within the realm of neurophysiological discourse we may construct a scheme to account for the functioning of the nervous system on the following lines. In the initial stages of an animal's development, the nervous system receives, as input, only the impulses from a large number of afferent nerve-fibres, among which, at any one time, some are active while others are not. No other information is available to it. Within the totality of this continually fluctuating array certain consistencies occur, and we may suppose certain cell groups to come, by the facilitation of repetitions, to develop consistent patterns of reaction. Localized associations within groups of such units lead to the set of contiguity relations constituting a 'field', such as might be represented, topologically, as a map. In visualizing the nature of this field we need to remember that the nervous system has no access to information enabling it to distinguish the origin of the afferents, e.g. as cutaneous, proprioceptive, retinal and so on, or of the nature of the stimulus, such as deformation or illumination, that preferentially excites certain receptors. Classification of afferents on this kind of basis must depend on the detection of associations of one kind or another between the activity patterns of specific individual afferents. The process that must underly any classification consists in the formation and 'recognition' of associations between input patterns. This occurs as a result of changes in the efficacy of the synaptic connections within functionally isolated networks of neurons, just as the training of an artificial neural network occurs by changing the weights of the linkages between the units of the network.

The relations of contiguity within the field of afferents lead to higher order distinctions such as between left and right, between above and below (on the map), between close and distant, and between more and less intense. These distinctions give structure to the map. The mechanism for discrimination described in detail above for the visual system can be applied equally to other modalities also, to locate activity in certain areas of the skin in the same way as on the retina, and to detect movement and orientation. Consistencies detected in these discriminations allow the formation of such concepts as separable objects, being associations between consistently related features.

It is not easy to see how it comes about that activities in certain afferents are associated with the 'qualities' that distinguish the modalities of sensation that we recognize in the mental domain, such as colour, warmth, sound, and so on. Perhaps this will have to remain a mystery. It is at least clear that we can have no knowledge of the nature of the sensations experienced by people other than ourselves, let alone by animals. A related difficulty arises when we wish to distinguish 'voluntary' activity from behaviour not consciously initiated. 'Consciousness' and the 'will' are terms for mental events, and the feeling that we are an active agent, rather than an automaton, is also a mental event. In the neurophysiological domain perhaps the best we can do is to distinguish a class of actions for which we can assign no obvious cause and to call this class 'voluntary behaviour', with the caution that the use of this convenient label is not to imply any commitment to a particular view as to the possible relationship between mental and neurophysiological events.

The actions of the neuromodulators and of the hormones may be invoked to account for the specific patterns of behaviour that we refer to as 'drives', such as the appetites for food, sex, domination, understanding and so on. They may also be taken to account for 'moods' such as gratification, satiety, aversion, elation, despair, and the recognition of the relevance of a reward or of a punishment.

The effect of these states on motor activity can be accounted for by supposing that some of the networks involved contain motoneurons as well as interneurons. Activity in such a network may produce certain patterns of motor output in response to specific inputs, which will include influences from other parts of the nervous system as well as more direct connections to afferent nerve-fibres. The connections within such a network will become modified by learning processes which start from the patterns of motor response that we see in the reflexes of reduced preparations, but which become progressively modified by reward sequences as the animal's experience progresses. With such a scheme it is not necessary to postulate that at any stage there should occur any discrimination of any of the quantitative physical measures that we use to describe experimental situations, such as muscle tensions or joint angles.

Any particular pattern of motor output will generate further input, by afferents of the proprioceptive system, and one can envisage cell groups whose function is to develop what amounts to expectations that certain motor activity will be accompanied, or followed, by particular patterns of afferent activity. Deviations from expectation will arise when a movement encounters an obstacle, leading to the excitation of cutaneous receptors. In this way new expectations can be built up to form a set associated with the boundaries of the animal's own body.

Unexpectedness leads to another kind of activity that can be referred to as 'attention'. This involves exercising selection on the types of input to be scrutinized, which will usually be limited to a small fraction of the total input, with different fractions being selected at different times. This process can lead to association between different sets of afferent input, to form 'concepts', which are collections of associated expectations. The concept of 'own body', as opposed to 'environment', is one such concept, as are those indicating separable objects in the environment, and the discrimination between unobstructed and obstructed possible paths for locomotion. An important concept in the context of balance and locomotion concerns the relevance of certain forms of self-motion to the expectation of the punishing effects of a fall.

We must suppose that concepts, or sequences of concepts, can lead to motor activity. As foreshadowed in earlier parts of this book, this motor activity can be achieved by affecting the synaptic efficacy of parts of the internal network of interconnections within those cell groups that contain motoneurons. In this way, the higher levels of motor control override the reflex mechanisms operated by the lower levels. When the higher levels are put out of action, as in a reduced preparation, the underlying mechanisms remain and can be revealed by appropriate experimental procedures. The mechanisms thus revealed, however, do not truly represent what actually takes place in the intact animal.

The motor pattern developed at any one time will be such as to provide gratification of whatever drives happen to be particularly clamant at that time, together with the avoidance of any perils in the environment that have currently been detected. Each combination of circumstances will generate a motor pattern that satisfies these criteria. There will, in general, be many motor patterns, differing among themselves in detail, which satisfactorily meet the current requirements. If one pattern encounters unexpected obstacles, another will be substituted to take account of the change in input.

At the basic reflex level we suppose certain cell groups to have a tendency, as a consequence of genetic influences operating in early development, to recognize certain patterns of afferent input and to generate specific motor patterns in response. It is unlikely that the details, either of the input patterns or of the output patterns, will be specified with any great precision in view of the multiplicity of relevant sensory channels that are available and of the very variable pattern of impulse traffic in each channel. The system has also to be able to draw on a repertoire of motor units, each of which can make some contribution to the overall response. We may suppose that the task of distinguishing the presence of the 'adequate stimulus', as well as that of formulating the appropriate motor response, is shared between a number of cell groups. With such an arrangement, the initiation of the reflex response depends on the recognition of a relevant gestalt, where a 'gestalt' is a pattern that can be identified even when some of its defining constituents are missing.

Both the input pattern recognized as the adequate stimulus and the output pattern of reflex motor response will be composed of separable elements, each of which may be recognized by cell groups at a higher level of organization. At this level new groupings of elements of motor activity may come to be brought into play with an appearance of spontaneity, as in the exploratory movements of the newborn. As a result, new associations are formed between proprioceptive and cutaneous afferent discharges. This reinforces the mapping of the cutaneous field by the rewarding, by gratification, of successful coordination between limb activity and messages from the skin indicating contact between a digit and a particular site on the face or body. In this process the rewarding function may be served by the recognition of a correlation between the sensory consequences of a motor action with a diminution in the strength of one of the drives.

When the baby emerges from the womb, it suddenly becomes important for it to associate cutaneous information with proprioceptive information about stress gradients, in order to ensure that the nostrils are kept clear of the substrate and thus to preserve an unobstructed airway. This leads to distinctions between 'own body' and 'supporting substrate', and eventually to righting and the formation of a functional concept of the behavioural vertical, as well as to the recognition of the condition of 'imminence of falling'. Coordination with eye movements leads to classification of parts of the substrate as more suitable than others for a supporting function, and to the discrimination and classification of separable objects.

Consistent rewarding by the gratification arising from successful co-ordination of motor patterns with expectations of afferent input patterns leads to consolidation of specific motor patterns. Subsequent training to cues leads to the regular performance of motor acts appropriate to current conditions. An important class of such learned responses to cues is that of the 'anticipatory pre-emptive actions' already referred to in Chapter 6.

ANTICIPATORY PRE-EMPTIVE ACTIONS

In some of these actions, the pattern of motor behaviour may have an effect similar to that of a specific reflex response. The components of the motor output will, however, differ between the two cases. The trigger for the anticipatory pre-emptive action is the recognition of a developing trend in the afferent input. The execution of the motor pattern alters the afferent pattern so that the trend is opposed. As a result, the conditions never develop to the point at which an adequate stimulus becomes detectable, and the related reflex response is consequently not elicited. The importance of this mechanism is that it enables corrective action to be taken very early, since it is set off by recognition of a trend. The response then does not have to wait while messages are passed, by impulse propagation and synaptic transmission, from the receptors that generate the signal indicating the presence of the adequate stimulus for reflex activity. The result is a great improvement in the smoothness of the stabilizing effect of motor activity.

Apart from the initial learning stages in infancy, and some unusual situations such as are involved when the supporting surface is moving, most of balancing behaviour is performed without the need for particular attention.

HABITS AND SKILLS

Patterns of learned behaviour that, after many repetitions, come to be performed without detailed attention may be classified as 'habits'. Once a habit has been formed it may prove difficult to change it. This is because the actions are triggered by a gestalt recognition process that is operating on sensory input of which the subject may be quite unaware. He may only realize that he is performing a habitual action when the sensory consequences of that action come to his attention. Some habitual actions, such as inappropriate grooming movements – rubbing the nose, scratching the head, grimacing, and the like – are comparatively harmless. Other habits may lead to chemical addiction, and here there may be an urgent need to avoid habitual behaviour that appears to be out of control.

If an attempt is to be made to change a person's habit, two things appear to be essential. The first is an adequate desire, on the part of the subject, to make the change. To achieve this, the helper needs to use his ingenuity to build up a suitable degree of motivation in the subject. The second requirement, and one which is much more difficult to meet, is that the person with the habit has to be brought to a condition in which he is aware of the 'feel' of that changing condition which will, if allowed to proceed, eventually lead to the production of the habitual movement. It is only after he has learned to recognize this crucial moment that he can take action to interpose an effective alternative pattern of behaviour.

The learned patterns of behaviour classified as habits are performed almost automatically and are carried to completion without supervision. This is in contrast with another group of learned behaviour patterns that require close supervision at every stage, as in the skilled control of a sharp tool. During the development of a skill a variety of motor patterns are tried out. The more successful of these come to form a repertoire from which appropriate versions can be selected in turn as the immediate requirements of the task unfold during its performance. Most everyday actions are made up of a mixture of motor elements, some habitual, some skilled, and some spontaneous.

A POSSIBLE SYNTHESIS

In the earlier parts of this chapter we have surveyed a number of the tasks that the central processor in the nervous system is called upon to perform. We have seen how unusual circumstances can produce noticeable differences in behaviour, and how advances in our detailed knowledge of neuroanatomy can begin to be married with advances in neurochemistry to set up a scheme of central nervous organization. This scheme, based on a hierarchy of relatively independent cell groups each with multiple internal interconnections, is radically different from the hitherto conventional view, which has called for close scrutiny, in ever finer detail, of the anatomy and pharmacology of individual neurons.

Further progress is made possible by the development of supercomputers, in which large numbers of independent processors can be arranged to interact continually with one another over any chosen complex network of interconnections. The whole enterprise of developing a conceptual scheme of how the central nervous system carries out its tasks is dependent on an understanding of how patterns of neuronal activity become appropriately modified without the intervention of any external agency that can operate as a 'teacher'. New light on this topic has come from advances in synaptic chemistry, including the behaviour of postsynaptic receptors of the type sensitive to N-methyl-dextro-aspartite (NMDA), and the role of nitric oxide in developing synchronized activity among neighbouring neurons.

Much of the recent development has concentrated on the visual system, partly because vision plays such a large part in perceptual experience and partly because visual stimuli are readily manipulated and controlled. The cell groups that operate as feature extractors in vision and which, for this purpose, need to have comparatively large receptive fields, communicate by re-entrant connections with cell groups that have more restricted receptive fields. This arrangement makes it possible to build up associations between specific features and precise locations. (Here 'features' correspond to the 'qualities' of subjective experience.) This type of association is needed for the discrimination of separate objects in the external world. We may suppose also that, on the motor side, a somewhat similar arrangement relates cell groups concerned with the control of a limb as a whole with other cell groups having more restricted influence, as in the control of individual pools of motor units. We may expect that comparable feature extractors to those found in the visual system will eventually be discovered in the proprioceptive field, detecting the positions and motions of the body parts together with the stresses in them.

It is appropriate to remember that the visual system serves other functions as well as that of providing the basis for conscious visual perception. This fact is highlighted by cases of what is called 'blindsight'. This expression refers to the condition of patients who have suffered localized damage to the primary visual cortex, but in whom the retina is intact, together with its connections to other parts of the brain. These patients report that they cannot see, recognize, or describe, objects presented in certain parts of their visual field. They appear to be totally blind in these areas. However, if asked to pick up a named object from a group of objects all of which are placed in the affected area of their visual field, they can reach out, with appropriate adjustment of the attitude of the fingers, and successfully grasp the named object. This means that, although they have no conscious experience of objects in the 'blind' area of their visual field, a considerable amount of visual detail is available to their central nervous systems. Comparable detail has to be available to the motor system. This is provided from proprioception, where there is a corresponding absence of conscious awareness.

We can envisage that components of reflex motor patterns are assembled into a repertoire from which, by new associations of components, fresh patterns of motor activity can be constructed as the responses to new configurations of sensory input.

The newly discovered fine anatomy of the neural connections within the visual system has been combined with realistic schemes for the mechanism of synaptic modification to set up large-scale models on a supercomputer. One such model, constructed by Gerald Edelman and his colleagues at the Institute of Neuroscience in New York, contains 10 000 units, each with its own set of types of connection. These units are divided into nine functionally segregated areas with three parallel anatomical streams, one each for form, colour and motion. The different areas are linked by about 1 000 000 connections: between areas at different levels (both forwards and backwards), between areas at the same level (lateral), and within an area (intrinsic). The model receives input from a colour camera. Random values are initially assigned to the synaptic efficacies of the various connections, and the algorithm for adjusting these efficacies is based on a realistic version of the way synaptic modification occurs in the nervous system.

Such a model spontaneously develops mosaics of related groups of units corresponding to the columnar organization of the primary visual cortex, together with a variety of complex feature extractors corresponding to those found in other cortical areas. It successfully discriminates a moving pattern from its background, using various cues to establish coherence between the parts of the pattern, and performs many of the other functions of the mammalian visual system, including the binding of colour cues with motion cues in the discrimination of objects.

The model can be provided with an output corresponding to the control of eye movement to bring an object of interest to the centre of attention, and a 'saliency system' with diffuse projection that serves as the reward function needed for operant conditioning. Such a system can exhibit learned discriminatory behaviour.

It is claimed that such models are also capable of processes comparable to concept-formation and to many other stages in what has, hitherto, been regarded as the domain of mental events, including the detection of illusory boundaries in certain optical illusions. It seems reasonable to suppose that feature extractors, similar to those found in the visual system but operating on signals from proprioceptors, discriminate overall limb positions, together with the magnitudes of the forces exerted against the supports. In addition, we may postulate higher order systems that detect the 'imminence of overbalancing', which may be regarded as a concept that includes both a direction and a rate-of-change. Other feature extractors record what patterns of motor activity produce limb thrusts of specific direction and force. A memory system stores the effectiveness of each thrust pattern in reducing the urgency of the imminence of overbalancing. Operant conditioning then builds up, from this type of experience, a repertoire of thrust patterns appropriate to each of a variety of conditions of imminence of overbalancing. What is now required is a mechanism operating, like a feature extractor in reverse, to formulate patterns of activation of motor units in order to achieve a specific direction and force of thrust. Mechanisms of this sort must be available for any form of voluntary movement to be possible.

It may be noted that the direction of the behavioural vertical itself is not something that can be directly sensed. It has the status of a concept of the limiting condition in which the imminence of overbalancing is reduced to zero. It is built up from experience of the effectiveness of various thrusts that have been exerted in the past. Its direction, in relation to the trunk, is continually changing, for reasons that have been explained earlier in this book. For stability, we aim to reduce the risk of overbalancing, while to initiate locomotion, we may develop a thrust that deliberately leads to overbalancing, so that a horizontal acceleration in a desired direction can be obtained from the interaction with gravity.

OVERALL SUMMARY AND CONCLUSIONS

Balance is maintained by exerting appropriate forces against the available supports. These forces are distributed through the springy lattice structure of the body, which consists of a framework of loosely-jointed struts (the bones of the skeleton) stiffened by ties (the muscles and tendons), from which the soft parts are suspended. In contrast with the forces in an inert system, the forces in the body of a man or of an animal vary continuously throughout life because of the brief time-course of the mechanical responses of skeletal muscle cells to activation through the motor nerves. Furthermore, any change in posture, including the inevitable swaying caused by respiratory and cardiac movements, entails a widespread readjustment of the supporting forces.

A number of automatic and semi-automatic nervous 'reactions' contribute to the organization of motor activity in certain specific conditions, including the cyclic changes in conditions involved in the various modes of locomotion. The initiation of these reactions depends on information derived from a variety of proprioceptive sense organs, in combination with signals from movement detectors in the peripheral retina. In each case the sensory signal is not directly related to any of those simple measures of the conditions at the receptor that one might speak of as 'physicist's variables', such as degree of deformation, stress gradient, or their rates-of-change. Instead, the signals appear to reflect a mixture of components, each with a different time-course, from which the simpler measures are not easily recovered.

Another factor that complicates the formulation of any input–output relationship between sensory information and force-generation is that the tension resulting from the activation of a particular set of muscle cells is very much dependent on the conditions of loading as well as on the pattern of neural activation. It follows that the central processing that organizes the motor commands to suit the incoming sensory information must involve gestalt recognition acts of two kinds:

1. a determination of the state of affairs in terms of the appropriateness of a particular moment for the emission of a specific command;
2. a selection of the necessary pattern of output messages to the muscles to achieve the desired change.

Conventional neuroanatomy, even when supported by recent advances in our knowledge of synaptic mechanisms, does not provide us with any adequate scheme to account for the way the central nervous system carries out its signal-processing task. On the other hand, certain developments in computer engineering, involving multiply-interconnected parallel processors, now make it possible to envisage how the extremely intricate interconnections between the vast numbers of neurons involved may come to be organized in such a way as to perform the necessary acts of recognition.

From what we now know, from computer simulations, of how interconnected groups of neurons can be expected to behave, we appear to be approaching a position in which we can account for the way the central nervous system organizes the strategic choice of sequences of offset thrusts by which we maintain our balance and perform acts of locomotion.

Sources of figures

Full details of the sources to which brief reference is made in the captions to the figures. The numbers in square brackets indicate the relevant figures in each case.

Bessou, P., Emonet-Dénand, F. and Laporte, Y. (1965) Motor fibres innervating extrafusal and intrafusal muscle fibres in the cat, *J. Physiol.*, **180**, 649–72. [8.6]

Boyd, I.A. (1962) The structure and innervation of the nuclear bag muscle fibre system and the nuclear chain muscle fibre system in mammalian muscle spindles, *Phil. Trans. Roy. Soc.*, B, **245**, 81–136. [8.5]

Boyd, I.A. (1980) The isolated mammalian muscle spindle, *Trends Neurosci.*, **3**, 258–65. [8.9]

Boyd, I.A. and Roberts, T.D.M. (1953) Proprioceptive discharges from stretch-receptors in the knee-joint of the cat, *J. Physiol.*, **122**, 38–58. [8.1]

Burke, R.E., Levine, D.N., Salcman, M. and Tsairis, P. (1974) Motor units in cat soleus muscle: physiological, histochemical and morphological characteristics, *J. Physiol.*, **238**, 503–14. [9.4]

Cajal, S. Ramon y (1952) *Histologie du Système Nerveux de l'Homme et des Vertébrés*, Vol. I, Consejo Superior de Investigaciones Cientificas, Instituto Ramon y Cajal, Madrid. [9.2]

Crosby, E.C., Humphrey, T. and Lauer, E.W. (1962) *Correlative Anatomy of the Nervous System*, Macmillan, New York. [9.5]

Curtin, N.A. and Davies, R.E. (1972) Chemical and mechanical changes during stretching of activated frog skeletal muscle, *Cold Spring Harbor Symp. Quant. Biol.*, **37**, 619–26. [4.10]

Gordon, A.M., Huxley, A.F. and Julian, F.J. (1966) The variation in isometric tension with sarcomere length in vertebrate muscle fibres, *J. Physiol.*, **184**, 170–92. [4.9]

Gray, A.A. (1907) *The Labyrinth of Animals, including mammals, birds, reptiles and amphibians*, (2 Vols), Churchill, London. [8.10]

Hill, A.V. (1953) The mechanics of active muscle, *Proc. Roy. Soc.*, B, **141**, 104–17. [4.8]

Lindeman, H.H. (1969) Studies on the morphology of the sensory regions of the vestibular apparatus, *Ergebn. Anat. Entwickl.–Gesch.*, **42**, 4–13. [8.10, 8.13]

Lowenstein, O. and Roberts, T.D.M. (1949) The equilibrium function of the otolith organs of the Thornback Ray (*Raja clavata*), *J. Physiol.*, **110**, 392–415. [8.17, 8.18, 8.19, 8.20]

McDonald, D.A. (1961) How does a man twist in the air? *New Scientist*, **10**, 501–3. [7.28]

McWilliam, P.N. (1975) The motor control of muscle spindles in the hindlimb of the cat, Ph.D. Thesis, Glasgow University. [8.8]

Muybridge, E. (1893) *Descriptive Zoopraxography, or the Science of Animal Locomotion Made Popular*, University of Pennsylvania. [7.17, 7.18, 7.19, 7.21, 7.23, 7.25]

Purdon Martin, J. (1967) *The Basal Ganglia and Posture*. Pitman, London. [6.34, 6.35, 6.36]

Rademaker, G.G.J. (1931) *Das Stehen*. Springer, Berlin. [6.13, 6.14, 6.15, 6.29, 6.30]

Reinking, R.M., Stephens, J.A. and Stuart, D.G. (1975) The tendon organs of cat medial gastrocnemius: significance of motor unit type and size for the activation of Ib afferents, *J. Physiol.*, **250**, 491–512. [8.2]

Retzius, G. (1881, 1884) *Das Gehörorgan der Virbelthiere*, Vols I and II, Samson & Wallin, Stockholm. [8.10]

Roberts, T.D.M. (1963) Rhythmic excitation of a stretch reflex, revealing (a) hysteresis and (b) a difference between the responses to pulling and to stretching, *Quart. J. Exp. Physiol.*, **48**, 328–45. [4.18]

Roberts, T.D.M. (1971) Standing with a bent knee, *Nature (Lond.)*, **230**, 499–501. [3.20, 3.21]

Roberts, T.D.M. and Murray-Smith, D.J. (1970) Method for the analysis of the neural mechanisms for postural adjustments, in *Principles and Practice of Bionics (AGARD Conference Proceedings, No. 44)* (eds. H.E. von Gierke, W.E. Keidel and H.L. Oestreicher), Technivision Services, Slough, pp. 371–87. [8.6, 8.7]

Swett, J.E. and Schoultz, T.W. (1975) Mechanical transduction in the Golgi tendon organ: a hypothesis, *Arch. Ital. Biol.*, **113**, 374–80. [8.3]

Szentágothai, J. (1967) Synaptic architecture of the spinal motoneurone pool, in *Recent Advances in Clinical Neurophysiology; Electroenceph. Clin. Neurophysiol.*, *Supp. 25*. (ed. L. Widén), Elsevier, Amsterdam, pp. 4–19. [9.1]

Whittaker, V.P. and Gray, E.G. (1962) The synapse: biology and morphology, *Brit. Med. Bull.*, **18**, 223–8. [9.3]

Index

Page numbers appearing in **bold** refer to figures and page numbers appearing in *italic* refer to tables.